American Joint Committee on Cancer

AJCC CANCER STAGING MANUAL

Fifth Edition

EDITORS

IRVIN D. FLEMING, M.D.
Professor of Surgery
University of Tennessee
St. Jude Children's Research Hospital
Memphis, Tennessee

JAY S. COOPER, M.D.
Professor, Department of Radiation Oncology
New York University Medical Center
New York, New York

DONALD EARL HENSON, M.D.
U.S. Public Health Service
Division of Cancer Prevention and Control
National Cancer Institute
Bethesda, Maryland

ROBERT V. P. HUTTER, M.D.
Clinical Professor, Department of Pathology
St. Barnabas Medical Center
Livingston, New Jersey
Professor of Pathology (Adjunct)
Columbia University College of Physicians and Surgeons
New York, New York

B. J. KENNEDY, M.D.
Regents' Professor of Medicine, Emeritus
Masonic Professor of Oncology, Emeritus
University of Minnesota
Minneapolis, Minnesota

GERALD P. MURPHY, M.D., D.S.c.
Professor, Department of Urology
Northwest Hospital
University of Washington
Pacific Northwest Cancer Foundation
Seattle, Washington

BRIAN O'SULLIVAN, M.B., F.R.C.P.C., F.R.C.P.I.
Associate Professor, Department of Radiation Oncology
The Princess Margaret Hospital
University of Toronto
Toronto, Ontario, Canada

LESLIE H. SOBIN, M.D.
Chief, Department of Gastrointestinal Pathology
Armed Forces Institute of Pathology
Washington, District of Columbia

JOHN W. YARBRO, M.D., Ph.D.
Professor Emeritus, Department of Medicine
University of Missouri
Editor, Seminars in Oncology
Columbia, Missouri

AJCC CANCER STAGING MANUAL

Fifth Edition

AMERICAN JOINT COMMITTEE ON CANCER

Executive Office
55 East Erie Street
Chicago, Illinois 60611

FOUNDING ORGANIZATIONS

American Cancer Society
National Cancer Institute
College of American Pathologists
American College of Physicians
American College of Radiology
American College of Surgeons

SPONSORING ORGANIZATIONS

American Cancer Society
American College of Surgeons

This manual was prepared and published through the support of the American Cancer Society and the American College of Surgeons

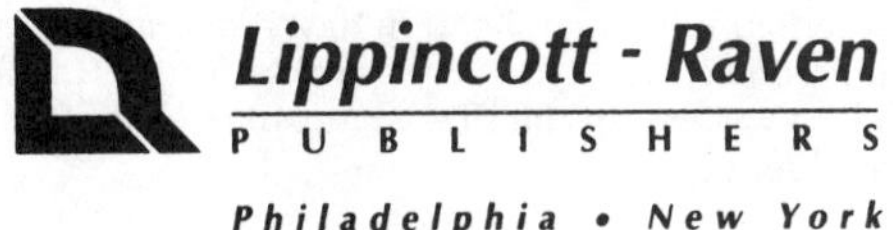

Manufacturing Manager: Dennis Teston
Production Manager: Jodi Borgenicht
Production Editor: Raeann Touhey
Cover Designer: Patricia Gast
Compositor: Tapsco, Inc.
Printer: Victor Graphics

FIFTH EDITION

First printing 1977
Revised and reprinted 1978
Reprinted 1979
Second edition 1983
Third edition 1988
Fourth edition 1992

Printed in the United States of America

9 8 7 6 5 4 3

Library of Congress Cataloging-in-Publication Data
AJCC cancer staging manual/American Joint Committee on Cancer.—5th ed.
p. cm.
Rev. ed. of: Manual of staging of cancer/American Joint Committee on Cancer. 4th ed. c1992.
"Founding organizations, American Cancer Society, et al.; sponsoring organizations, American Cancer Society, American College of Surgeons."
Includes bibliographical references.
ISBN 0-397-58414-8
1. Tumors—Classification—Handbooks, manuals, etc. I. American Joint Committee on Cancer. II. American Cancer Society. III. American College of Surgeons. IV. Manual for staging of cancer.
[DNLM: 1. Neoplasm Staging. 2. Neoplasms—classification. QZ 241 A312 1997]
RC258.M36 1997
616.99'4'0012—dc21
DNLM/DLC
for Library of Congress

Care has been taken to confirm the accuracy of the information presented and to describe generally accepted practices. However, the editors and publisher are not responsible for errors or omissions or for any consequences from application of the information in this book and make no warranty, express or implied, with respect to the contents of the publication.

The editors and publisher have exerted every effort to ensure that drug selection and dosage set forth in this text are in accordance with current recommendations and practice at the time of publication. However, in view of ongoing research, changes in government regulations, and the constant flow of information relating to drug therapy and drug reactions, the reader is urged to check the package insert for each drug for any change in indications and dosage and for added warnings and precautions. This is particularly important when the recommended agent is a new or infrequently employed drug.

Some drugs and medical devices presented in this publication have Food and Drug Administration (FDA) clearance for limited use in restricted research settings. It is the responsibility of the health care provider to ascertain the FDA status of each drug or device planned for use in their clinical practice.

FIFTH EDITION

Dedicated to Oliver Howard Beahrs, M.D.

Dr. Beahrs is known internationally for his kindness, humanitarianism, infinite enthusiasm, and unsurpassed knowledge. Dr. Oliver H. Beahrs (Ollie to those who know him) has demonstrated time and again his devotion to and deep concern for cancer patients and their families. His many attributes have established him as a leader in the fields of surgery and oncology.

Dr. Beahrs received his medical degree in 1949 from Northwestern University in Evanston, Illinois and served his entire career at the Mayo Clinic in Rochester, Minnesota. His commitment to public service is evident in his appointments as president or chairman of various clinical and surgical societies and organizations, including Chairman (1975–1980) and Executive Director (1980–1993) of the American Joint Committee on Cancer, Chairman of the Board of Regents (1984–1987) and President (1988–1989) of the American College of Surgeons, and Honorary Life Member of the American Cancer Society's Board of Directors.

Dr. Beahrs was instrumental in the work and publications of the AJCC. Previous editions of the *AJCC Manual for Staging of Cancer* have come to be known as "the Beahrs Manual;" this Fifth Edition will likely be similarly known.

FOURTH EDITION

Dedicated to the memory of Harvey Baker, M.D., Chairman of the American Joint Committee on Cancer from 1982 to 1985.

THIRD EDITION

Dedicated to the memory of
W. A. D. Anderson, M.D.
Marvin Pollard, M.D.
Paul Sherlock, M.D.

SECOND EDITION

Dedicated to the memory of
Murray M. Copeland, M.D.

The first chairman of the American Joint Committee on Cancer Staging and End-Results Reporting.

Preface

The editors of the Fifth Edition of the *Cancer Staging Manual* of the American Joint Committee on Cancer wish to recognize the contributions of hundreds of participants who have volunteered their time over 38 years in the evolution of the recommendations for staging cancer. The process began with retrospective studies at selected anatomic sites. In addition, reviews of available literature and information from personal experience of participants, as well as reviews of staging recommendations previously brought forward by others, were incorporated in deliberations for a comprehensive staging reference. This resulted in the First Edition of the manual in 1977.

Subsequently, the Committee has continued to review its definitions and fine tune the recommendations and stage groupings for all anatomic sites with the hope that staging of cancer will be most helpful in arriving at decisions regarding appropriate treatment of malignant tumors and in determining prognosis and end results.

Recommendations regarding staging of cancer by individual researchers, specialists, committees, and other groups had not been uniform in the past. This was also true in some instances in the published reports of the TNM Committee of the International Union Against Cancer (UICC) and the American Joint Committee on Cancer (AJCC). Under the leadership of Dr. Harvey Baker as Chairman of the AJCC from 1982 to 1985, discussions were first undertaken with the UICC TNM Committee to reach uniform recommendations of the two groups so that one system of staging might be used worldwide. These efforts have been actively pursued under the subsequent chairmanships of Drs. Robert Hutter and Donald Henson with the cooperation of Dr. Leslie Sobin, Chairman of the TNM Committee, and with the aid of Professor Paul Hermanek and his associates.

Through multiple meetings with worldwide input, agreements have been reached on all definitions of T, N, and M and on stage groupings for cancers at all anatomic sites. The recommendations of the AJCC in the Third Edition of the manual and the publications of the UICC, published in 1987, are identical. Thus, an international system of staging cancer is available. The use of this system facilitates appropriate decisions regarding treatment and, more important, evaluation of end results and comparability of data.

Although recommendations for staging at most anatomic sites remain as those published in the Fourth Edition, those for the gynecologic sites have been modified and are consistent with the recommendations of the Federation Internationale de Gynecologie et d'Obstetrique (FIGO). Likewise, the prostate staging recommendations have changed so that they will be consistent with recommendations of urologists. The site codes listed at the beginning of each chapter were revised in 1992 in accordance with the International Classification of Diseases for Oncology (ICD-O), Second Edition (1990). New chapters on staging of fallopian tube cancer and gestational trophoblastic tumors have been added to this edition. Staging for cancers of the head and neck, lung, soft tissue sarcoma, testis, and brain have been revised. General agreement on the staging of pediatric cancers has not been reached, and those chapters are not included in this edition.

Credit is due to all members of the American Joint Committee on Cancer and its Task Forces for individual anatomic sites. Special credit in preparation of the Fifth Edition is given to those in leadership positions and to staff support persons, in particular, Rosemarie Clive, Joanne Sylvester, Lisa Richards, and Deirdre McAllister. We are also grateful for the assistance provided by members of the Surveillance, Epidemiology, and End Results Program of the National Cancer Institute and the National Tumor Registrars Association. Personnel of Lippincott-Raven Publishers have been most cooperative and helpful. The interest and help of the publisher is greatly appreciated.

Irvin D. Fleming, M.D.
Jay S. Cooper, M.D.
Donald Earl Henson, M.D.
Robert V.P. Hutter, M.D.
B. J. Kennedy, M.D.
Gerald P. Murphy, M.D., D.SC.
Brian O'Sullivan, M.B., F.R.C.P.C., F.R.C.P.I.
Leslie H. Sobin, M.D.
John W. Yarbro, M.D., Ph.D.

Introduction

This manual brings together all currently available information on staging of cancer at various anatomic sites as developed by the American Joint Committee on Cancer (AJCC) in cooperation with the TNM Committee of the International Union Against Cancer (UICC). All of the schemes included here are uniform between the two organizations. The manual permits consistency in describing the extent of the neoplastic diseases in different anatomic parts, systems, or organs.

Proper classification and staging of cancer will allow the physician to determine treatment more appropriately, to evaluate results of management more reliably, and to compare worldwide statistics reported from various institutions on a local, regional, and national basis more confidently.

Staging of cancer is not a fixed science. As new information becomes available about etiology and various diagnostic and treatment methods, the classification and staging of cancer will change. Periodically, this manual will be revised to reflect the changing knowledge and new technology, but revisions will occur only at reasonable periods. At the present time the anatomic extent of the cancer is the primary basis for staging; the histopathologic grade and the age of the patient are also factors in some tumors. In the future, biologic markers, molecular, genetic, and other prognostic indicators may play a part.

It is intended that the staging recommendations included in this manual will be used as published so that consistency in data gathering will be possible. The recommendations in the manual are to be used in the cancer programs approved by the multidisciplinary Approvals Committee of the Commission on Cancer of the American College of Surgeons and is being considered as a requirement by the Joint Commission on Accreditation of Health Care Organizations in recordkeeping. Also, future reports by the Surveillance, Epidemiology, and End-Results Program (SEER) of the National Cancer Institute (NCI) will be based on the classifications recommended by the AJCC.

The AJCC was first organized on January 9, 1959, as the American Joint Committee for Cancer Staging and End-Results Reporting (AJC), for the purpose of developing a system of clinical staging for cancer acceptable to the American medical profession. The sponsoring organizations are the American College of Surgeons, the American College of Radiology, the College of American Pathologists, the American College of Physicians, the American Cancer Society, and the National Cancer Institute. Each of the sponsoring organizations designates three representatives to the Committee. The American College of Surgeons serves as administrative sponsor. Subcommittees, called "task forces," have been established to consider malignant neoplasms of selected anatomic sites in order to develop or review current classifications. Each task force is composed of committee members and other professional appointees whose special interests and skills are appropriate to the site under consideration.

During its 38 years of activity, various special consultants have worked with the Committee, as well as liaison representatives from the American Society of Clinical Oncology, the Centers for Disease Control and Prevention, the American Urological Association, the Association of American Cancer Institutes, the National Cancer Registrars Association, the Society of Gynecologic Oncologists, the Society of Urologic Oncology, and the SEER program of the NCI. More than 400 individuals have contributed to the work of the various task forces. Dr. Murray Copeland was Chairman from the inception until 1969, Dr. W. A. D. Anderson from 1969 to 1974, Dr. Oliver H. Beahrs from 1974 to 1979, Dr. David T. Carr from 1979 to 1982, Dr. Harvey W. Baker from 1982 to 1985, Dr. Robert V. P. Hutter from 1985 to 1990, and Dr. Donald E. Henson from 1990 to 1995. The current Chairman is Dr. Irvin D. Fleming.

Pioneer work on the clinical classification of cancer was done by the League of Nations Health Organization (1929), the International Commission on Stage Grouping and Presentation of Results (ICPR) of the International Congress of Radiology (1953), and the International Union Against Cancer (Union Internationale Contre le Cancer, UICC). The latter organization became most active in the field through its Committee on Clinical Stage Classification and Applied Statistics (1954), later known as the UICC TNM Committee.

The AJCC decided to use the TNM system, when applicable, to describe the anatomic extent of the cancer at the time of diagnosis (before the application of definitive treatment), and from this to develop classification into stages, which would serve as a guide for treatment and prognosis and for comparing the end results of treatment. Subsequently, the system has been extended to other periods during the natural history and treatment of a cancer. Task forces to accomplish this extension were established to focus on particular sites of cancer. Retrospective studies have resulted in recommendations for stage classifications for cancer at various sites or systems, which have been published and distributed in separate fascicles and articles.

The AJCC sponsored a National Cancer Conference on Classification and Staging in Atlanta on March 27–28, 1976. This conference delineated the accomplishments to that time and brought into focus future needs and activities.

In January 1970, a revised statement of the "Objectives, Rules and Regulations of the American Joint Committee" was adopted. This statement broadened the scope of the Committee by including in its objectives the formulation and publication of systems of classification of cancer, not limited to, but including staging and end-results reporting.

It was recognized that for cancer of certain sites the information made available by observation at the time of a surgical procedure, as well as information from the pathologic examination of the surgically removed cancer, could form the basis for useful classifications. From this evolved a "surgical evaluative staging" and a "postsurgical treatment-pathologic staging." Surgical evaluative staging has subsequently been dropped. Information obtained during surgical exploration may be used for clinical staging.

Further consideration of the chronology of staging has led to two main time periods. First is the Clinical Stage, which uses all data available to the first definitive treatment. Second is the Pathologic Stage, which can be established if a completely resected specimen of the lesion is available.

It is also evident that for certain organs (e.g., thyroid), the biologic potential of different histologic types of cancer is such that different types cannot be mixed together in a meaningful classification. Therefore, cases should be analyzed separately by histologic type. In some cancers, such as soft-tissue sarcomas, histologic grading is of such significance that it becomes a necessary component of the classification system. For certain cancers, widely used and accepted classifications, such as the Ann Arbor classification of Hodgkin's disease and the Federation Internationale de Gynecologie et d'Obstetrique (FIGO) classifications for carcinomas of the gynecological sites, are considered in the recommendations. Whenever possible, established and accepted classifications are considered.

The various data published previously in individual-site fascicles, with revisions and the addition of other material, were brought together to form a Manual for Staging of Cancer, the First Edition of which was published in 1977. A second printing, slightly revised, appeared in 1978. The Second Edition of the manual (1983) updated the earlier publications and included additional sites. Also, the recommendations were brought more closely in conformity with those of the TNM Committee.

The need for a staging form for use in the staging system of each site has been recognized for some years. Such forms ensure the uniform recording of data necessary for stage classification. Recent emphasis has been given to the development of a data form for each cancer site for which there is a stage classification and to the availability of such data forms as a part of each staging recommendation.

The expanding role of the Committee in a variety of cancer classifications, including its significance and value and the promotion of indicated usage in cancer diagnosis and therapy, suggested that the original name of the Committee no longer portrayed the broader scope of its interests and activities. The name was therefore changed in June, 1980 to the American Joint Commitee on Cancer (AJCC). The publication of this new edition of the manual reflects the widening interests and activities of the Committee.

The TNM Committee of the UICC and the AJCC have been working along similar lines and with similar objectives. In the past, points of view and methods have occasionally differed. Since 1982, cooperation between the two groups has resulted in uniform and identical definitions and stage grouping of cancers for all anatomic sites so that a universal system is now available. The TNM classification and stage grouping in this revision correspond exactly with those appearing in the Fifth Edition of the UICC TNM Classification of Malignant Tumors.

Members of the AJCC, its task forces and its committees, as well as the sponsoring organizations, owe a debt of gratitude to the many physicians and others who have voluntarily contributed to this effort in the hope that patients with cancer would survive and that the quality of life of the cancer patient could be as near normal as possible. The contributions of the TNM Committee of the UICC and other international organizations are gratefully acknowledged.

Contents

PART I

General Information on Cancer Staging and End-Results Reporting

PART II

Staging of Cancer at Specific Anatomic Sites

PART I

General Information on Cancer Staging and End-Results Reporting

1

Purposes and Principles of Staging

Philosophy of Classification and Staging by the TNM System

A classification scheme for cancer must encompass all attributes of the tumor that define its life history. The American Joint Committee on Cancer (AJCC) classification is based on the premise that cancers of the same anatomic site and histology share similar patterns of growth and extension.

The size of the untreated primary cancer (T) increases progressively, and at some point in time regional lymph node involvement (N) and/or distant metastasis (M) occur. A simple classification scheme, which can be incorporated into a form for staging and universally applied, is the goal of the TNM system as proposed by the AJCC. This classification is identical to that of the Union Internationale Contre le Cancer (UICC) and is a distillate of several existing systems.

As the primary tumor (T) increases in size over time, local invasion occurs, followed by spread to the regional lymph nodes draining the area of the tumor and/or to other sites via blood vessel invasion. The period when this spread is manifest or discernible by available methods of clinical examination is thus another significant marker in the progression of the cancer (N). It is usually later, either in the middle or older period of the cancer life span, that distant spread, i.e., distant metastasis (M), becomes evident from clinical examination. Thus, distant metastasis (M) is ordinarily the third time marker.

These three significant events in the life history of a cancer—local tumor growth (T), spread to regional lymph nodes (N), and metastasis (M)—are used as they appear (or do not appear) on clinical examination, before definitive therapy begins, to indicate the anatomic extent of the cancer. This shorthand method of indicating the extent of disease (TNM) at a particular designated time is an expression of the stage of the cancer at that time in its progression.

Events such as spread to regional lymph nodes and/or distant metastasis occur before they are discernible by clinical examination. Thus, examination during the surgical procedure and histologic examination of the surgically removed tissues may identify significant additional indicators of the life history of the cancer, i.e., the prognosis of the patient, (T, N, and M) as different from what could be discerned clinically before therapy. Since this is the pathologic (pTNM) classification and stage grouping (based on examination of a surgically resected specimen with sufficient tissue to evaluate the highest T, N, or an M classification), it is recorded in addition to the clinical classification. It does not replace the clinical classification. Both should be maintained in the patient's permanent medical record. The clinical stage is used as a guide to the selection of primary therapy. The pathologic stage can be used as a guide for the need for adjuvant therapy, for estimation of prognosis, and for reporting end results.

Therapeutic procedures, even if not curative, may alter the course and life history of a cancer patient. Although cancers that recur after therapy may be staged with the same criteria as are used in pretreatment clinical staging, the significance of these criteria may not be the same. Hence the "restage" classification of recurrent cancer (rTNM) is considered separately for therapeutic guidance, estimation of prognosis, and end-results reporting at that time in the patient's clinical course.

The significance of the criteria for defining anatomic extent of disease differs for tumors at different anatomic sites and of different histologic types. Therefore, the criteria for T, N, and M must be defined for tumors of each anatomic site to attain validity. With certain types of tumors, such as Hodgkin's disease and lymphomas, a different system for designating the anatomic extent of the disease and for classifying its stage grouping is necessary to accomplish validity. In these exceptional circumstances other symbols or descriptive criteria are used in place of T, N, and M.

The combination of the T, N, and M classifications into stage groupings is, thus, a method of designating the anatomic extent of a cancer and is related to the natural course of the particular type of cancer. It is intended to provide a way by which this information can readily be communicated to others, to assist in therapeutic decisions, and estimate prognosis. Ultimately, it provides a mechanism for comparing similar groups of cases, in the evaluation of different potentially therapeutic procedures.

For most cancer sites the staging recommendations in this manual are concerned only with anatomic extent of disease, but in several instances histologic grade (soft-tissue sarcoma) and age (thyroid carcinoma) are factors that significantly influence prognosis and must be considered. In the future, biologic markers and other parameters may have to be included along with those of anatomic extent in classifying cancer, but they are supplements to and not necessarily components of the TNM stage based on anatomic extent of the cancer.

In addition to anatomic extent, the histologic classification and histologic grade of the tumor may be important prognostic determinants in the classification for staging. The histologic type of tumor and the histologic grade are also important variables affecting choices for treatment. For sarcomas, the tumor grade may prove to be the most important variable.

Philosophy of changes: The introduction of new types of therapeutic interventions or new technologies may require modification of the classification and staging systems. These dynamic processes may alter treatment and outcomes. It is essential to recognize the kinetics of change of staging systems. In the future, well-evaluated prognostic factors will be incorporated into the current classification and staging systems. As a first step towards this goal, in this edition serum biologic markers have been introduced as significant prognostic factors in the staging of testis cancer. At the present time, additional prognostic factors under study are not sufficiently validated to be incorporated into the staging systems; however, future modifications of other anatomic sites can be anticipated.

Nomenclature of the Morphology of Cancer

Cancer therapy decisions are made after an assessment of the patient and tumor, using many methods that often include sophisticated technical procedures. For most types of cancer, the anatomic extent to which the disease has spread is probably the most important factor determining prognosis and must be given prime consideration in evaluating and comparing different therapeutic regimens.

Staging classifications are based on documentation of the anatomic extent of disease, and their design requires a thorough knowledge of the natural history of each type of cancer. Such knowledge has been and continues to be derived primarily from morphologic studies, which also provide us with the definitions and classifications of tumor types.

An accurate histologic diagnosis, therefore, is an essential element in a meaningful evaluation of the tumor. In certain types of cancer, biochemical, molecular, genetic, or immunologic measurements of normal or abnormal cellular function have become important elements in classifying tumors precisely. Increasingly, definitions and classifications should include function as a component of the pathologist's anatomic diagnosis. One may also anticipate that special techniques as histochemistry, tissue culture, cytogenetics, and molecular biology will be used more routinely for typing and characterizing tumors and their behavior.

The most complete and best known English language compendium of tumor macroscopic and microscopic characteristics and their associated behavior is the Atlas of Tumor Pathology series, published in many volumes by the Armed Forces Institute of Pathology in Washington, D.C. These are revised periodically and are used as a basic reference by pathologists throughout the world.

No acceptable staging system has yet been developed for primary tumors of the central nervous system. Pediatric tumors are not included in this manual.

Related Classifications

Since 1958 the World Health Organization (WHO) has had a program aimed at providing internationally acceptable criteria for the histologic classification of tumors of various anatomic sites. This has resulted in the International Histological Classification of Tumours which contains, in an illustrated 25-volume series, definitions, descriptions and multiple illustrations of tumor types and proposed nomenclature. The series of books in the second edition is now being published.

The WHO International Classification of Diseases for Oncology (ICD-O), second edition, is a numerical coding system for neoplasms by topography and morphology. The coded morphology nomenclature is identical to the morphology field for neoplasms in the Systematized Nomenclature of Medicine (SNOMED) published by the College of American Pathologists.

In the interest of promoting national and international collaboration in cancer research and specifically to facilitate appropriate comparison of data among different clinical investigations, use of the International Histological Classification of Tumours for classification and definition of tumor types, and the ICD-O codes for storage and retrieval of data are recommended.

BIBLIOGRAPHY

Atlas of tumor pathology, third series: Washington, DC, Armed Forces Institute of Pathology, 1991–

Hermanek P, Gospodarowicz MK, Henson DE, et al: Prognostic factors in cancer. Berlin-Heidelberg-New York: Springer-Verlag, 1995

World Health Organization: ICD-O International classification of diseases for oncology, 2nd ed. Geneva: WHO, 1990

World Health Organization: International histological classification of tumours, 2nd ed. Berlin-Heidelberg-New York: Springer-Verlag, 1988 to 1997

General Rules for Staging of Cancer

The practice of dividing cancer cases into groups according to "stage" arose from the fact that survival rates were higher for cases in which the disease was localized than for those in which the disease has extended beyond the organ or site of origin. These groups were often referred to as "early cases" and "late cases," implying some regular progression with time. Actually, the stage of disease at the time of diagnosis may be a reflection not only of the rate of growth and extension of the neoplasm but also of the type of tumor and of the tumor-host relationship.

The staging of cancer, a hallowed tradition, is used to analyze and compare groups of patients. It is preferable to reach agreement on the recording of accurate information on the anatomic extent of the disease for each site because the precise clinical description and histopathologic classification of malignant neoplasms may serve a number of related objectives, such as: (1) selection of primary and adjuvant therapy, (2) estimation of prognosis, (3) assistance in evaluation of the results of treatment, (4) facilitation of the exchange of information among treatment centers, (5) contribution to the continuing investigation of human cancers.

The principal purpose served by international agreement on the classification of cancer cases by anatomic extent of disease, however, is to provide a method of conveying clinical experience to others without ambiguity.

There are many bases or axes of classification; for example, the anatomic site and the clinical and pathologic anatomic extent of disease; the reported duration of symptoms or signs, the sex and age of the patient, and the histologic type and grade. All of these represent variables that are known to have an influence on the outcome of the patient. Classification by anatomic extent of disease as determined clinically and histopathologically (when possible) is the classification to which the attention of the AJCC and the UICC is primarily directed.

The clinician's immediate task is to select the most effective course of treatment and estimate the prognosis. This decision and this judgment require, among other things, an objective assessment of the anatomic extent of the disease.

To meet these stated objectives, a system of classification is needed that (1) has basic principles applicable to all anatomic sites regardless of treatment, and (2) in which clinical appraisal can be supplemented by later information from surgery, histopathology, and/or other technologies. The TNM system meets these requirements.

General Rules of the TNM System

The TNM system is an expression of the anatomic extent of disease and is based on the assessment of three components:

T The extent of the primary tumor
N The absence or presence and extent of regional lymph node metastasis
M The absence or presence of distant metastasis

The use of numerical subsets of the TNM components indicates the progressive extent of the malignant disease.

T0, T1, T2, T3, T4 N0, N1, N2, N3 M0, M1

In effect, the system is a shorthand notation for describing the clinical and pathologic anatomic extent of a particular malignant tumor.

General rules applicable to all sites follow:

1. All cases must be confirmed microscopically for TNM classification (including clinical classification).
2. Four classifications are described for each site, namely:

   Clinical Classification, designated cTNM or TNM. Clinical classification is based on evidence acquired before primary treatment. Such evidence arises from physical examination, imaging, endoscopy, biopsy, surgical exploration, and other relevant findings. In other words, all information available prior to first definitive treatment.

   Pathologic Classification, designated pTNM. Pathologic classification includes the evidence acquired before treatment, supplemented or modified by the additional evidence acquired during and from surgery, particularly from pathologic examination. The pathologic assessment of the primary tumor (pT) entails resection of the primary tumor sufficient in extent to evaluate the highest pT category. The pathologic assessment of the regional lymph nodes (pN) also entails removal of a sufficient number of lymph nodes to evaluate the highest pN category. Included in the N classification is a nodule in the fat adjacent to a colorectal carcinoma, greater than 3 mm in largest extent, without evidence of residual lymph node tissue. This is classified as a regional lymph node metastasis. If the nodule is less than 3 mm it is classified as a discontinuous extension of the primary carcinoma (pT3).

   For early stages of disease (Stage I, II) pathologic classification of the extent of the primary tumor (T) and lymph nodes (N) is essential. Pathologic staging depends on the proven anatomic extent of disease whether or not the primary lesion has been completely removed. Furthermore, when dealing with Stage III or IV disease, in instances when a biopsied primary tumor technically cannot be removed, or when it is unreasonable to remove it, and if the highest T and N, or the M1 category of the tumor can be confirmed microscopically, the criteria for pathologic classification and staging have been satisfied without total removal of the primary cancer.

   Retreatment Classification. Retreatment classification is used after a disease-free interval when further treatment (such as hemotherapy) is planned for recurrent cancer. All information available at the time of retreatment should be used in determining the stage of the recurrent tumor (rTNM). Biopsy confirmation of the cancer is required.

   Autopsy Classification. If classification of a cancer is done after the death of a patient by postmortem examination, the classification of the stage is identified as aTNM.
3. After assigning cT, cN, and cM and/or pT, pN, and pM categories, these may be grouped into stages. Both TNM classifications and stage groupings, once established, remain in the medical record. The clinical stage is essential to select and evaluate primary therapy, and the pathologic stage provides additional precise data to estimate prognosis and calculate end results. Therefore, each should remain in the medical record. The pathologic stage does not replace the clinical stage.
4. If there is doubt concerning the correct T, N, or M classification to which a particular case should be allotted, then the lower (less advanced) category is chosen. This also applies to the stage grouping.
5. In the case of multiple, simultaneous tumors in one organ, the tumor with the highest T category is the one selected for classification and staging, and the multiplicity or the number of tumors is indicated in parentheses: for example, T2(m), or T2(5). In the circumstance of simultaneous bilateral cancers in paired organs, each tumor is classified separately as an independent tumor in different organs. In the case of tumors of the thyroid, liver, and ovary, multiplicity is a criterion of T classification.
6. Definitions of TNM categories and stage grouping may be telescoped (expanded as subsets of existing classifications) for research purposes as long as the original definitions are not changed. For instance, any of the published T, N, or M classifications can be divided into subgroups for testing, and if validated may be submitted to the

American Joint Committee on Cancer to be evaluated for inclusion into the classification system.

7. In the case of a primary of unknown origin, staging will be based on clinical suspicion of the primary origin (e.g., T0 N1 M0).

ANATOMIC REGIONS AND SITES

The sites in this classification are listed by code number of the International Classification of Diseases for Oncology, Second Edition (ICD-O, World Health Organization, 1990). Each chapter is constructed according to the following outline:

Introduction
Anatomy
  Primary site
  Regional lymph nodes
  Metastatic sites
Rules for Classification
  Clinical (TNM or cTNM)
  Pathologic (pTNM)
Definitions of TNM for each specific anatomic site
  T: Primary tumor size/extent
  N: Regional lymph node involvement: number/extent
  M: Distant metastasis absent/present
Stage Grouping
Histopathologic Type
Histopathologic Grade

TNM CLINICAL CLASSIFICATION

The following general definitions are used throughout:

Primary Tumor (T)

TX	Primary tumor cannot be assessed
T0	No evidence of primary tumor
Tis	Carcinoma *in situ*
T1, T2, T3, T4	Increasing size and/or local extent of the primary tumor

Regional Lymph Nodes (N)

NX	Regional lymph nodes cannot be assessed
N0	No regional lymph node metastasis
N1, N2, N3	Increasing involvement of regional lymph nodes

Note: Direct extension of the primary tumor into a lymph node(s) is classified as a lymph node metastasis.

Note: Metastasis in any lymph node other than regional is classified as a distant metastasis.

Note: A microscopically confirmed tumor nodule up to 3 mm in greatest extent, is classified in the T category, as discontinuous extension of the primary tumor. If the tumor nodule is greater than 3 mm, without evidence of residual lymph node tissue, it is classified as a regional lymph node metastasis.

Distant Metastasis (M)

MX	Distant metastasis cannot be assessed
M0	No distant metastasis
M1	Distant metastasis

Note: For pathologic stage grouping, if sufficient tissue has been removed for pathologic examination to evaluate the highest T and highest N categories, M1 may be either (cM1) or pathologic (pM1). However, if only a metastasis has had microscopic confirmation, the classification is pathologic (pM1) and the stage is pathologic.

The category M1 may be further specified according to the following notation:

Pulmonary PUL
Osseous OSS
Hepatic HEP
Brain BRA
Lymph Nodes LYM
Bone Marrow MAR
Pleura PLE
Peritoneum PER
Adrenals ADR
Skin SKI
Other OTH

Subdivisions of TNM. Subdivisions of some main categories are available for those who need greater specificity (e.g., T1a, 1b or N2a, 2b as with Breast and Prostate)

HISTOPATHOLOGIC TYPE

The histopathologic type is a *qualitative* assessment whereby a tumor is categorized (typed) according to the normal tissue type or cell type it most closely resembles (e.g., lobular carcinoma, osteosarcoma, squamous cell carcinoma). In general the World Health Organization Histologic Typing of Tumors, published in several anatomic site-specific editions, may be used for histopathologic typing.

HISTOPATHOLOGIC GRADE (G)

The histopathologic grade is a qualitative assessment of the differentiation of the tumor expressed as the extent to which a tumor resembles the normal tissue at that site, expressed in numerical grades of differentiation from most differentiated (Grade 1) to least differentiated (Grade 4), e.g., squamous cell carcinoma, moderately differentiated, Grade 2.

GX Grade cannot be assessed
G1 Well differentiated
G2 Moderately differentiated
G3 Poorly differentiated
G4 Undifferentiated

If there is evidence of more than one grade of differentiation of the tumor, the least differentiated is recorded as the histopathologic grade, using only G2 through G4. For example, a colonic adenocarcinoma that is partially well differentiated, and partially moderately differentiated is coded as grade 2 (G2). The growing edge of a tumor is not generally assessed in grading as it may appear to be a high grade.

For some anatomic sites, grade 3 and grade 4 are combined into a single grade: poorly differentiated to undifferentiated, G3-4. The combination is valid, for example, for carcinomas of the uterine corpus, ovary, prostate, urinary bladder, kidney, renal pelvis, ureter, and urethra. Only three grades are used for melanoma of the conjunctiva and uvea. Such grading does not apply to carcinomas of the thyroid, eyelids, retinoblastoma, malignant testicular tumors, and melanoma of the skin.

The use of G4 is reserved only for those tumors that show no specific differentiation that would identify the cancer as arising from its site of origin. In some sites, the WHO histologic classification includes undifferentiated carcinomas, for example, in the stomach or gallbladder. In these cases, the tumor is graded as undifferentiated, G4.

Some histologic tumor types are by definition, listed as G4. These include:

Undifferentiated carcinoma, any site
Small cell carcinoma, any site
Large cell carcinoma of lung
Ewing's sarcoma of bone and soft tissue
Rhabdomyosarcoma of soft tissue

ADDITIONAL DESCRIPTORS

For identification of special cases of TNM or pTNM classifications, the "m" suffix and y, r, and a prefixes are used. Although they do not affect the stage grouping, they indicate cases needing separate analysis.

m Suffix. Indicates the presence of multiple primary tumors in a single site and is recorded in parentheses: pT(m)NM

y Prefix. In those cases in which classification is performed during or following initial multimodality therapy, for example, neoadjuvant therapy which might alter the original pathology, the TNM or pTNM categories are identified by a y prefix: ypTNM

r Prefix. A recurrent tumor, when staged after a disease-free interval, is identified by the r prefix: rTNM

a Prefix. Designates the stage determined at autopsy: aTNM

OTHER DESCRIPTORS

Lymphatic Vessel Invasion (L)

LX Lymphatic vessel invasion cannot be assessed
L0 No lymphatic vessel invasion
L1 Lymphatic vessel invasion

Venous Invasion (V)

VX Venous invasion cannot be assessed
V0 No venous invasion
V1 Microscopic venous invasion
V2 Macroscopic venous invasion

Residual Tumor (R)

The absence or presence of residual tumor after treatment is described by the symbol R.

TNM and pTNM describe the anatomic extent of cancer in general without consideration of treatment. The TNM and pTNM can be supplemented by the R classification which deals with the tumor status after treatment. It reflects the effects of therapy, influences further therapeutic procedures, and is a strong predictor of prognosis.

The R categories are:

RX Presence of residual tumor cannot be assessed
R0 No residual tumor
R1 Microscopic residual tumor
R2 Macroscopic residual tumor

STAGE GROUPING

Classification by the TNM system achieves reasonably precise description and recording of the anatomic extent of disease. A tumor with four categories of T, three categories of N, and two categories of M has 24 TNM categories. For purposes of tabulation and analysis, except in very large series, it is necessary to condense these categories into a convenient number of TNM stage-groupings.

The grouping adopted ensures, as far as possible, that each stage group is relatively homogeneous with respect to survival, and that the survival rates of these stage groupings for each cancer site are distinctive. Carcinoma *in situ* is categorized Stage 0; a case with distant metastasis is categorized Stage IV. Stages I, II, and III indicate relatively greater anatomic extent of cancer within the range from Stage 0 to Stage IV.

Cancer Staging Data Form

Each anatomic site staging form is to be used to record the TNM classification and the stage of the cancer. The specific anatomic site of the cancer is recorded, as well as the histologic type and grade. The appropriate period of the chronology of classification must be recorded, such as at the time of primary therapy or at the time of recurrence. If a cancer is staged during several time periods, a separate form is used for each time period; or if all are recorded on a single form, the stage for each period is clearly identified.

The T, N, and M classifications can be checked opposite the appropriate definitions of the extent of the primary tumor, the regional lymph nodes, and distant metastasis. The lesion(s) can be marked on a diagram and, finally, the stage can be checked according to the grouping of TNM. In some instances information regarding other characteristics of the tumor (not included in the stage) might be requested. These data may be pertinent in deciding management of the patient. On the reverse side of the staging form are information and definitions that are important in the proper classification of a cancer.

The cancer staging form is a specific additional document in the patient's record indicating anatomic extent of disease. It is not a substitute for history, treatment, or follow-up records. The data forms in this manual may be duplicated for individual or institutional use without permission from the AJCC or the publisher.

2

Cancer Survival Analysis

Analyses of cancer survival data and related outcomes are quantitative tools commonly used to assess the experience of cancer treatment programs and to monitor the progress of regional and national cancer control programs. In this chapter the most common survival analysis methodology will be illustrated, basic terminology will be defined, and the essential elements of data collection and reporting will be described. Although the underlying principles are applicable to both, the focus of this discussion will be on use of survival analysis to describe data typically available in cancer registries rather than to analyze research data obtained from clinical trials or laboratory experimentation. Discussion of statistical principles and methodology will be limited. Persons interested in statistical underpinnings or research applications are referred to textbooks that explore these topics at length (Kalbfleisch and Prentice, 1980; Kleinbaum, 1996; Lee, 1980).

BASIC CONCEPTS

A survival *rate* is a statistical index which summarizes the probable frequency of specific outcomes for a group of patients at a particular point in time. A survival *curve* is a summary display of the pattern of survival rates over time. The basic concept is simple. For example, for a certain category of patient, one might ask what proportion are likely to be alive at the end of a specified interval, such as five years? The greater the proportion surviving, the more effective the program. Survival analysis, however, is somewhat more complicated than it first might appear. If one were to measure the length of time between diagnosis and death or record the vital status when last observed for every patient in a selected patient group, one might be tempted to describe the survival of the group as the proportion alive at the end of the period under investigation. This simple measure will be informative, however, only if all of the patients were observed for the same length of time.

In most real situations it is not the case that all members of the group are observed for the same amount of time. Patients diagnosed near the end of the study period are more likely to be alive at last contact and will have been followed for less time than those diagnosed earlier. Even though it was not possible to follow these persons as long as the others, the length of their survival might eventually have proved to be just as long or longer. Another difficulty is that it usually is not possible to know the outcome status of all of the persons who were in the group at the beginning. People move or change names and are lost to follow-up. Some of these persons may have died and others could be still living. Thus, if a survival rate is to accurately describe the outcomes for an entire group, there must be some means to deal with the fact that different persons in the group are observed for different lengths of time and, for others, their vital status is not known at the time of analysis. In the parlance of survival analysis, subjects who are observed until they reach the end point of interest (e.g., death) are called *uncensored* cases, and those who survive beyond the end of the follow-up or who are lost to follow-up at some point, are termed *censored* cases or observations.

Two basic survival procedures that enable one to determine overall group survival, taking into account both censored and uncensored observations, are the life table (Berkson and Gage, 1950) and Kaplan-Meier (Kaplan and Meier, 1958) methods. The life table method was the first method generally used to describe cancer survival results and this came to be known as the actuarial method because of its similarity to the work done by actuaries in the insurance industry. The subsequently developed Kaplan-Meier procedure is similar to the life table method in that regard and, for this reason, it is no longer as informative to describe the method of survival analysis only as actuarial. The specific method of computation, i.e., life table or Kaplan-Meier, should always be indicated to avoid any confusion associated with the use of less precise terminology. Rates computed by different methods are not directly comparable with each other, and when the survival experiences of different patient groups are compared, the different rates must be computed by the same method.

These commonly used survival methods can be calculated by hand and previous editions (Beahrs et al., 1992) of this manual describe the procedures for doing this for the simplest procedures. Hand calculation can be tedious and the wide availability of statistical programs suitable for use on personal computers now makes such effort unnecessary. Identical results can be obtained with the survival routines included in different tumor registry data management software as well as most commonly used statistical packages. Most computer software packages also have the capability to generate graphs and this feature is very useful for visually interpreting and reporting results.

The illustrations in this chapter are based on data obtained from the public use files of the National Cancer Institute Surveillance, Epidemiology, and End Results (SEER) program. The cases selected are a 1% random sample of the total number for the selected sites and years of diagnosis. Follow-up of these patients continued through the end of 1993. Thus, for the earliest patients, there can be as much as nine years of follow-up; but for those diagnosed at the end of the study period, there can be as little as one year of follow-up. These data are used because they are realistic in terms of both the actual survival rates they yield, as well as encompassing a number of cases that might be seen in a single large tumor registry over a comparable number of years. They are intended only to illustrate the methodology. SEER results are more fully described elsewhere (Kosary et al., 1995) and these illustrations should not be regarded as an adequate description of the total or current United States patterns of breast or lung cancer survival.

THE LIFE TABLE METHOD

The life table method involves dividing the total period over which a group is observed into fixed intervals, usually months or years. For each interval, the proportion surviving to the end of the interval is calculated based on the number known to have experienced the endpoint event (e.g., death) during the interval and the number estimated to have been at risk at the start of the interval. For each succeeding interval a cumulative survival rate may be calculated. The cumulative survival rate is the probability of surviving the most recent interval multiplied by the probabilities of surviving all of the prior intervals. Thus, if the percent of the patients surviving the first interval is 90% and is the same for the second and third intervals, the cumulative survival percentage is 72.9% ($.9 \times .9 \times .9 = .729$).

Results from the life table method for calculating survival for the breast cancer illustration are shown in Figure 2-1. One thousand five hundred forty-three (1,543) patients diagnosed between 1983 and 1992 were followed through 1993. Following the life table calculation method for each year after diagnosis, the one year survival rate is 94.5%. The five year cumulative survival rate is 73.1%. At ten years, the cumulative survival is 56.1%.

The lung cancer data show a much different survival pattern (Fig. 2-2). At one year following diagnosis the survival rate is only 41.2%. By five years it has fallen to 10.3% and only 5.1% of lung cancer patients are estimated to have survived for ten years following diagnosis. For lung cancer patients the *median survival time* is 10.2 months. Median survival time is the amount of time required to pass so that half the patients have experienced the endpoint event and half the patients remain event free. If the cumulative survival does not fall below 50% it is not possible to estimate median survival from the data, as is the case in the breast cancer data.

In the case of breast cancer, the ten year survival rate is important because such a large proportion of patients live more than five years past their diagnosis. The ten year time frame for lung cancer is less meaningful since such a large proportion of this patient group dies well before that much time passes.

The power of the actuarial approach on which the life table method is based is demonstrated by the fact that even though only those patients diagnosed before 1983 actually could be observed for as long as ten years, the method provides valid ten year survival estimates that describe the entire population; including even those diagnosed too recently to permit the full ten years of observation.

An important assumption of all actuarial survival methods is that censored cases do not dif-

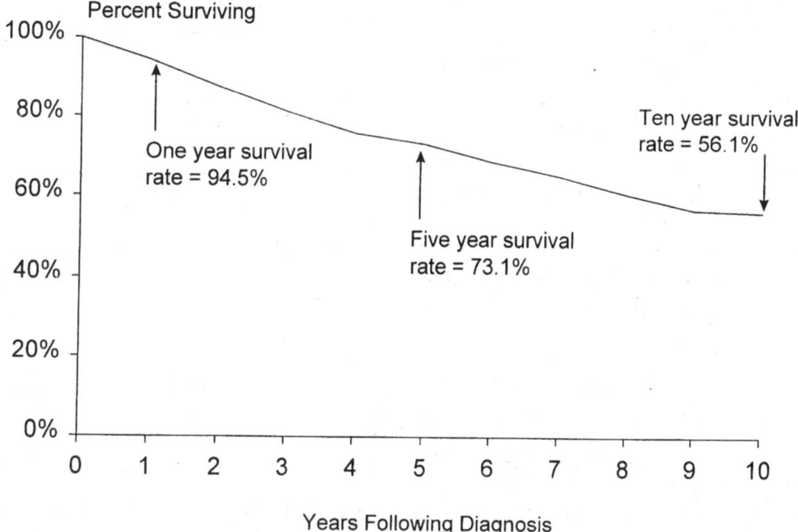

FIG. 2-1. Ten-year survival of 1,543 breast cancer patients from the Surveillance, Epidemiology, and End Results Program of the National Cancer Institute, 1983–1992. Calculated by the life table method.

fer from the entire collection of uncensored cases in any systematic manner that would affect their survival. For example, if the more recently diagnosed cases in Figure 2-1, i.e., those who were most likely not to have died yet, tended to be detected with earlier stage disease than the uncensored cases; or were treated differently, the assumption about comparability of censored and uncensored cases would not be met and the result for the group as a whole would be inaccurate. Thus, it is important when patients are included in a life table analysis one be reasonably confident differences in the amount of information available about survival are not related to differences that might affect survival.

THE KAPLAN-MEIER METHOD

These same data can be analyzed using the Kaplan-Meier method. It is similar to the life table method but provides for calculating the proportion surviving to each point in time that a death occurs rather than at fixed intervals. The

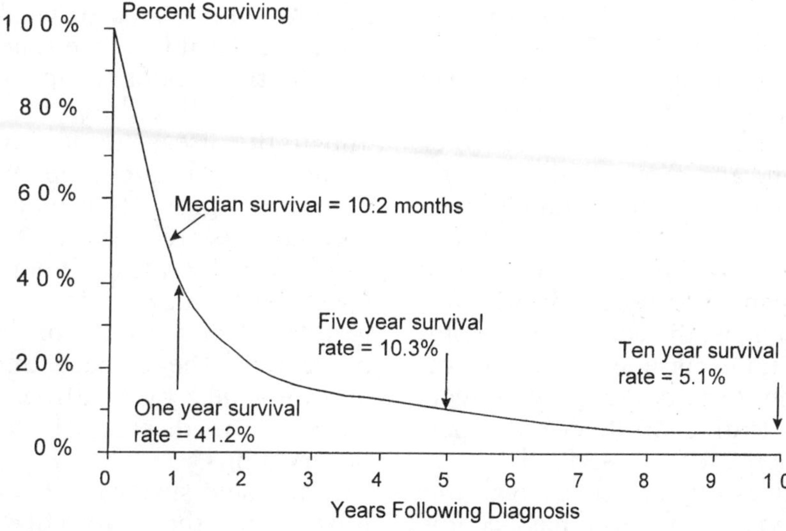

FIG. 2-2. Ten-year survival of 1,275 lung cancer patients from the Surveillance, Epidemiology, and End Results Program of the National Cancer Institute, 1983–1992. Calculated by the life table method.

principal difference evident in a survival curve is that the stepwise changes in the cumulative survival rate appear to occur independently of the intervals on the time of follow-up axis. The life table and Kaplan-Meier methods will give identical results only in the absence of censored observations.

PATIENT, DISEASE, TREATMENT-SPECIFIC SURVIVAL

Although overall group survival is informative, comparisons of the overall survival between two groups often are confounded by differences in the patients, their tumors, or the treatments they received. For example, it would be misleading to compare the overall survival depicted in Figure 2-1 with the overall survival of other breast cancer patients who tend to be diagnosed with more advanced disease whose survival would be presumed to be poorer. The simplest approach to accounting for possible differences between groups is it provide survival results which are specific to the categories of patient, disease, or treatment that may affect results. In most cancer applications the most important variable by which survival results should be subdivided is the stage of disease. In Figure 2-3 the *stage-specific* five year survival curves of the same breast cancer patients described earlier are shown. These data show that breast cancer patient survival differs markedly according to the stage of the tumor at the time of diagnosis.

Almost any variable can be used to sub-classify survival rates but some are more meaningfui than others. For example, it would be possible to provide season-of-diagnosis specific (i.e., Spring, Summer, Winter, Fall) survival rates, but the season of diagnosis probably has no biologic association with the length of a breast cancer patient's survival. On the other hand, the age-specific and race-specific survival rates shown in Figures 2-4 and 2-5 suggest that both of these variables are related to breast cancer survival. Whites have the highest survival and African-Americans the poorest. In the case of age, these data suggest that it is only the oldest aged patients who experience poor survival and it would be helpful to consider the effects of other causes of death that affect older persons using adjustments to be described.

Although the factors that affect survival may be unique to each type of cancer, it has become conventional that a basic description of survival for a specific cancer should include stage, age, and race specific survival results. Treatment is

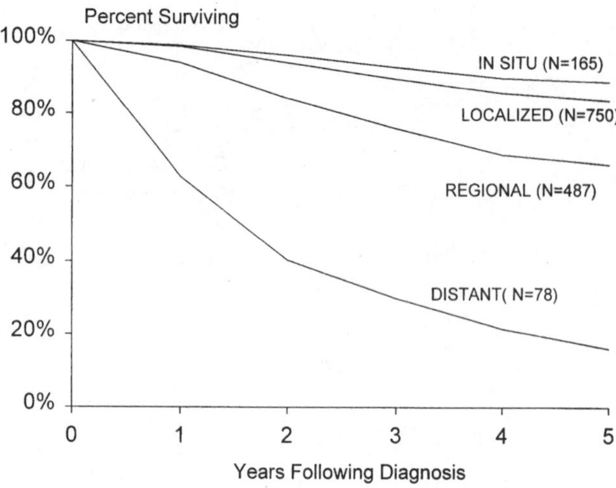

FIG. 2-3. Five-year survival by stage of disease at diagnosis of 1,480 breast cancer patients from the Surveillance, Epidemiology, and End Results Program of the National Cancer Institute, 1983–1992. Excludes 63 patients with unknown stage of disease. Calculated by the life table method. (*Note*: SEER uses extent of disease [EOD] staging. For TNM survival curves for breast cancer, see Chapter 25.)

a fourth factor by which survival is commonly subdivided but it must be kept in mind that selection of treatment is usually related to some other factors which exert influence on survival. For example, in cancer care the choice of treatment is often dependent on the stage of disease at diagnosis.

ADJUSTED SURVIVAL RATE

The survival rates depicted in the illustrations account for all deaths, regardless of cause. This is known as *observed* survival rate. Although observed survival is a true reflection of total mortality in the patient group, we frequently are interested in describing mortality attributable only to the disease under investigation. The *adjusted* survival rate is the proportion of the initial patient group that escaped death due to a specific cause (e.g., cancer) if no other cause of death was operating. Whenever reliable information on cause of death is available, an adjustment can be made for deaths due to causes other than the disease under study. This is accomplished by treating patients who died without the disease of interest as censored observations.

If adjusted survival rates were calculated for lung cancer, the pattern of survival would show little difference between observed and adjusted rates because lung cancer usually is the cause of death for patients with the diagnosis. For dis-

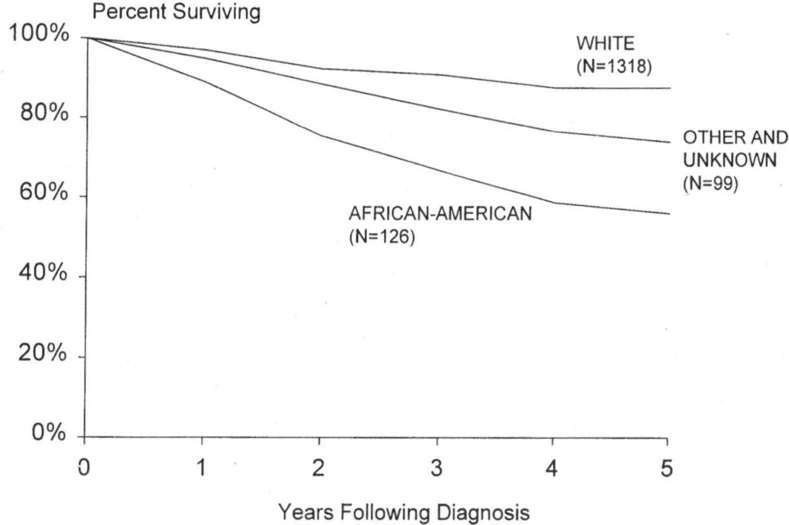

FIG. 2-4. Five-year survival by race of 1,543 breast cancer patients from the Surveillance, Epidemiology, and End Results Program of the National Cancer Institute, 1983–1992. Calculated by the life table method.

eases with more favorable survival patterns, such as breast cancer, patients live long enough to be at risk of other causes of death and, in these instances, adjusted survival rates will tend to be higher than observed survival and give a clearer picture of the specific effects of the diagnosis under investigation. Adjusted rates can be calculated for either life table or Kaplan-Meier results.

RELATIVE SURVIVAL

Information on cause of death is sometimes unavailable or unreliable. Under such circumstances, it is not possible to compute an adjusted survival rate. However, it is possible to partially adjust for differences in the risk of dying from causes other than the disease under study. This can be done by means of the relative survival rate which is the ratio of the observed survival rate to the expected rate for a group of people in the general population similar to the patient group with respect to race, sex, and age. The relative survival rate is calculated using a procedure described by Ederer, Axtell, and Cutler (1961).

The relative survival rate represents the likelihood that a patient will not die from causes associated specifically with their cancer at some specified time after diagnosis. It is always larger than the observed survival rate for the same group of patients. If the group is sufficiently large and the patients are roughly representative of the population of the United States (taking race, sex, and age into account), the relative survival rate provides a useful estimate of the probability of escaping death from the specific cancer under study. However, if reliable information on cause of death is available, it is preferable to use the adjusted rate. This is particularly true if the series is small or if the patients are largely drawn from a particular socioeconomic segment of the population. Relative survival rates may be derived from life table or Kaplan-Meier results.

MULTIVARIATE METHODS

Examining survival within specific patient, disease or treatment categories is the simplest way of studying multiple factors possibly associated with survival. This approach, however, is limited to factors into which patients may be broadly grouped. This approach does not lend itself to studying the effects of measures that vary on an interval scale. There are many examples of interval variables in cancer such as number of positive nodes, cell counts and, laboratory marker values. If the patient population were to be divided up into each interval value, too few subjects would be in each analysis to be meaningful. In addition, when more than one factor is considered, the number of curves that result provide so many comparisons that the effects of the factors defy interpretation.

Multiple regression analysis is a conventional statistical method to study the joint effects of multiple variables on a single outcome, but

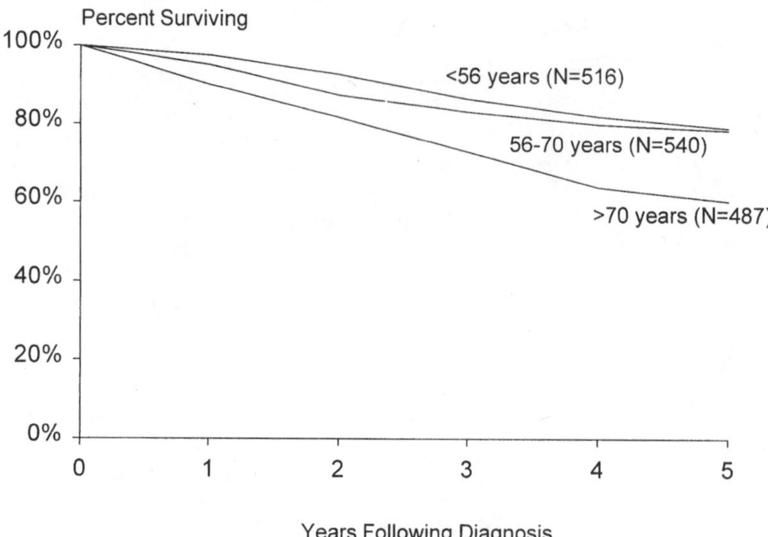

FIG. 2-5. Five-year survival by age of 1,543 breast cancer patients from the Surveillance, Epidemiology, and End Results Program of the National Cancer Institute, 1983–1992. Calculated by the life table method.

multiple regression analysis is incapable of dealing with censored observations. For this reason other statistical methods have had to be developed to assess the relationship of survival time to a number of variables simultaneously. The most commonly used is the Cox proportional hazards regression model (Cox, 1972; Meier, 1985). This model provides a method for estimating the influence of multiple covariates on the survival distribution from data that includes censored observations. Covariates are the multiple factors to be studied in association with survival. In the Cox proportional hazards regression model the covariates may be categorical variables such as race or interval measures such as age, or laboratory test results.

Specifics of multivariate methodology are beyond the scope of this chapter. Fortunately, many readily accessible computer packages for statistical analysis now permit the methods to be applied quite easily by the knowledgeable analyst. Although much useful information can be derived from multivariate survival models, they generally do require additional assumptions about the shape of the survival curve and the nature of the effects of the covariates. One must always examine the appropriateness of the model that is used relative to the assumptions required.

STANDARD ERROR OF A SURVIVAL RATE

Survival rates that describe the experience of the specific group of patients are frequently used to generalize to larger populations. The existence of true population values is postulated and these values are estimated from the group under study, which is only a sample of the larger population. If a survival rate were calculated from a second sample taken from the same population, it is unlikely that the results would be exactly the same. The difference between the two results is called the sampling variation (chance variation or sampling error). The *standard error* is a measure of the extent to which sampling variation influences the computed survival rate. In repeated observations under the same conditions, the true or population survival rate will lie within the range of two standard errors on either side of the computed rate about 95 times in 100. This range is called the *95% confidence interval.*

COMPARISON OF SURVIVAL BETWEEN PATIENT GROUPS

In comparing survival rates of two patient groups, the statistical significance of the observed difference is of interest. The essential question is: What is the probability that the observed difference may have occurred by chance? The standard error of the survival rate provides a simple means for appraising this question. If the 95% confidence intervals of two survival rates do not overlap, the observed difference would be customarily considered as statistically significant, that is, unlikely to be due to chance.

It is possible that the differences between two groups at each comparable time of follow-up do not differ significantly but when the survival curves are considered in their entirety, the individual insignificant differences combine to yield a significantly different pattern of survival. The most common statistical test that examines the whole pattern of differences between survival curves is the *log rank test.* This test equally weights the effects of differences occurring throughout the follow-up and is the appropriate choice for most situations. Other tests weight the differences according to the numbers of persons at risk at different points and can yield different results depending on whether deaths tend more to occur early or later in the follow-up.

Care must be exercised in the interpretation of tests of statistical significance. For example, if differences exist in the patient and disease characteristics of two treatment groups, a statistically significant difference in survival results may primarily reflect differences in the two patient series, rather than differences in efficacy of the treatment regimens. The more definitive approach to therapy evaluation requires a randomized clinical trial that helps to ensure comparability of the two treatment groups and their disease.

DEFINITION OF STUDY STARTING POINT

The starting time for determining survival of patients depends on the purpose of the study. For example, the starting time for studying the natural history of a particular cancer might be defined in reference to the appearance of the first symptom. Various reference dates are commonly used as starting times for evaluating the effects of therapy. These include (1) date of diagnosis; (2) date of first visit to physician or clinic; (3) date of hospital admission; and (4) date of treatment initiation. If the time to recurrence of a tumor after apparent complete remission is being studied, the starting time is the date of apparent complete remission. The specific reference date used should be clearly specified in every report.

The date of initiation of therapy should be used as the starting time for evaluating therapy. For untreated patients, the most comparable date is the time at which it was decided that no tumor-directed treatment would be given. For both treated and untreated patients, the above times from which survival rates are calculated will usually coincide with the date of the initial staging of cancer.

VITAL STATUS

At any given time the vital status of each patient is defined as alive, dead, or unknown (i.e., lost to follow-up). The end point of each patient's participation in the study is either (1) a specified "terminal event" such as death, (2) survival to the completion of the study, or (3) loss to follow-up. In each case, the observed follow-up time is the time from the starting point to the terminal event, to the end of the study, or to the date of last observation. This observed follow-up may be further described in terms of patient status at the end point such as:

Alive; tumor-free; no recurrence
Alive; tumor-free; after recurrence
Alive with persistent, recurrent, or metastatic disease
Alive with primary tumor
Dead; tumor-free
Dead; with cancer (primary, recurrent, or metastatic disease)
Dead; postoperative
Unknown; lost to follow-up

Completeness of the follow-up is crucial in any study of survival because even a small number of patients lost to follow-up may lead to inaccurate or biased results. The maximum possible effect of bias from patients lost to follow-up may be ascertained by calculating a maximum survival rate, assuming that all lost patients lived to the end of the study. A minimum survival rate may be calculated by assuming that all patients lost to follow-up died at the time they were lost.

TIME INTERVALS

The total survival time is often divided into intervals in units of weeks, months, or years. The survival curve for these intervals provides a description of the population under study with respect to the dynamics of survival over a specified time. The time interval used should be selected with regard to the natural history of the disease under consideration. In diseases with a long natural history, the duration of study could be 5 to 20 years and survival intervals of 6 to 12 months will provide a meaningful description of the survival dynamics. If the population being studied has a very poor prognosis (e.g., patients with carcinoma of the esophagus or pancreas), the total duration of study may be 2 to 3 years and the survival intervals described in terms of 1 to 3 months. In interpreting survival rates one must also take into account the number of individuals entering a survival interval.

SUMMARY

This chapter has reviewed the rudiments of survival analysis as it is often applied to cancer registry data. Complex analysis of data and exploration of research hypotheses demands greater knowledge and expertise than could be conveyed herein. Survival analysis is now performed automatically in many different registry data management and statistical analysis programs available for use on personal computers. Persons with access to these programs are encouraged to explore the different analysis features they have available do demonstrate for themselves the insight on cancer registry data that survival analysis can provide.

BIBLIOGRAPHY

Beahrs OH, Henson DE, Hutter RVP, Kennedy BJ, (Eds.): American Joint Committee on Cancer: manual for staging of cancer, 4th ed. Philadelphia: JB Lippincott, 1992

Berkson J, Gage RP: Calculation of survival rates for cancer. Proc Staff Meet Mayo Clin 25:270–286, 1950

Cox DR: Regression models and life tables. J R Stat Soc B 34:187–220, 1972

Ederer F, Axtell LM, Cutler SJ: The relative survival rate: a statistical methodology. Natl Cancer Inst Monogr 6:101–121, 1961

Kalbfleisch JD, Prentice RL: The statistical analysis of failure time data. New York: John Wiley and Sons; 321, 1980

Kaplan EL, Meier P: Nonparametric estimation from incomplete observations. J Am Stat Assn 53:457–481, 1958

Kleinbaum DG: Survival analysis: a self learning text. New York: Springer-Verlag, 1996

Kosary CL, Ries LAG, Miller BA, et al (Eds.): SEER cancer statistics review, 1973–1992: tables and graphs, National Cancer Institute. Bethesda, Maryland: National Institutes of Health, NIH Pub. No. 96-2789. 1995

Lee ET: Statistical methods for survival data analysis. Belmont, California: Wadsworth, Inc, 1980

Mantel N: Evaluation of survival data and two new rank order statistics arising in its consideration. Cancer Chemother Rep 50:163–170, 1966

Meier P: Anatomy and interpretation of the Cox regression model. ASAIO J 8:3–12, 1985

PART II

Staging of Cancer at Specific Anatomic Sites

HEAD AND NECK SITES

Cancers of the head and neck may arise from any of the lining membranes of the upper aerodigestive tract. The T classifications indicating the extent of the primary tumor are generally similar but differ in specific details for each site because of anatomic considerations. The N classification for cervical lymph node metastasis is uniform for all mucosal sites except nasopharynx. The N classification for thyroid and nasopharynx are unique to those sites and are based upon tumor behavior and prognosis. The staging systems presented in this section are all clinical staging, based on the best possible estimate of the extent of the disease before first treatment. Imaging techniques (computed tomography [CT], magnetic resonance imaging [MRI], ultrasonography) may be applied, and in more advanced tumor stages, have added to the accuracy of primary (T) and nodal (N) staging, especially in the nasopharyngeal, paranasal sinuses and regional lymph nodal areas. Appropriate imaging studies should be obtained whenever the clinical findings are uncertain. Fine needle aspiration biopsy (FNAB), may confirm the presence of tumor and its histopathologic nature, but cannot prove the absence of tumor.

Any diagnostic information which contributes to the overall accuracy of the pretreatment assessment should be considered in clinical staging and treatment planning. When surgical treatment is carried out, cancer of the head and neck can be staged (pathologic stage [pTNM]) using all information available from clinical assessment as well as from the pathologic study of the resected specimen. The pathologic stage does not replace the clinical stage, which should be reported as well.

In reviewing the staging systems, minor changes in the T classifications have been made. A major revision of the nasopharynx classification has been stimulated by clinical experience from several Asian sources.

This section presents the staging classification for six major head and neck sites: the oral cavity, the pharynx (nasopharynx, oropharynx, hypopharynx), the larynx, the paranasal sinuses, the salivary glands, and the thyroid gland.

Regional Lymph Nodes. The status of the regional lymph nodes in head and neck cancer is of such prognostic importance that the cervical nodes must be assessed for each patient and tumor. The lymph nodes may be subdivided into specific anatomic subsites and grouped into seven levels for ease of description.

Level I:	Submental
	Submandibular
Level II:	Upper jugular
Level III:	Mid-jugular
Level IV:	Lower jugular
Level V:	Posterior triangle (Spinal accessory)
	(Upper, mid and lower, corresponding to the levels that define upper, mid, and lower jugular nodes)
Level VI:	Prelaryngeal (Delphian)
	Pretracheal
	Paratracheal
Level VII:	Upper mediastinal

Other groups: Retropharyngeal
- Buccinator (facial)
- Intraparotid
- Preauricular
- Postauricular
- Suboccipital

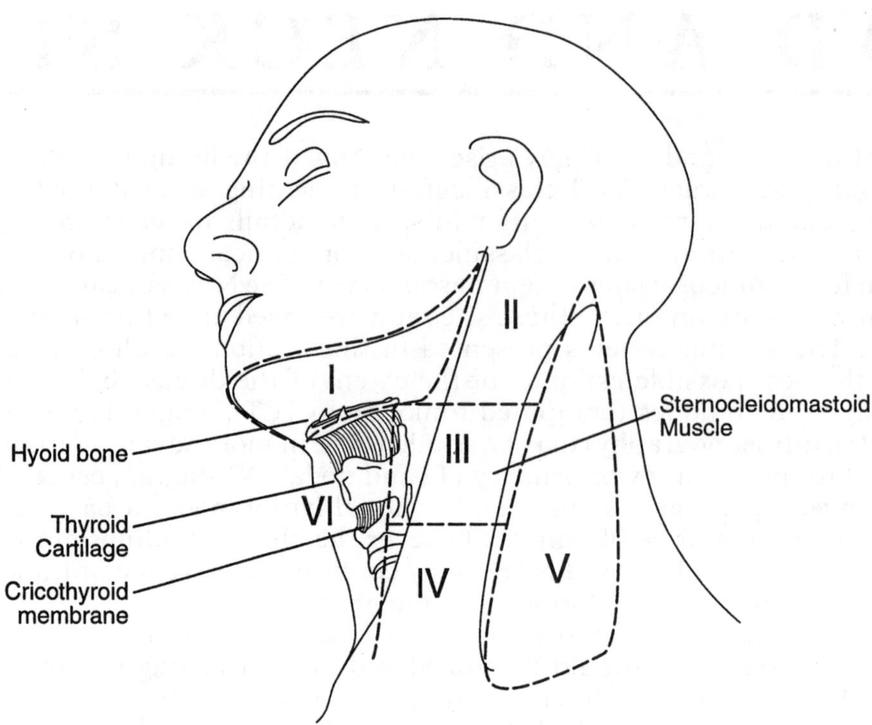

FIG. 1. Schematic diagram indicating the location of the lymph node levels in the neck as described in the text.

The location of the lymph node levels conforms to the following clinical descriptions which also correlate with surgical landmarks at the time of surgical neck exploration (Fig. 1).

Level I: Contains the submental and submandibular triangles bounded by the posterior belly of the digastric muscle, the hyoid bone inferiorly and the body of the mandible superiorly.

Level II: Contains the upper jugular lymph nodes and extends from the level of the hyoid bone inferiorly to the skull base superiorly.

Level III: Contains the middle jugular lymph nodes from the hyoid bone superiorly to the cricothyroid membrane inferiorly.

Level IV: Contains the lower jugular lymph nodes from the cricothyroid membrane superiorly to the clavicle inferiorly.

Level V: Contains the lymph nodes in the posterior triangle bounded by the anterior border of the trapezius posteriorly, the posterior border of the sternocleidomastoid muscle anteriorly, and the clavicle inferiorly.

For descriptive purposes Level V may be further subdivided into upper, middle, or lower levels corresponding to the superior and inferior planes that define levels II, III, and IV.

Level VI: Contains the lymph nodes of the anterior compartment from the hyoid bone superiorly to the suprasternal notch inferiorly. On each side the lateral border is formed by the medial border of the carotid sheath.

Level VII: Contains the lymph nodes inferior to the suprasternal notch in the upper mediastinum.

The pattern of the lymphatic drainage varies for different anatomic sites. The natural history of and response to treatment of cervical nodal metastases from nasopharynx primary sites is different, impacts upon prognosis, and justifies a different "N" classification scheme. Regional node metastases from well-differentiated thyroid cancer do not significantly impact upon the ultimate prognosis and, therefore, justify a unique staging system for thyroid cancers.

Histopathologic examination is necessary to exclude the presence of tumor in lymph nodes. No imaging study (as yet) can identify microscopic tumor foci in regional nodes or distinguish between small reactive nodes and small malignant nodes without radiographic inhomogeneity.

When enlarged lymph nodes can be detected, the actual size of the nodal mass(es) should be measured. It is recognized that most masses over 3 cm in diameter are not single nodes but are confluent nodes or tumor in soft tissues of the neck. Imaging studies showing amorphous spiculated margins of involved nodes or involvement of internodal fat resulting in loss of normal oval to round nodal shape strongly suggest extracapsular (extranodal) tumor spread. Pathologic examination is necessary for documentation of such disease extent.

Metastatic Sites. The most common sites of distant spread are in the lungs and bones; hepatic metastases occur less often. Mediastinal lymph node metastases are considered distant metastases.

BIBLIOGRAPHY

Cooper JS, Farnan NC, Asbell SO, et al: Recursive partitioning analysis of 2105 patients treated in Radiation Therapy Oncology Group studies of head and neck cancer. Cancer 77:1905–1911, 1996

Deleyiannis FW, Thomas DB, Vaughan TL, et al: Alcoholism: independent predictor of survival in patients with head and neck cancer. J Natl Cancer Inst 88:542–549, 1996

Faye-Lund H, Abdelnoor M. Prognostic factors of survival in a cohort of head and neck cancer patients in Oslo. Eur J Cancer B Oral Oncol 2:83–90, 1996

Grandi C, Alloisio M, Moglia D, et al: Prognostic significance of lymphatic spread in head and neck carcinomas: therapeutic implications. Head Neck Surg 8:67–73, 1985

Harnsberger HR: Squamous cell carcinoma: nodal staging. In Handbook of head and neck imaging, 2nd ed. St Louis: Mosby; 283–298, 1995

Hillsamer PJ, Schuller DE, McGhee RB, et al: Improving diagnostic accuracy of cervical metastases with CT and MR imaging. Arch Otolaryngol Head Neck Surg 116:1297–1301, 1990

Kalnins IK, Leonard AG, Sako K, et al: Correlation between prognosis and degree of lymph node involvement in carcinoma of the oral cavity. Am J Surg 34:450–454, 1977

Mancuso AA, Harnsberger HR, Muraki AS, et al: Computed tomography of cervical and retropharyngeal lymph nodes: normal anatomy, variants of normal, and application in staging head and neck cancer. II. Pathology. Radiology 148:715–723, 1983

Medina JE: A rational classification of neck dissections. Otolaryngol Head Neck Surg 100:169–176, 1989

Piccirillo JF: Inclusion of comorbidity in a staging system for head and neck cancer. Oncology 9:831–836, 1995

Richard JM, Sancho-Garnier H, Michaeu C, et al: Prognostic factors in cervical lymph node metastasis in upper respiratory and digestive tract carcinomas: study of 1713 cases during a 15-year period. Laryngoscope 97:97–101, 1987

Robbins KT: Neck dissection: classification and incisions. In Shockley WW, Pillsbury HC, (Eds.), The neck: diagnosis and surgery. St Louis: Mosby; 381–391, 1994

Som PM: Detection of metastasis in cervical lymph nodes: CT And MR criteria and differential diagnosis. AJR 158:961–969, 1992

Stell PM, Morton RP, Singh SD: Cervical lymph node metastases: the significance of the level of the lymph node. Clin Oncol 9:101–107, 1983

Stevens MH, Harnsberger HR, Mancuso AA: Computed tomography of cervical lymph nodes: staging and management of head and neck cancer. Arch Otolaryngol 11:735–739, 1985

Strong EW, Kasdorf H, Henk JM: Squamous cell carcinoma of the head and neck. In Hermanek P, Gospodarowicz MK, Henson DE, et al (Eds.), Prognostic factors in cancer, UICC Geneva. Berlin-New York: Springer-Verlag; 23–27, 1995

Yousem DM, Som PM, Hackney DB, et al: Central nodal necrosis and extracapsular neoplastic spread in cervical lymph nodes: MR imaging versus CT. Radiology 182:753–759, 1992

3

Lip and Oral Cavity

(Nonepithelial tumors such as those of lymphoid tissue, soft tissue, bone, and cartilage are not included.)

C00.0 External upper lip
C00.1 External lower lip
C00.2 External lip, NOS
C00.3 Mucosa of upper lip
C00.4 Mucosa of lower lip
C00.5 Mucosa of lip, NOS
C00.6 Commissure
C00.8 Overlapping lesion
C00.9 Lip, NOS

C02.0 Dorsal surface of tongue, NOS
C02.1 Border of tongue
C02.2 Ventral surface of tongue, NOS
C02.3 Anterior two-thirds of tongue, NOS
C02.8 Overlapping lesion
C02.9 Tongue, NOS

C03.0 Upper gum
C03.1 Lower gum
C03.9 Gum, NOS

C06.2 Retromolar gingiva (gum)

C04.0 Anterior floor of mouth
C04.1 Lateral floor of mouth
C04.8 Overlapping lesion
C04.9 Floor of mouth, NOS

C05.0 Hard palate

C05.8 Overlapping lesion
C05.9 Palate, NOS

C06.0 Cheek mucosa
C06.1 Vestibule of mouth
C06.2 Retromolar area
C06.8 Overlapping lesion of other and unspecified parts of mouth
C06.9 Mouth, NOS

ANATOMY

Primary Site. The oral cavity extends from the skin-vermilion junction of the lips to the junction of the hard and soft palate above and to the line of circumvallate papillae below and is divided into the following specific areas:

Mucosal Lip. The lip begins at the junction of the vermilion border with the skin and includes only the vermilion surface or that portion of the lip that comes into contact with the opposing lip. It is well defined into an upper and lower lip joined at the commissures of the mouth.

Buccal Mucosa. This includes all the membrane lining of the inner surface of the cheeks and lips from the line of contact of the opposing lips to the line of attachment of mucosa of the alveolar ridge (upper and lower) and pterygomandibular raphe.

Lower Alveolar Ridge. This refers to the mucosa overlying the alveolar process of the mandible which extends from the line of attachment of mucosa in the buccal gutter to the line of free mucosa of the floor of the mouth. Posteriorly it extends to the ascending ramus of the mandible.

Upper Alveolar Ridge. This refers to the mucosa overlying the alveolar process of the maxilla which extends from the line of attachment of mucosa in the upper gingival buccal gutter to the junction of the hard palate. Its posterior margin is the upper end of the pterygopalatine arch.

Retromolar Gingiva (Retromolar Trigone). This is the attached mucosa overlying the ascending ramus of the mandible from the level of the posterior surface of the last molar tooth to the apex superiorly, adjacent to the tuberosity of the maxilla.

Floor of the Mouth. This is a semilunar space over the myelohyoid and hyoglossus muscles, extending from the inner surface of the lower alveolar ridge to the undersurface of the tongue. Its posterior boundary is the base of the anterior pillar of the tonsil. It is divided into two sides by the frenulum of the tongue and contains the ostia of the submaxillary and sublingual salivary glands.

Hard Palate. This is the semilunar area between the upper alveolar ridge and the mucous membrane covering the palatine process of the maxillary palatine bones. It extends from the inner surface of the superior alveolar ridge to the posterior edge of the palatine bone.

Anterior Two-Thirds of the Tongue (Oral Tongue). This is a freely mobile portion of the tongue that extends anteriorly from the line of circumvallate papillae to the undersurface of the tongue at the junction of the floor of the mouth. It is composed of four areas: the tip, the lateral borders, the dorsum, and the undersurface (nonvillous ventral surface of the tongue). The undersurface of the tongue is considered as a separate category by the World Health Organization (WHO).

Regional Lymph Nodes. Mucosal cancer of the oral cavity may spread to regional lymph node(s). Tumors of each anatomic site have their own predictable patterns of regional spread. The risk of regional metastasis generally relates to T category and probably more importantly to the depth of infiltration of the primary tumor. Cancer of the lip carries a low metastatic risk and initially involves adjacent submental and submandibular nodes, then jugular nodes. Cancers of the hard palate and alveolar ridge likewise have a low metastatic potential and involve buccinator, submandibular, jugular and occasionally retropharyngeal nodes. Other oral cancers will primarily spread to submandibular and jugular nodes, uncommonly posterior triangle/supraclavicular nodes. Cancer of the anterior oral tongue may spread directly to lower jugular nodes. The closer to the midline the primary is, the greater the risk of bilateral cervical nodal spread. Any previous treatment to the neck, surgical and/or radiation, may alter normal lymphatic drainage patterns resulting in unusual distribution of regional spread of disease to the neck (cervical) lymph nodes. In general, cervical lymph node involvement from oral cavity primary sites is predictable and orderly, spreading from the primary to upper, then middle, and subsequently lower cervical nodes. However, disease in the anterior oral cavity may also spread directly to the midcervical lymph nodes. The risk of distant metastasis is more dependent upon the "N" than the "T" status of the head and neck cancer. Midline nodes are considered ipsilateral. In addition to the components to describe the N-category, regional lymph nodes should also be described according to the level of the neck that is involved.

For pN, a selective neck dissection will ordinarily include 6 or more lymph nodes and a radical or modified radical neck dissection will ordinarily include 10 or more lymph nodes.

Metastatic Sites. The lungs are the commonest site of distant metastases; skeletal or hepatic metastases occur less often. Mediastinal lymph node metastases are considered distant metastases.

RULES FOR CLASSIFICATION

Clinical Staging. The assessment of the primary tumor is based upon inspection and palpation of the oral cavity and neck. Additional studies may include CT or MRI. When imaging is utilized one study will generally suffice to evaluate primary and nodal tumor extent. Clinical assessment of extent of mucosal involvement is more accurate than is radiographic assessment. The radiographic estimate of deep tissue extent and of regional lymph node involvement is usually more accurate than the clinical. MRI is generally more revealing of extent of soft tissue, perivascular and perineural spread, skull base involvement and intracranial tumor. High resolution CT with contrast will often provide similar information if carefully done, will better image bone and larynx detail and be minimally affected by motion. CT or MR imaging may be more useful in more advanced tumor for assessment of bone invasion (mandible or maxilla) and deep tissue invasion (deep extrinsic tongue muscles, midline tongue, soft tissues of neck). If imaging is undertaken for primary tumor evaluation, radiologic assessment of nodal involvement should also be done simultaneously. For lesions of an advanced extent appropriate screening for distant metastases should be considered. Ultrasonography may be helpful in assessment of major vascular invasion as an adjunctive test. The tumor must be confirmed histologically. All clinical, imaging, and pathologic data available prior to first definitive treatment may be used for clinical staging.

Pathologic Staging. Complete resection of the primary site and/or regional nodal dissections followed by pathologic examination of the resected specimen(s) allow the use of this designation for pT and/or pN, respectively. Specimens that are resected after radiation or chemotherapy need to be identified and considered in context. pT is derived from the actual measurement of the unfixed tumor in the surgical specimen. It represents additional and important information and should be included as such in staging but does not supplant clinical staging as the primary staging scheme.

DEFINITION OF TNM

Primary Tumor (T)

- TX Primary tumor cannot be assessed
- T0 No evidence of primary tumor
- Tis Carcinoma *in situ*
- T1 Tumor 2 cm or less in greatest dimension
- T2 Tumor more than 2 cm but not more than 4 cm in greatest dimension
- T3 Tumor more than 4 cm in greatest dimension
- T4 (lip) Tumor invades adjacent structures (e.g., through cortical bone, inferior alveolar nerve, floor of mouth, skin of face)
- T4 (oral cavity) Tumor invades adjacent structures (e.g., through cortical bone, into deep [extrinsic] muscle of tongue, maxillary sinus, skin. Superficial erosion alone of bone/tooth socket by gingival primary is not sufficient to classify as T4)

Regional Lymph Nodes (N)

- NX Regional lymph nodes cannot be assessed
- N0 No regional lymph node metastasis
- N1 Metastasis in a single ipsilateral lymph node, 3 cm or less in greatest dimension
- N2 Metastasis in a single ipsilateral lymph node, more than 3 cm but not more than 6 cm in greatest dimension; or in multiple ipsilateral lymph nodes, none more than 6 cm in greatest dimension; or in bilateral or contralateral lymph nodes, none more than 6 cm in greatest dimension
  - N2a Metastasis in single ipsilateral lymph node more than 3 cm but not more than 6 cm in greatest dimension
  - N2b Metastasis in multiple ipsilateral lymph nodes, none more than 6 cm in greatest dimension
  - N2c Metastasis in bilateral or contralateral lymph nodes, none more than 6 cm in greatest dimension
- N3 Metastasis in a lymph node more than 6 cm in greatest dimension

Distant Metastasis (M)

- MX Distant metastasis cannot be assessed
- M0 No distant metastasis
- M1 Distant metastasis

STAGE GROUPING

Stage 0	Tis	N0	M0
Stage I	T1	N0	M0
Stage II	T2	N0	M0
Stage III	T3	N0	M0
	T1	N1	M0
	T2	N1	M0
	T3	N1	M0
Stage IVA	T4	N0	M0
	T4	N1	M0
	Any T	N2	M0
Stage IVB	Any T	N3	M0
Stage IVC	Any T	Any N	M1

HISTOPATHOLOGIC TYPE

The predominant cancer is squamous cell carcinoma. Nonepithelial tumors such as those of lymphoid tissue, soft tissue, bone and cartilage are not included. Histologic confirmation of diagnosis is required. Histopathologic grading of squamous carcinoma is recommended; the grade is subjective and uses a descriptive as well as numerical form, i.e., well, moderately well, and poorly differentiated, depending upon the degree of closeness to or deviation from squamous epithelium in mucosal sites. Also recommended where feasible, is a quantitative evaluation of depth of invasion of the primary tumor and the presence or absence of vascular/perineural invasion. Although the grade of the tumor does not enter into staging of the tumor, it should be recorded. The pathologic description of any lymphadenectomy specimen should describe the size, number, and position of involved lymph node(s).

HISTOPATHOLOGIC GRADE (G)

GX Grade cannot be assessed
G1 Well differentiated
G2 Moderately differentiated
G3 Poorly differentiated

PROGNOSTIC FACTORS

In addition to the importance of the TNM factors outlined previously, the overall health of these patients clearly influences outcome. Comorbidity can be classified by more general measures, such as the Karnofsky performance score, or more specific measures, such as the Kaplan-Feinstein Index.

Continued exposure to carcinogens, such as alcohol and tobacco smoke, likely also affects patients' outcome adversely.

BIBLIOGRAPHY

Byers RM, Weber RS, Andrews T, et al: Frequency and therapeutic implications of "skip metastases" in the neck from squamous carcinoma of the oral tongue. Head Neck 19:14–19, 1997

Cooper JS, Farnan NC, Asbell SO, et al: Recursive partitioning analysis of 2105 patients treated in Radiation Therapy Oncology Group studies of head and neck cancer. Cancer 77:1905–1911, 1996

Cruse CW, Radocha RF: Squamous carcinoma of the lip. Plast Reconst Surg 80:787–791, 1987

Deleyiannis FW, Thomas DB, Vaughan TL, et al: Alcoholism: independent predictor of survival in patients with head and neck cancer. J Natl Cancer Inst 88:542–549, 1996

Evans JF, Shah JP: Epidermoid carcinoma of the palate. Am J Surg 142:451–455, 1981

Faye-Lund H, Abdelnoor M: Prognostic factors of survival in a cohort of head and neck cancer patients in Oslo. Eur J Cancer B Oral Oncol 2:83–90, 1996

Franceschi D, Gupta R, Spiro RH, et al: Improved survival in the treatment of squamous carcinoma of the oral tongue. Am J Surg 166:360–365, 1992

Kaplan MH, Feinstein AR: The importance of classifying initial co-morbidity in evaluating the outcome of diabetes mellitus. J Chron Dis 27:387–404, 1974

Karnofsky DA, Abelman WH, Craver LF, Burchenal JH: The use of the nitrogen mustards in the palliative treatment of carcinoma. Cancer 1:634–656, 1948

Krishnan-Nair M, Sankaranarayanan N, Padmanabhan T: Evaluation of the role of radiotherapy in the management of carcinoma of the buccal mucosa. Cancer 61:1326–1331, 1988

Petrovich Z, Krusk H, Tobochnik N, et al: Carcinoma of the lip. Arch Otolaryngol 105:187–191, 1979

Piccirillo JF: Inclusion of comorbidity in a staging system for head and neck cancer. Oncology 9:831–836, 1995

Rodgers LW, Stringer SP, Mendenhall WH, et al: Management of squamous carcinoma of the floor of the mouth. Head Neck 15:16–19, 1993

Shaha AR, Spiro RH, Shah JP, et al: Squamous carcinoma of the floor of the mouth. Am J Surg 148:455–459, 1984

Soo KC, Spiro RH, King W, et al: Squamous carcinoma of the gums. Am J Surg 156:281–285, 1988

Spiro RH, Spiro JD, Strong EW: Surgical approaches to squamous carcinoma confined to the tongue and floor of the mouth. Head Neck 9:27–31, 1986

Totsuka Y, Usui Y, Tei K, et al: Mandibular involvement by squamous cell carcinoma of the lower alveolus: analysis and comparative study of the histologic and radiologic features. Head Neck 13:40–50, 1991

Urist M, O'Brien CJ, Soong SJ, et al: Squamous cell carcinoma of the buccal mucosa: analysis of prognostic factors. Am J Surg 154:411–414, 1987

Wendt CD, Peters LJ, Delclos L, et al: Primary radiotherapy in the treatment of Stage I and II oral tongue cancer: importance of the proportion of therapy delivered with interstitial therapy. Int J Radiation Oncology Biol Phys 18:1287–1292, 1990

Data Form for Cancer Staging

Patient identification
Name ______
Address ______
Hospital or clinic number ______
Age ____ Sex ____ Race ______

Institution identification
Hospital or clinic ______
Address ______

Oncology Record

Anatomic site of cancer ______
Histologic type ______
Grade (G) ______
Date of classification ______

DEFINITIONS

Primary Tumor (T)

Clin	Path		
[ ]	[ ]	TX	Primary tumor cannot be assessed
[ ]	[ ]	T0	No evidence of primary tumor
[ ]	[ ]	Tis	Carcinoma *in situ*
[ ]	[ ]	T1	Tumor 2 cm or less in greatest dimension
[ ]	[ ]	T2	Tumor more than 2 cm but not more than 4 cm in greatest dimension
[ ]	[ ]	T3	Tumor more than 4 cm in greatest dimension
[ ]	[ ]	T4	(lip) Tumor invades adjacent structures (e.g., through cortical bone, inferior alveolar nerve, floor of mouth, skin of face)
[ ]	[ ]	T4	(oral cavity) Tumor invades adjacent structures (e.g., through cortical bone, into deep [extrinsic] muscle of tongue, maxillary sinus, skin. Superficial erosion alone of bone/tooth socket by gingival primary is not sufficient to classify as T4.)

Regional Lymph Nodes (N)

Clin	Path		
[ ]	[ ]	NX	Regional lymph nodes cannot be assessed
[ ]	[ ]	N0	No regional lymph node metastasis
[ ]	[ ]	N1	Metastasis in a single ipsilateral lymph node, 3 cm or less in greatest dimension
[ ]	[ ]	N2	Metastasis in a single ipsilateral lymph node, more than 3 cm but not more than 6 cm in greatest dimension; or in multiple ipsilateral lymph nodes, none more than 6 cm in greatest dimension; or in bilateral or contralateral lymph nodes, none more than 6 cm in greatest dimension
[ ]	[ ]	N2a	Metastasis in a single ipsilateral lymph node more than 3 cm but not more than 6 cm in greatest dimension
[ ]	[ ]	N2b	Metastasis in multiple ipsilateral lymph nodes, none more than 6 cm in greatest dimension
[ ]	[ ]	N2c	Metastasis in bilateral or contralateral lymph nodes, none more than 6 cm in greatest dimension
[ ]	[ ]	N3	Metastasis in a lymph node more than 6 cm in greatest dimension

Distant Metastasis (M)

Clin	Path		
[ ]	[ ]	MX	Distant metastasis cannot be assessed
[ ]	[ ]	M0	No distant metastasis
[ ]	[ ]	M1	Distant metastasis

Stage Grouping

Clin	Path	Stage	T	N	M
[ ]	[ ]	0	Tis	N0	M0
[ ]	[ ]	I	T1	N0	M0
[ ]	[ ]	II	T2	N0	M0
[ ]	[ ]	III	T3	N0	M0
			T1	N1	M0
			T2	N1	M0
			T3	N1	M0
[ ]	[ ]	IVA	T4	N0	M0
			T4	N1	M0
			Any T	N2	M0
[ ]	[ ]	IVB	Any T	N3	M0
[ ]	[ ]	IVC	Any T	Any N	M1

Staged by ______ M.D.
______ Registrar
Date ______

(continued on next page)

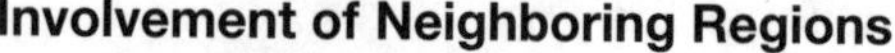

Location of Tumor

[ ] Lips: Upper
Lower
[ ] Buccal mucosa
[ ] Floor of mouth
[ ] Oral tongue
[ ] Hard palate
[ ] Gingivae: Upper
Lower
Retromolar trigone

Characteristics of Tumor

[ ] Exophytic
[ ] Superficial
[ ] Moderately infiltrating
[ ] Deeply infiltrating
[ ] Ulcerated
[ ] Extends to or overlies bone
[ ] Gross erosion of bone
[ ] Radiographic destruction of bone

Involvement of Neighboring Regions

[ ] Tonsillar pillar or soft palate
[ ] Nasal cavity or antrum
[ ] Nasopharynx
[ ] Pterygoid muscles
[ ] Soft tissues or skin of neck

Histopathologic Type

The predominant cancer is squamous cell carcinoma. Nonepithelial tumors such as those of lymphoid tissue, soft tissue, bone, and cartilage are not included in this system.

Histopathologic Grade (G)

[ ] GX Grade cannot be assessed
[ ] G1 Well differentiated
[ ] G2 Moderately differentiated
[ ] G3 Poorly differentiated

Illustrations

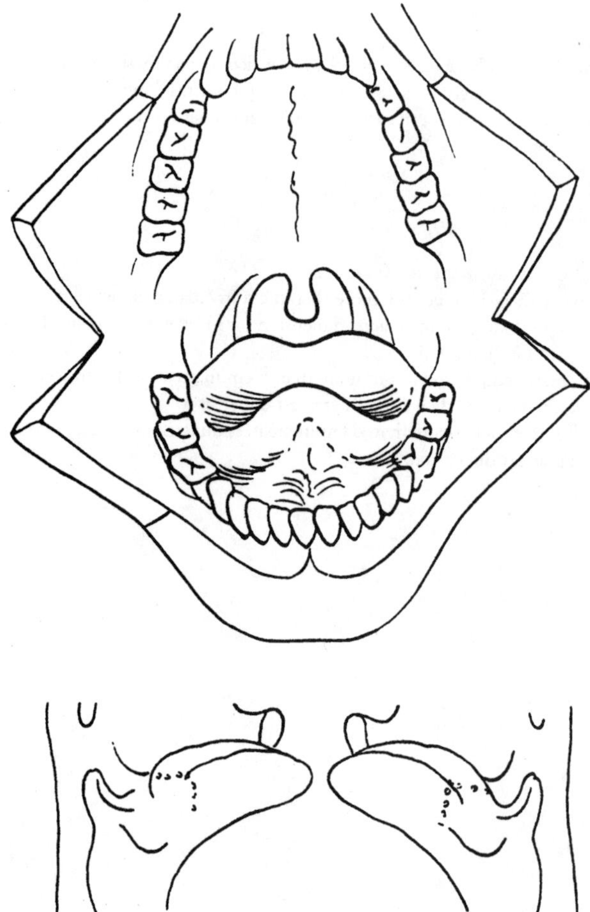

Indicate location of tumor.
Maximum tumor size: _____ cm

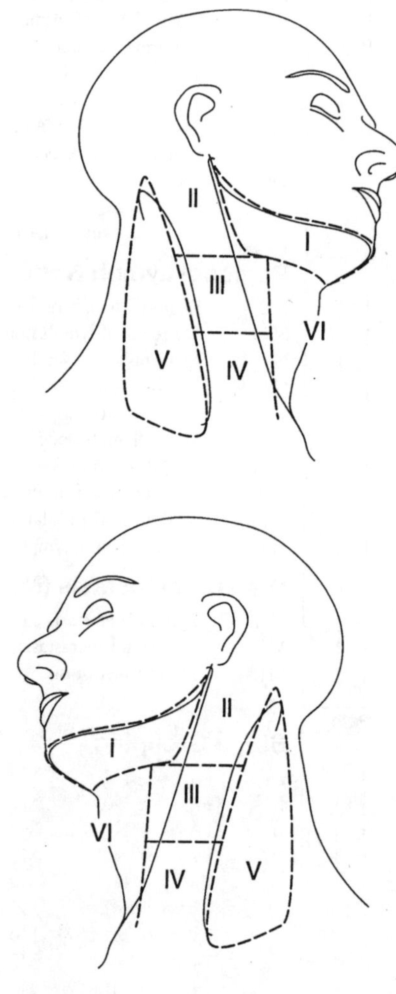

Indicate on diagram regional nodes involved.

4

Pharynx (Including Base of Tongue, Soft Palate, and Uvula)

(Nonepithelial tumors such as those of lymphoid tissue, soft tissue, bone, and cartilage are not included.)

C01.9 Base of tongue, NOS

C02.4 Lingual tonsil

C05.1 Soft palate, NOS
C05.2 Uvula

C09.0 Tonsillar fossa
C09.1 Tonsillar pillar
C09.8 Overlapping lesion
C09.9 Tonsil, NOS

C10.0 Vallecula
C10.2 Lateral wall of oropharynx
C10.3 Posterior wall of oropharynx
C10.4 Branchial cleft
C10.8 Overlapping lesion
C10.9 Oropharynx, NOS

C11.0 Superior wall of nasopharynx
C11.1 Posterior wall of nasopharynx
C11.2 Lateral wall of nasopharynx
C11.3 Anterior wall of nasopharynx
C11.8 Overlapping lesion
C11.9 Nasopharynx, NOS

C12.9 Pyriform sinus

C13.0 Postcricoid region
C13.1 Hypopharyngeal aspect of aryepiglottic fold
C13.2 Posterior wall of hypopharynx
C13.8 Overlapping lesion
C13.9 Hypopharynx, NOS

C14.0 Pharynx, NOS
C14.1 Laryngopharynx
C14.2 Waldeyer's ring
C14.8 Overlapping lesion of lip, oral cavity and pharynx

ANATOMY

Primary Sites and Subsites. The pharynx (including base of tongue, soft palate, and uvula) is divided into three regions: nasopharynx, oropharynx and hypopharynx (Fig. 4-1). Each region is further subdivided into specific sites as summarized in the following:

Nasopharynx. The nasopharynx begins anteriorly at the posterior choana and extends along the plane of the airway to the level of the free border of the soft palate. It includes the vault, the lateral walls including the fossae of Rosenmuller and the mucosa covering the torus tubarius forming the eustachian tube orifice, and the posterior wall. The floor is the superior surface of the soft palate. The posterior margins of the choanal orifices and of the nasal septum are included in the nasal fossa. Parapharyngeal involvement denotes postero-lateral infiltration of tumor beyond the pharyngobasilar fascia. Involvement of the infratemporal fossa denotes extension of tumor beyond the anterior surface of the lateral pterygoid muscle, or lateral exten-

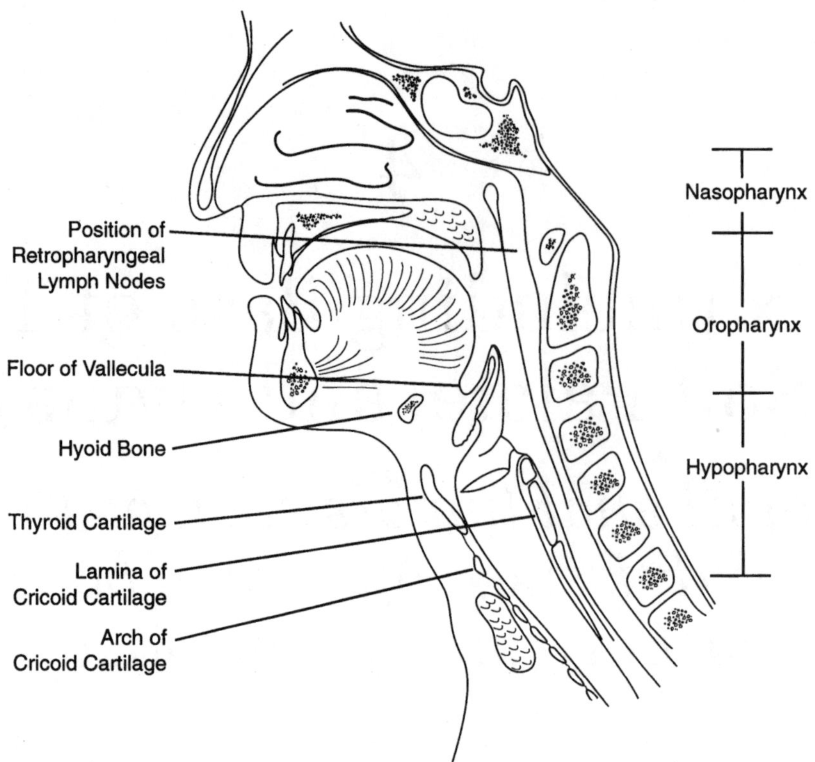

FIG. 4-1. Sagittal view of the face and neck depicting the subdivisions of the pharynx as described in the text.

sion beyond the postero-lateral wall of the maxillary antrum, pterygo-maxillary fissure.

Oropharynx. The oropharynx is that portion of the continuity of the pharynx extending from the plane of the inferior surface of the soft palate to the plane of the superior surface of the hyoid bone (or floor of the vallecula) and includes the base of tongue, the inferior surface of the soft palate and the uvula, the anterior and posterior tonsillar pillars, the glossotonsillar sulci, the pharyngeal tonsils; the lateral and posterior walls.

Hypopharynx. The hypopharynx is that portion of the pharynx extending from the plane of the superior border of the hyoid bone (or floor of the vallecula) to the plane corresponding to the lower border of the cricoid cartilage and includes the pyriform fossae (right and left), the lateral and posterior hypopharyngeal walls, and the postcricoid region.

The postcricoid area extends from the level of the arytenoid cartilages and connecting folds to the inferior border of the cricoid cartilage and connects the two pyriform sinuses thus forming the anterior wall of the hypopharynx. The pyriform sinus extends from the pharyngoepiglottic fold to the upper end of the esophagus at the lower border of the cricoid cartilage and is bounded laterally by the inner surface of the thyroid cartilage and medially by the hypopharyngeal surface of the aryepiglottic fold, arytenoid and cricoid cartilages. The posterior pharyngeal wall extends from the superior level of the hyoid bone (or floor of the vallecula) to the inferior border of the cricoid cartilage and from the apex of one pyriform sinus to the other.

Regional Lymph Nodes. The risk of regional nodal spread from cancers of the pharynx is high. Primary nasopharyngeal tumors commonly spread to retropharyngeal, upper jugular, and spinal accessory nodes, often bilaterally. Oropharyngeal cancers involve upper and mid-jugular lymph nodes, less likely submental/submandibular nodes. Hypopharyngeal cancers spread to adjacent parapharyngeal, paratracheal and mid- and lower jugular nodes. Bilateral lymphatic drainage is common.

In clinical evaluation the maximum size of the nodal mass should be measured. It is recognized that most masses over 3 cm in diameter are not single nodes but are confluent nodes or tumor in soft tissues of the neck. There are three categories of clinically involved nodes for the nasopharynx, oropharynx and hypopharynx: N1, N2, and N3. The use of subgroups a, b, and c is not required, but is recommended. Midline nodes are considered ipsilateral nodes. In addition to the components to describe the N-category, regional lymph nodes should also be described according to the level of the neck that is involved. It is recognized that the level of involved nodes in the neck is prognostically significant (lower is worse) as is the presence of extracapsular extension of metastatic tumor from individual nodes. Imaging studies showing amorphous spiculated margins of involved nodes or involvement of internodal fat resulting in loss of normal oval-to-round nodal shape strongly suggest extracapsular (extranodal) tumor spread; however, pathologic examination is necessary for documentation of such disease extent. No imaging study (as yet) can identify microscopic-sized foci in regional nodes or distinguish between small reactive nodes and small malignant nodes (unless central radiographic inhomogeneity is present).

For pN, a selective neck dissection will ordinarily include 6 or more lymph nodes and a radical or modified radical neck dissection will ordinarily include 10 or more lymph nodes.

Metastatic Sites. The lungs are the commonest sites of distant metastases; skeletal or hepatic metastases occur less often. Mediastinal lymph node metastases are considered distant metastases.

RULES FOR CLASSIFICATION

Clinical Staging. Clinical staging is generally employed for squamous cell carcinomas of the pharynx. Assessment is based primarily on inspection, and by indirect and direct endoscopy. Palpation of sites (when feasible) and of neck nodes is essential. Neurologic evaluation of all cranial nerves is required. Imaging studies are essential in clinical staging of pharynx tumors. Cross-sectional imaging in nasopharyngeal cancer is mandatory to complete the staging process. Magnetic resonance imaging (MRI) often is the study of choice because of its multiplanar capability, superior soft tissue contrast and its sensitivity to skull base and intracranial tumor spread. Computed tomography (CT) staging with axial and coronal thin section technique with contrast is an alternative. Radiologic nodal staging should be done to assess adequately the retropharyngeal and cervical nodal status.

Cross-sectional imaging in oropharyngeal carcinoma is recommended when the deep tissue extent of the primary tumor is in question. CT or MRI may be employed. Radiologic nodal staging should also be done simultaneously. Cross-sectional imaging of hypopharyngeal carcinoma is recommended when the extent of the primary tumor is in doubt, particularly its deep extent in relationship to adjacent structures (i.e., larynx, thyroid, cervical vertebrae, and carotid sheath). CT is preferred currently because of less motion artifact than MRI. Radiologic nodal staging should be done simultaneously. Complete endoscopy, usually under general anesthesia, is generally performed after completion of other staging studies, to accurately assess, document and facilitate biopsy of the surface extent of the tumor and to assess deep involvement by palpation, free of muscle resistance. A careful search for other primary tumors of the upper aerodigestive tract is indicatedbecause of the incidence of multiple independent primary tumors occurring simultaneously.

Pathologic Staging. Pathologic staging requires the use of all information obtained in clinical staging in addition to histologic study of the surgically resected specimen. The surgeon's evaluation of gross unresected residual tumor must also be included. Thepathologic description of any lymphadenectomy specimen should describe the size, number and level of any involved nodes.

DEFINITION OF TNM

Primary Tumor (T)

TX Primary tumor cannot be assessed
T0 No evidence of primary tumor
Tis Carcinoma *in situ*

Nasopharynx

T1 Tumor confined to the nasopharynx
T2 Tumor extends to soft tissues of oropharynx and/or nasal fossa
  T2a without parapharyngeal extension
  T2b with parapharyngeal extension
T3 Tumor invades bony structures and/or paranasal sinuses
T4 Tumor with intracranial extension and/or involvement of cranial nerves, infratemporal fossa, hypopharynx, or orbit

Oropharynx

T1 Tumor 2 cm or less in greatest dimension
T2 Tumor more than 2 cm but not more than 4 cm in greatest dimension
T3 Tumor more than 4 cm in greatest dimension
T4 Tumor invades adjacent structures (e.g., pterygoid muscle[s], mandible, hard palate, deep muscle of tongue, larynx)

Hypopharynx

T1 Tumor limited to one subsite of hypopharynx and 2 cm or less in greatest dimension
T2 Tumor involves more than one subsite of hypopharynx or an adjacent site, or measures more than 2 cm but not more than 4 cm in greatest diameter without fixation of hemilarynx
T3 Tumor measures more than 4 cm in greatest dimension or with fixation of hemilarynx
T4 Tumor invades adjacent structures (e.g., thyroid/cricoid cartilage, carotid artery, soft tissues of neck, prevertebral fascia/muscles, thyroid and/or esophagus)

Definition

Supraclavicular zone or fossa. This is relevant to the staging of nasopharyngeal carcinoma and is the triangular region originally described by Ho. It is defined by three points: (1) the superior margin of the sternal end of the clavicle; (2) the superior margin of the lateral end of the clavicle; (3) the point where the neck meets the shoulder (see Fig. 4-2). Note that this would include caudal portions of Levels IV and V. All cases with lymph nodes (whole or part) in the fossa are considered N3b.

Regional Lymph Nodes (N): Nasopharynx

The distribution and the prognostic impact of regional lymph node spread from nasopharynx cancer, particularly of the undifferentiated type, is different than that of other head and neck mucosal cancers and justifies use of a different N classification scheme.

NX Regional lymph nodes cannot be assessed
N0 No regional lymph node metastasis
N1 Unilateral metastasis in lymph node(s), 6 cm or less in greatest dimension, above the supraclavicular fossa
N2 Bilateral metastasis in lymph node(s), 6 cm or less in greatest dimension, above the supraclavicular fossa
N3 Metastasis in a lymph node(s)
 N3a greater than 6 cm in dimension
 N3b extension to the supraclavicular fossa

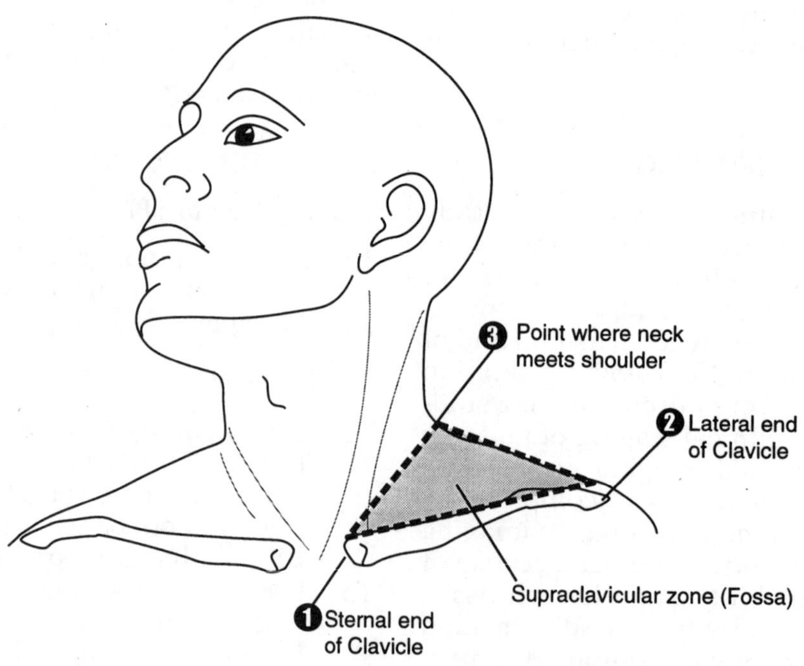

FIG. 4-2. Shaded triangular area corresponds to the supraclavicular fossa used in staging carcinoma of the nasopharynx.

Regional Lymph Nodes (N): Oropharynx and Hypopharynx

NX Regional lymph nodes cannot be assessed
N0 No regional lymph node metastasis
N1 Metastasis in a single ipsilateral lymph node, 3 cm or less in greatest dimension
N2 Metastasis in a single ipsilateral lymph node, more than 3 cm but not more than 6 cm in greatest dimension, or in multiple ipsilateral lymph nodes, none more than 6 cm in greatest dimension, or in bilateral or contralateral lymph nodes, none more than 6 cm in greatest dimension
  N2a Metastasis in a single ipsilateral lymph node more than 3 cm but not more than 6 cm in greatest dimension
  N2b Metastasis in multiple ipsilateral lymph nodes, none more than 6 cm in greatest dimension
  N2c Metastasis in bilateral or contralateral lymph nodes, none more than 6 cm in greatest dimension
N3 Metastasis in a lymph node more than 6 cm in greatest dimension

Distant Metastasis (M)

MX Distant metastasis cannot be assessed
M0 No distant metastasis
M1 Distant metastasis

STAGE GROUPING: Nasopharynx

Stage 0	Tis	N0	M0
Stage I	T1	N0	M0
Stage IIA	T2a	N0	M0
Stage IIB	T1	N1	M0
	T2	N1	M0
	T2a	N1	M0
	T2b	N0	M0
	T2b	N1	M0
Stage III	T1	N2	M0
	T2a	N2	M0
	T2b	N2	M0
	T3	N0	M0
	T3	N1	M0
	T3	N2	M0
Stage IVA	T4	N0	M0
	T4	N1	M0
	T4	N2	M0
Stage IVB	Any T	N3	M0
Stage IVC	Any T	Any N	M1

Table 4-1. Classification of Nasopharyngeal Carcinoma

WHO CLASSIFICATION	FORMER TERMINOLOGY
Type 1. Squamous cell carcinoma	Squamous cell carcinoma
Type 2. Nonkeratinizing carcinoma without lymphoid stroma with lymphoid stroma	Transitional cell carcinoma intermediate cell carcinoma Lymphoepithelial carcinoma (Regaud)
Type 3. Undifferentiated carcinoma without lymphoid stroma with lymphoid stroma	Anaplastic carcinoma, clear cell carcinoma Lymphoepithelial carcinoma (Schminke)

STAGE GROUPING: Oropharynx, Hypopharynx

Stage 0	Tis	N0	M0
Stage I	T1	N0	M0
Stage II	T2	N0	M0
Stage III	T3	N0	M0
	T1	N1	M0
	T2	N1	M0
	T3	N1	M0
Stage IVA	T4	N0	M0
	T4	N1	M0
	Any T	N2	M0
Stage IVB	Any T	N3	M0
Stage IVC	Any T	Any N	M1

HISTOPATHOLOGIC TYPE

The predominant cancer type is squamous cell carcinoma for all pharyngeal sites. Nonepithelial tumors such as those of lymphoid tissue, soft tissue, bone and cartilage are not included in this system. For nasopharyngeal carcinomas it is recommended that the World Health Organization (WHO) Classification be used (Table 4-1). Histologic diagnosis is required to use this classification.

HISTOPATHOLOGIC GRADE (G): Oropharynx, Hypopharynx

GX Grade cannot be assessed
G1 Well differentiated
G2 Moderately differentiated
G3 Poorly differentiated

PROGNOSTIC FACTORS

In addition to the importance of the TNM factors outlined previously, the overall health of these patients clearly influences outcome. Comorbidity can be classified by more general measures, such as the Karnofsky performance score, or more specific measures, such as the Kaplan-Feinstein Index.

Continued exposure to carcinogens, such as alcohol and tobacco smoke, likely also affects patients' outcome adversely.

BIBLIOGRAPHY

Archer CR, Yeager VL, Herbold DR: CT versus histology of laryngeal cancer: the value in predicting laryngeal cartilage invasion. Laryngoscope 93:140–147, 1983

Bataini JP, Bernier J, Brugere J, et al: Natural history of neck disease in patients with squamous cell carcinoma of the oropharynx and pharyngolarynx. Radiother and Oncol 3:245–255, 1985

Byers RM, Krueger WW, Saxton J: Use of surgery and postoperative radiation therapy in treatment of advanced squamous carcinoma of the pyriform sinus. Am J Surg 138:597–603, 1979

Chua DT, Sham JS, Kwong DL, et al: Prognostic value of paranasopharyngeal extension of nasopharyngeal carcinoma. A significant factor in local control and distant metastasis. Cancer 78:202–210, 1996

Cooper JS, Farnan NC, Asbell SO, et al: Recursive partitioning analysis of 2105 patients treated in Radiation Therapy Oncology Group studies of head and neck cancer. Cancer 77:1905–1911, 1996

Deleyiannis FW, Thomas DB, Vaughan TL, et al: Alcoholism: independent predictor of survival in patients with head and neck cancer. J Natl Cancer Inst 88:542–549, 1996

Faye-Lund H, Abdelnoor M: Prognostic factors of survival in a cohort of head and neck cancer patients in Oslo. Eur J Cancer B Oral Oncol 2:83–90, 1996

Hart AMH, Mak-Kregar S, Hilgers FJM, et al: The importance of correct stage grouping in oncology: results of a nationwide study of oropharyngeal carcinoma in the Netherlands. Cancer 75:2656–2662, 1995

Ho JHC. Stage classification of nasopharyngeal carcinoma: a review in nasopharyngeal carcinoma, etiology, and control. *IARC Scientific Publications.* No. 20;99–113, 1978

Kaplan MH, Feinstein AR: The importance of classifying initial co-morbidity in evaluating the outcome of diabetes mellitus. J Chron Dis 27:387–404, 1974

Karnofsky DA, Abelman WH, Craver LF, Burchenal JH: The use of the nitrogen mustards in the palliative treatment of carcinoma. Cancer 1:634–656, 1948

Kraus DH, Vastola AP, Huvos AG, et al: Surgical management of squamous cell carcinoma of the base of the tongue. Am J Surg 166:384–388, 1993

Lee AWM, Foo W, Law CK, et al: N-Staging of nasopharyngeal carcinoma: discrepancy between UICC/AJCC and Ho systems. Clin Oncol 8:155–159, 1996

Lee AWM, Foo W, Poon YF, et al: Staging of nasopharyngeal carcinoma: evaluation of N-Staging by Ho and UICC/AJCC systems. Clin Oncol 8:146–154, 1996

Lee AW, Poon YF, Foo W, et al: Retrospective analysis of 5037 patients with nasopharyngeal carcinoma treated during 1976–1985: overall survival and patterns of failure. Int J Radiation Oncology Biol Phys 23:261–270, 1992

Lo K, Fletcher GH, Byers RM, et al: Results of irradiation in the squamous cell carcinoma of the anterior faucial pillar-retromolar trigone. Int J Radiation Oncology Biol Phys 13:969–974, 1987

Marks JE, Smith PG, Sessions DG: Pharyngeal wall cancer: a reappraisal after comparison of treatment methods. Arch Otolaryngol 111:79–85, 1985

Muraki AS, Mancuso AA, Harnsberger HR, et al: CT of the oropharynx, tongue base, floor of mouth: normal anatomy and range of variations, and applications in staging carcinoma. Radiology 148: 725–731, 1983

Perez CA, Carmichael T, Devineni VR, et al: Carcinoma of the tonsillar fossa: a nonrandomized comparison of irradiation alone or combined with surgery: long-term results. Head Neck 13:282–290, 1991

Piccirillo, JF: Inclusion of comorbidity in a staging system for head and neck cancer. Oncology 9:831–836; 1995

Schaefer SD, Merkel M, Diehl J: CT assessment of squamous cell carcinoma of the oral and pharyngeal cavities. Arch Otolaryngol 108:688–692, 1982

Sham JST, Choy D: Prognostic value of paranasopharyngeal extension of nasopharyngeal carcinoma on local control and short-term survival. Head Neck 13:298–310, 1991

Shanmugaratnam K: Histological typing of tumours of the upper respiratory tract and ear. WHO international histological classification of tumors, 2nd ed. Berlin-New York: Springer-Verlag, 1991

Strong EW, Kasdorf H, Henk JM: Squamous cell carcinoma of the head and neck. In Hermanek P, Gospodarowicz MK, Henson DE, Hutter RVP, Sobin LH (Eds.) Prognostic factors in cancer, UICC, Geneva. Berlin-New York: Springer-Verlag; 23–27, 1995

Teo PML, Leung SF, Yu P, Tsao SY, Foo W, Shiu W. A comparison of Ho, International Union against Cancer, and American Joint Committee stage classifications for nasopharyngeal carcinoma. Cancer 67:434–439, 1991

Teo PML, Tsao SY, Ho JHC, Yu P: A proposed modification of the Ho stage-classification for nasopharyngeal carcinoma. Radiother Oncol 21:11–23, 1991

Teresi LM, Lufkin RB, Vinuela F, et al: MR imaging of the nasopharynx and floor of the middle cranial fossa. Part II. Malignant tumors. Radiology 164:187–821, 1987

Data Form for Cancer Staging

Patient identification
Name ______
Address ______
Hospital or clinic number ______
Age ____ Sex ____ Race ______

Institution identification
Hospital or clinic ______
Address ______

Oncology Record

Anatomic site of cancer ______
Histologic type ______
Grade (G) ______
Date of classification ______

DEFINITIONS

Primary Tumor (T)

Clin	Path		
[ ]	[ ]	TX	Primary tumor cannot be assessed
[ ]	[ ]	T0	No evidence of primary tumor
[ ]	[ ]	Tis	Carcinoma *in situ*

Nasopharynx

Clin	Path		
[ ]	[ ]	T1	Tumor confined to the nasopharynx
[ ]	[ ]	T2	Tumor extends to soft tissues of oropharynx and/or nasal fossa
[ ]	[ ]	T2a	without parapharyngeal extension
[ ]	[ ]	T2b	with parapharyngeal extension
[ ]	[ ]	T3	Tumor invades bony structures and/or paranasal sinuses
[ ]	[ ]	T4	Tumor with intracranial extension and/or involvement of cranial nerves, infratemporal fossa, hypopharynx, or orbit

Oropharynx

Clin	Path		
[ ]	[ ]	T1	Tumor 2 cm or less in greatest dimension
[ ]	[ ]	T2	Tumor more than 2 cm but not more than 4 cm in greatest dimension
[ ]	[ ]	T3	Tumor more than 4 cm in greatest dimension
[ ]	[ ]	T4	Tumor invades adjacent structures (e.g., pterygoid muscle[s], mandible, hard palate, deep muscle of tongue, larynx)

Hypopharynx

Clin	Path		
[ ]	[ ]	T1	Tumor limited to one subsite of hypopharynx and 2 cm or less in greatest dimension
[ ]	[ ]	T2	Tumor involves more than one subsite of hypopharynx or an adjacent site, or measures more than 2 cm but not more than 4 cm in greatest diameter without fixation of hemilarynx
[ ]	[ ]	T3	Tumor measures more than 4 cm in greatest dimension or with fixation of hemilarynx
[ ]	[ ]	T4	Tumor invades adjacent structures (e.g., thyroid/cricoid cartilage, carotid artery, soft tissues of neck, prevertebral fascia/muscles, thyroid and/or esophagus)

Regional Lymph Nodes (N): Nasopharynx

The distribution and the prognostic impact of regional lymph node spread from nasopharynx cancer, particularly of the undifferentiated type, is different from that of other head and neck mucosal cancers and justifies use of a different N classification scheme.

Clin	Path		
[ ]	[ ]	NX	Regional lymph nodes cannot be assessed
[ ]	[ ]	N0	No regional lymph node metastasis
[ ]	[ ]	N1	Unilateral metastasis in lymph node(s), 6 cm or less in greatest dimension, above the supraclavicular fossa
[ ]	[ ]	N2	Bilateral metastasis in lymph node(s), 6 cm or less in greatest dimension, above the supraclavicular fossa
[ ]	[ ]	N3	Metastasis in a lymph node(s)
[ ]	[ ]	N3a	greater than 6 cm in dimension
[ ]	[ ]	N3b	in the supraclavicular fossa

Regional Lymph Nodes (N): Oropharynx and Hypopharynx

Clin	Path		
[ ]	[ ]	NX	Regional lymph nodes cannot be assessed
[ ]	[ ]	N0	No regional lymph node metastasis
[ ]	[ ]	N1	Metastasis in a single ipsilateral lymph node, 3 cm or less in greatest dimension
[ ]	[ ]	N2	Metastasis in a single ipsilateral lymph node, more than 3 cm but not more than 6 cm in greatest dimension, or in multiple ipsilateral lymph nodes, none more than 6 cm in greatest dimension, or in bilateral or contralateral lymph nodes, none more than 6 cm in greatest dimension

(continued on next page)

Clin	Path		
[ ]	[ ]	N2a	Metastasis in a single ipsilateral lymph node more than 3 cm but not more than 6 cm in greatest dimension
[ ]	[ ]	N2b	Metastasis in multiple ipsilateral lymph nodes, none more than 6 cm in greatest dimension
[ ]	[ ]	N2c	Metastasis in bilateral or contralateral lymph nodes, none more than 6 cm in greatest dimension
[ ]	[ ]	N3	Metastasis in a lymph node more than 6 cm in greatest dimension

Distant Metastasis (M)

Clin	Path		
[ ]	[ ]	MX	Distant metastasis cannot be assessed
[ ]	[ ]	M0	No distant metastasis
[ ]	[ ]	M1	Distant metastasis

Stage Grouping: Nasopharynx

Clin	Path	Stage	T	N	M
[ ]	[ ]	0	Tis	N0	M0
[ ]	[ ]	I	T1	N0	M0
[ ]	[ ]	IIA	T2a	N0	M0
[ ]	[ ]	IIB	T1	N1	M0
			T2	N1	M0
			T2a	N1	M0
			T2b	N0, N1	M0
[ ]	[ ]	III	T1	N2	M0
			T2a, T2b	N2	M0
			T3	N0, N1, N2	M0
[ ]	[ ]	IVA	T4	N0, N1, N2	M0
[ ]	[ ]	IVB	Any T	N3	M0
[ ]	[ ]	IVC	Any T	Any N	M1

Stage Grouping: Oropharynx, Hypopharynx

Clin	Path	Stage	T	N	M
[ ]	[ ]	0	Tis	N0	M0
[ ]	[ ]	I	T1	N0	M0
[ ]	[ ]	II	T2	N0	M0
[ ]	[ ]	III	T3	N0	M0
			T1	N1	M0
			T2	N1	M0
			T3	N1	M0
[ ]	[ ]	IVA	T4	N0	M0
			T4	N1	M0
			Any T	N2	M0
[ ]	[ ]	IVB	Any T	N3	M0
[ ]	[ ]	IVC	Any T	Any N	M1

Staged by ______________________________ M.D.

______________________________ Registrar

Date ______________________________

Histopathologic Grade (G): Oropharynx, Hypopharynx

[ ] GX Grade cannot be assessed
[ ] G1 Well differentiated
[ ] G2 Moderately differentiated
[ ] G3 Poorly differentiated

Classification of Nasopharyngeal Carcinoma

WHO Classification

Type 1. Squamous cell carcinoma
Type 2. Nonkeratinizing carcinoma
  Without lymphoid stroma
  With lymphoid stroma
Type 3. Undifferentiated carcinoma
  Without lymphoid stroma
  With lymphoid stroma

Former Terminology

Type 1. Squamous cell carcinoma
Type 2. Transitional cell carcinoma
  Intermediate cell carcinoma
Lymphoepithelial carcinoma (Regaud)
Type 3. Anaplastic carcinoma, clear cell carcinoma
Lymphoepithelial carcinoma (Schminke)

Location of Tumor

Oropharynx
[ ] Faucial arch
[ ] Tonsillar fossa, tonsil
[ ] Base of tongue
[ ] Pharyngeal wall
Nasopharynx
[ ] Posterosuperior wall
[ ] Lateral wall
Hypopharynx
[ ] Pyriform fossa
[ ] Postcricoid area
[ ] Posterior wall

Characteristics of Tumor

[ ] Superficial
[ ] Exophytic
[ ] Moderate infiltration
[ ] Deep infiltration

Histopathologic Type

The predominant cancer type is squamous cell carcinoma for all pharyngeal sites. Nonepithelial tumors such as those of lymphoid tissue, soft tissue, bone, and cartilage are not included in this system.

(continued on next page)

Illustrations

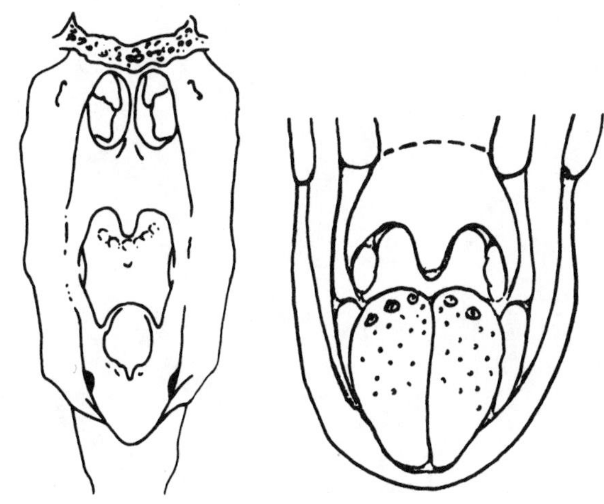

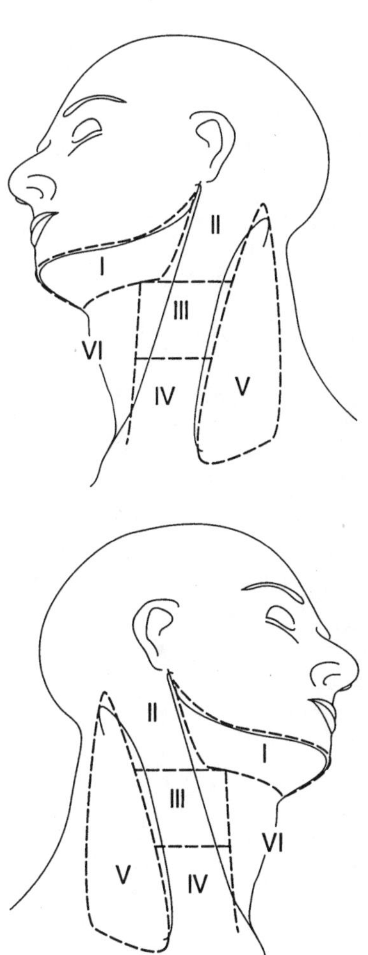

Indicate on diagram regional nodes involved.

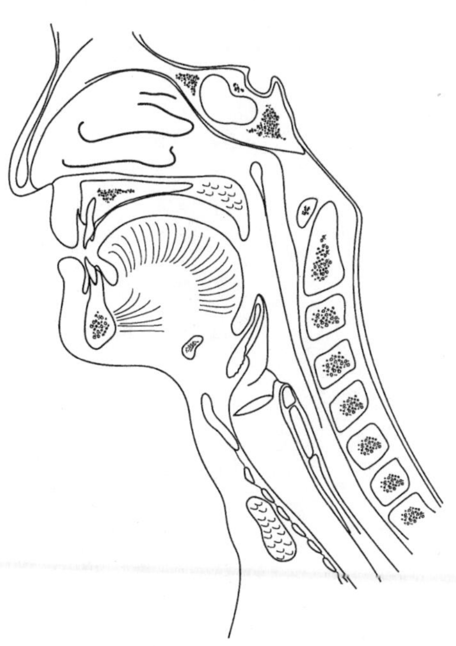

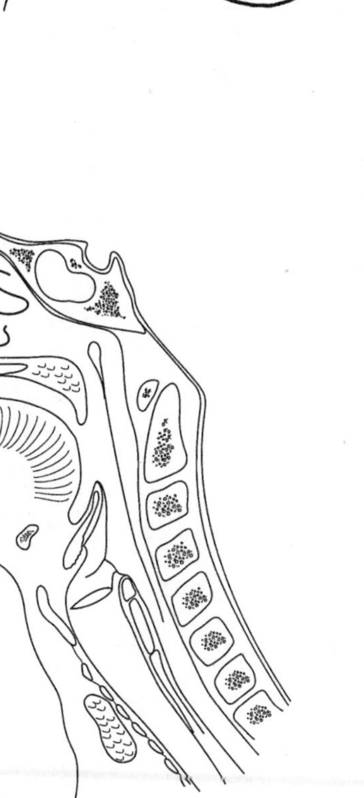

Indicate location of primary tumor.
Maximum tumor size: ____ cm.

5

Larynx

(Nonepithelial tumors such as those of lymphoid tissue, soft tissue, bone and cartilage are not included.)

C10.1 Anterior (lingual) surface of epiglottis

C32.0 Glottis
C32.1 Supraglottis (laryngeal surface)
C32.2 Subglottis
C32.3 Laryngeal cartilage
C32.8 Overlapping lesion
C32.9 Larynx, NOS

ANATOMY

Primary Site. The following anatomic definition of the larynx allows classification of carcinomas arising in the encompassed mucous membranes but excludes cancers arising on the lateral or posterior pharyngeal wall, pyriform fossa, postcricoid area, or base of tongue.

The anterior limit of the larynx is composed of the anterior or lingual surface of the suprahyoid epiglottis, the thyrohyoid membrane, the anterior commissure, and the anterior wall of the subglottic region, which is composed of the thyroid cartilage, the cricothyroid membrane, and the anterior arch of the cricoid cartilage.

The posterior and lateral limits include the laryngeal aspect of aryepiglottic folds, the arytenoid region, the interarytenoid space, and the posterior surface of the subglottic space, represented by the mucous membrane covering the surface of the cricoid cartilage.

The superolateral limits are composed of the tip and the lateral borders of the epiglottis. The inferior limits are made up of the plane passing through the inferior edge of the cricoid cartilage.

For purposes of this clinical stage classification, the larynx is divided into three regions: supraglottis, glottis, and subglottis. The supraglottis is composed of the epiglottis (both its lingual and laryngeal aspects), aryepiglottic folds (laryngeal aspect), arytenoids, and ventricular bands (false cords). The epiglottis is divided for staging purposes into suprahyoid and infrahyoid positions by a plane at the level of the hyoid bone. The inferior boundary of the supraglottis is a horizontal plane passing through the lateral margin of the ventricle at its junction with the superior surface of the vocal cord. The glottis is composed of the true vocal cords, including the anterior and posterior commissures, superior and inferior surfaces. It occupies a horizontal plane, 1 cm in thickness, extending inferiorly from the lateral margin of the ventricle. The subglottis is the region extending from the lower boundary of the glottis to the lower margin of the cricoid cartilage.

The division of the larynx is summarized in the following table:

Site	Subsite
Supraglottis	Suprahyoid epiglottis
	Infrahyoid epiglottis
	Aryepiglottic folds (laryngeal aspect)
	Arytenoids
	Ventricular bands (false cords)
Glottis	True vocal cords including anterior and posterior commissures
Subglottis	Subglottis

Regional Lymph Nodes. The incidence and distribution of cervical nodal metastases from cancer of the larynx varies with the site of origin and the "T" classification of the primary tumor. The true vocal cords are nearly devoid of lymphatics and tumors of that site alone rarely spread to regional nodes. On the contrary, the supraglottis has a rich and bilaterally interconnected lymphatic network and primary supraglottic cancers are commonly accompanied by regional nodal spread. Glottic tumors may spread directly to adjacent soft tissues and prelaryngeal, pretracheal, paralaryngeal and paratracheal nodes as well as upper, mid and lower jugular nodes. Supraglottic tumors commonly spread to upper and midjugular nodes, considerably less commonly to submental or submandibular nodes, but occasionally to retropharyngeal nodes. The rare subglottic primary tumors spread first to adjacent soft tissues and prelaryngeal, pretracheal, paralaryngeal and paratracheal nodes, then to mid and lower jugular nodes. Contralateral lymphatic spread is common.

In clinical evaluation the physical size of the nodal mass should be measured. It is recognized that most masses over 3 cm in diameter are not single nodes but are confluent nodes or tumor in soft tissues of the neck. There are three categories of clinically positive nodes: N1, N2, and N3. The use of subgroups a, b, and c is not required but is recommended. Midline nodes are considered ipsilateral nodes. In addition to the components to describe the N-category, regional lymph nodes should also be described according to the level of the neck that is involved. Pathologic examination is necessary for documentation of such disease extent. Imaging studies showing amorphous spiculated margins of involved nodes or involvement of internodal fat resulting in loss of normal oval-to-round nodal shape strongly suggest extracapsular (extranodal) tumor spread. No imaging study (as yet) can identify microscopic foci in regional nodes or distinguish between small reactive nodes and small malignant nodes without central radiographic inhomogeneity.

For pN, a selective neck dissection will ordinarily include 6 or more lymph nodes and a radical or modified radical neck dissection will ordinarily include 10 or more lymph nodes.

Metastatic Sites. Distant spread is common only for patients who have bulky adenopathy. When distant metastases occur spread to the lungs is most common; skeletal or hepatic metastases occur less often. Mediastinal lymph node metastases are considered distant metastases.

RULES FOR CLASSIFICATION

Clinical Staging. The assessment of the larynx is accomplished primarily by inspection, using indirect mirror and direct endoscopic examination. The tumor must be confirmed histologically, and any other data obtained by biopsies may be included. Cross-sectional imaging in laryngeal carcinoma is recommended when the primary tumor extent is in question based upon clinical examination. Radiologic nodal staging should be done simultaneously to supplement clinical examination.

Complete endoscopy, usually under general anesthesia, is generally performed after completion of other diagnostic studies to accurately assess, document and biopsy the tumor.

Pathologic Staging. All information used in clinical staging and in histologic studies of the surgically resected specimen is used for pathologic staging. The surgeon's evaluation of gross unresected residual tumor must also be included. The pathologic description of any lymphadenectomy specimen should describe the size, number, and level of involved lymph nodes.

DEFINITION OF TNM

Primary Tumor (T)

TX Primary tumor cannot be assessed
T0 No evidence of primary tumor
Tis Carcinoma *in situ*

Supraglottis

T1 Tumor limited to one subsite of supraglottis with normal vocal cord mobility
T2 Tumor invades mucosa of more than one adjacent subsite of supraglottis or glottis or region outside the supraglottis (e.g., mucosa of base of tongue, vallecula, medial wall of pyriform sinus) without fixation of the larynx
T3 Tumor limited to larynx with vocal cord fixation and/or invades any of the following: postcricoid area, pre-epiglottic tissues
T4 Tumor invades through the thyroid cartilage, and/or extends into soft tissues of the neck, thyroid, and/or esophagus

Glottis

T1 Tumor limited to the vocal cord(s) (may involve anterior or posterior commissure) with normal mobility
  T1a Tumor limited to one vocal cord
  T1b Tumor involves both vocal cords
T2 Tumor extends to supraglottis and/or subglottis, and/or with impaired vocal cord mobility
T3 Tumor limited to the larynx with vocal cord fixation
T4 Tumor invades through the thyroid cartilage and/or to other tissues beyond the larynx (e.g., trachea, soft tissues of neck, including thyroid, pharynx)

Subglottis

T1 Tumor limited to the subglottis
T2 Tumor extends to vocal cord(s) with normal or impaired mobility
T3 Tumor limited to larynx with vocal cord fixation
T4 Tumor invades through cricoid or thyroid cartilage and/or extends to other tissues beyond the larynx (e.g., trachea, soft tissues of neck, including thyroid, esophagus)

Regional Lymph Nodes (N)

NX Regional lymph nodes cannot be assessed
N0 No regional lymph node metastasis
N1 Metastasis in a single ipsilateral lymph node, 3 cm or less in greatest dimension
N2 Metastasis in a single ipsilateral lymph node, more than 3 cm but not more than 6 cm in greatest dimension, or in multiple ipsilateral lymph nodes, none more than 6 cm in greatest dimension, or in bilateral or contralateral lymph nodes, none more than 6 cm in greatest dimension
  N2a Metastasis in a single ipsilateral lymph node more than 3 cm but not more than 6 cm in greatest dimension
  N2b Metastasis in multiple ipsilateral lymph nodes, none more than 6 cm in greatest dimension
  N2c Metastasis in bilateral or contralateral lymph nodes, none more than 6 cm in greatest dimension
N3 Metastasis in a lymph node more than 6 cm in greatest dimension

Distant Metastasis (M)

MX Distant metastasis cannot be assessed
M0 No distant metastasis
M1 Distant metastasis

STAGE GROUPING

Stage 0	Tis	N0	M0
Stage I	T1	N0	M0
Stage II	T2	N0	M0
Stage III	T3	N0	M0
	T1	N1	M0
	T2	N1	M0
	T3	N1	M0
Stage IVA	T4	N0	M0
	T4	N1	M0
	Any T	N2	M0
Stage IVB	Any T	N3	M0
Stage IVC	Any T	Any N	M1

HISTOPATHOLOGIC TYPE

The predominant cancer type is squamous cell carcinoma. Nonepithelial tumors such as those of lymphoid tissue, soft tissue, bone and cartilage are not included. Histologic diagnosis is required to use this classification. Tumor grading of squamous carcinoma is recommended. The grade is subjective and uses a descriptive, as well as a numerical form; i.e., well, moderately well, and poorly differentiated, depending upon the degree of closeness to or deviation from squamous epithelium in normal mucosal sites. Also recommended where feasible is a quantitative evaluation of depth of invasion of the primary tumor and the presence or absence of vascular/perineural invasion.

HISTOPATHOLOGIC GRADE (G)

GX Grade cannot be assessed
G1 Well differentiated
G2 Moderately differentiated
G3 Poorly differentiated

PROGNOSTIC FACTORS

In addition to the importance of the TNM factors outlined previously, the overall health of these patients clearly influences outcome. Comorbidity can be classified by more general measures, such as the Karnofsky performance score, or more specific measures, such as the Kaplan-Feinstein Index.

Continued exposure to carcinogens, such as alcohol and tobacco smoke, likely also affects patients' outcome adversely.

BIBLIOGRAPHY

Archer CR, Yeager VL, Herbold DR: CT versus histology of laryngeal cancer: the value in predicting laryngeal cartilage invasion. Laryngoscope 93:140–147, 1983

Cooper JS, Farnan NC, Asbell SO, et al: Recursive partitioning analysis of 2105 patients treated in Radiation Therapy Oncology Group studies of head and neck cancer. Cancer 77:1905–1911, 1996

Deleyiannis FW, Thomas DB, Vaughan TL, et al: Alcoholism: independent predictor of survival in patients with head and neck cancer. J Natl Cancer Inst 88:542–549, 1996

Eibaud JD, Elias EG, Suter CM, et al: Prognostic factors in squamous cell carcinoma of the larynx. Am J Surg 158:314–317, 1989

Faye-Lund H, Abdelnoor M: Prognostic factors of survival in a cohort of head and neck cancer patients in Oslo. Eur J Cancer B Oral Oncol 2:83–90, 1996

Isaacs JJ, Mancuso AA, Mendenhall WM, et al: Deep spread patterns in CT staging of T2-4 squamous cell laryngeal carcinoma. Otolaryngol Head Neck Surg 99:455–464, 1988

Kaplan MH, Feinstein AR: The importance of classifying initial co-morbidity in evaluating the outcome of diabetes mellitus. J Chron Dis 27:387–404, 1974

Karnofsky DA, Abelman WH, Craver LF, Burchenal JH: The use of the nitrogen mustards in the palliative treatment of carcinoma. Cancer 1:634–656, 1948

Mafee MF, Schield JA, Valvassori GE, et al: CT of the larynx: correlation with anatomic and pathologic studies in cases of laryngeal carcinoma. Radiology 147:123–128, 1983

Mendenhall WM, Parsons JT, Stringer SP, et al: Carcinoma of the supraglottic larynx: a basis for comparing the results of radiotherapy and surgery. Head Neck 12:204–209, 1990

Piccirillo, JF. Inclusion of comorbidity in a staging system for head and neck cancer. Oncology 9:831–836, 1995

Rozack MS, Maipang T, Sabo K, et al: Management of advanced glottic carcinomas. Am J Surg 158:318–320, 1989

Strong EW: Cancer of the larynx and hypopharynx. Prob Gen Surg 5:166–189, 1988

Van Nostrand AWP, Brodarec I: Laryngeal carcinoma: modification of surgical techniques based upon an understanding of tumor growth characteristics. J Otolaryngol 11:186–192, 1982

Veterans Administration Laryngeal Study Group. Induction chemotherapy plus radiation compared to surgery plus radiation in patients with advanced laryngeal cancer. N Engl J Med 324:1685–1690, 1991

LARYNX

Data Form for Cancer Staging

Patient identification
Name ______
Address ______
Hospital or clinic number ______
Age ____ Sex ____ Race ______

Institution identification
Hospital or clinic ______
Address ______

Oncology Record

Anatomic site of cancer ______
Histologic type ______
Grade (G) ______
Date of classification ______

Clin	Path	DEFINITIONS	
		Primary Tumor (T)	
[ ]	[ ]	TX	Primary tumor cannot be assessed
[ ]	[ ]	T0	No evidence of primary tumor
[ ]	[ ]	Tis	Carcinoma *in situ*
		Supraglottis	
[ ]	[ ]	T1	Tumor limited to one subsite of supraglottis with normal vocal cord mobility
[ ]	[ ]	T2	Tumor invades mucosa of more than one adjacent subsite of supraglottis or glottis or region outside the supraglottis (e.g., mucosa of base of tongue, vallecula, medial wall of pyriform sinus) without fixation of the larynx
[ ]	[ ]	T3	Tumor limited to larynx with vocal cord fixation and/or invades any of the following: postcricoid area, pre-epiglottic tissues
[ ]	[ ]	T4	Tumor extends through the thyroid cartilage, and/or extends into soft tissues of the neck, thyroid and/or esophagus
		Glottis	
[ ]	[ ]	T1	Tumor limited to vocal cord(s) (may involve anterior or posterior commissures) with normal mobility
[ ]	[ ]	T1a	Tumor limited to one vocal cord
[ ]	[ ]	T1b	Tumor involves both vocal cords
[ ]	[ ]	T2	Tumor extends to supraglottis and/or subglottis, and/or with impaired vocal cord mobility
[ ]	[ ]	T3	Tumor limited to the larynx with vocal cord fixation
[ ]	[ ]	T4	Tumor invades through thyroid cartilage and/or to other tissues beyond the larynx, e.g., trachea, soft tissues of neck, including thyroid, pharynx
		Subglottis	
[ ]	[ ]	T1	Tumor limited to the subglottis
[ ]	[ ]	T2	Tumor extends to vocal cord(s) with normal or impaired mobility
[ ]	[ ]	T3	Tumor limited to larynx with vocal cord fixation
[ ]	[ ]	T4	Tumor invades through cricoid or thyroid cartilage and/or extends to other tissues beyond the larynx (e.g., trachea, soft tissues of neck, including thyroid, esophagus)
		Regional Lymph Nodes (N)	
[ ]	[ ]	NX	Regional lymph nodes cannot be assessed
[ ]	[ ]	N0	No regional lymph node metastasis
[ ]	[ ]	N1	Metastasis in a single ipsilateral lymph node, 3 cm or less in greatest dimension
[ ]	[ ]	N2	Metastasis in a single ipsilateral lymph node, more than 3 cm but not more than 6 cm in greatest dimension, or multiple ipsilateral lymph nodes, none more than 6 cm in greatest dimension, or bilateral or contralateral lymph nodes, none more than 6 cm in greatest dimension
[ ]	[ ]	N2a	Metastasis in a single ipsilateral lymph node more than 3 cm but not more than 6 cm in greatest dimension
[ ]	[ ]	N2b	Metastasis in multiple ipsilateral lymph nodes, none more than 6 cm in greatest dimension
[ ]	[ ]	N2c	Metastasis in bilateral or contralateral lymph nodes, none more than 6 cm in greatest dimension
[ ]	[ ]	N3	Metastasis in a lymph node more than 6 cm in greatest dimension
		Distant Metastasis (M)	
[ ]	[ ]	MX	Distant metastasis cannot be assessed
[ ]	[ ]	M0	No distant metastasis
[ ]	[ ]	M1	Distant metastasis

(continued on next page)

Stage Grouping

Clin	Path				
[ ]	[ ]	0	Tis	N0	M0
[ ]	[ ]	I	T1	N0	M0
[ ]	[ ]	II	T2	N0	M0
[ ]	[ ]	III	T3	N0	M0
			T1	N1	M0
			T2	N1	M0
			T3	N1	M0
[ ]	[ ]	IVA	T4	N0	M0
			T4	N1	M0
			Any T	N2	M0
[ ]	[ ]	IVB	Any T	N3	M0
[ ]	[ ]	IVC	Any T	Any N	M1

Staged by ______________________________ M.D.

______________________________ Registrar

Date ______________________________

Histopathologic Type

The predominant cancer type is squamous cell carcinoma. Nonepithelial tumors such as those of lymphoid tissue, soft tissue, bone and cartilage are not included in this system.

Illustrations

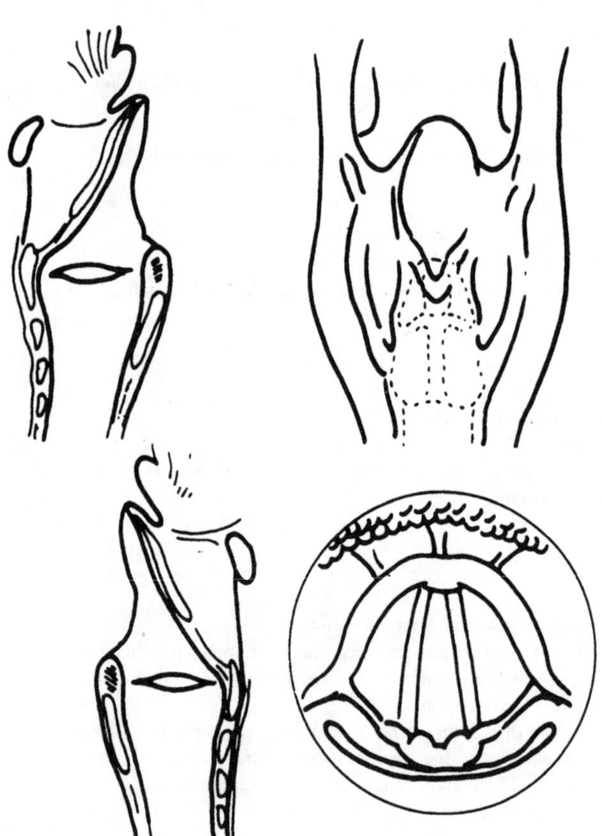

Indicate size and location of primary tumor.

Histopathologic Grade (G)

[ ] GX Grade cannot be assessed
[ ] G1 Well differentiated
[ ] G2 Moderately differentiated
[ ] G3 Poorly differentiated

Location of Tumor

Supraglottis
[ ] Suprahyoid epiglottis
[ ] Infrahyoid epiglottis
[ ] Aryepiglottic folds (laryngeal aspect)
[ ] Arytenoids
[ ] Ventricular bands (false cords)
Glottis
[ ] Right true vocal cord
[ ] Left true vocal cord
[ ] Anterior commissure
[ ] Posterior commissure
Subglottis
[ ] Subglottis

Involvement of Neighboring Structures

[ ] Oropharynx
[ ] Hypopharynx
[ ] Soft tissues or skin of neck

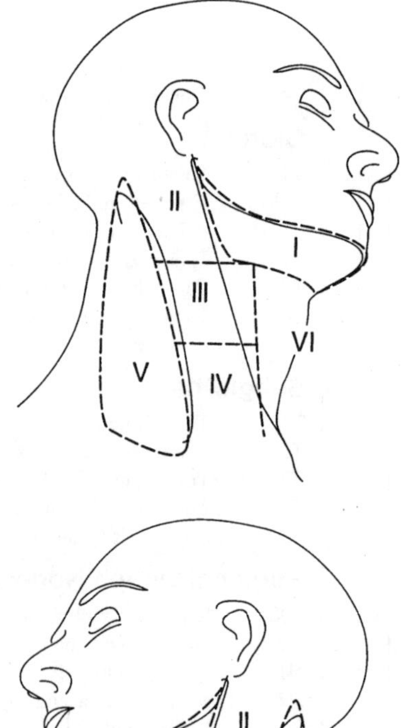

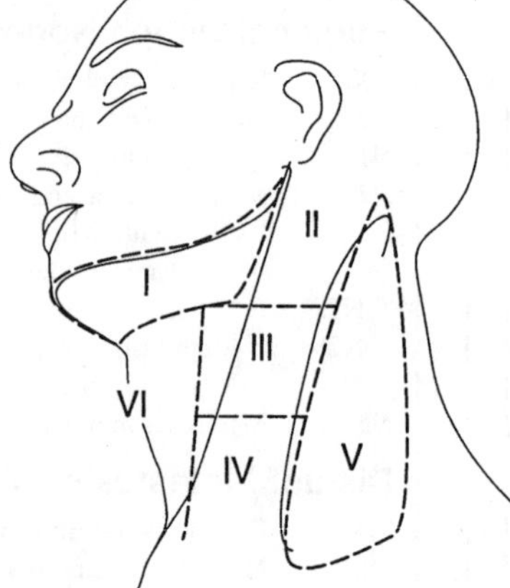

Indicate on diagram primary tumor and regional nodes involved.

6

Paranasal Sinuses

(Nonepithelial tumors such as those of lymphoid tissue, soft tissue, bone, and cartilage are not included.)

C31.0 Maxillary sinus
C31.1 Ethmoid sinus

ANATOMY

Primary Site. Cancer of the maxillary sinus is the most common of the paranasal sinus cancers. Ethmoid sinus cancers are less common. Tumors of the sphenoid and frontal sinuses are so rare as not to warrant staging.

Ohngren's line is a line joining the medial canthus of the eye with the angle of the mandible dividing the maxillary antrum into an anteroinferior portion (infrastructure) and a superoposterior portion (suprastructure) (Fig. 6-1). The location, as well as the extent, of the mucosal lesion within the antrum has prognostic significance.

Regional Lymph Nodes. Regional lymph node spread from cancer of paranasal sinus origin is relatively uncommon. Involvement of buccinator, submandibular, upper jugular and occasionally retropharyngeal nodes may occur with advanced maxillary sinus cancer, particularly those extending beyond the sinus walls to involve adjacent structures including soft tissues of the cheek, upper alveolus and palate, and buccal mucosa. Ethmoid sinus cancers are less prone to regional lymphatic spread. When only one side of the neck is involved, it should be considered ipsilateral. Bilateral spread may occur with advanced primary cancer, particularly with spread of the primary beyond the midline.

In clinical evaluation the physical size of the nodal mass should be measured. It is recognized that most masses over 3 cm in diameter are not single nodes but are confluent nodes or tumor in soft tissues of the neck. There are three categories of clinically positive nodes: N1, N2, and N3. The use of subgroups a, b, and c is not required but is recommended. Midline nodes are considered ipsilateral nodes. In addition to the components to describe the N-category, regional lymph nodes should also be described according to the level of the neck that is involved. Pathologic examination is necessary for documentation of such disease extent. Imaging studies showing amorphous spiculated margins of involved nodes or involvement of internodal fat resulting in loss of normal oval-to-round nodal shape strongly suggest extracapsular (extranodal) tumor spread. No imaging study (as yet) can identify microscopic foci in regional nodes or distinguish between small reactive nodes and small malignant nodes without central radiographic inhomogeneity.

For pN, a selective neck dissection will ordinarily include 6 or more lymph nodes and a radical or modified radical neck dissection will ordinarily include 10 or more lymph nodes.

Metastatic Sites. Distant spread to lungs is most common; occasionally there is spread to bone.

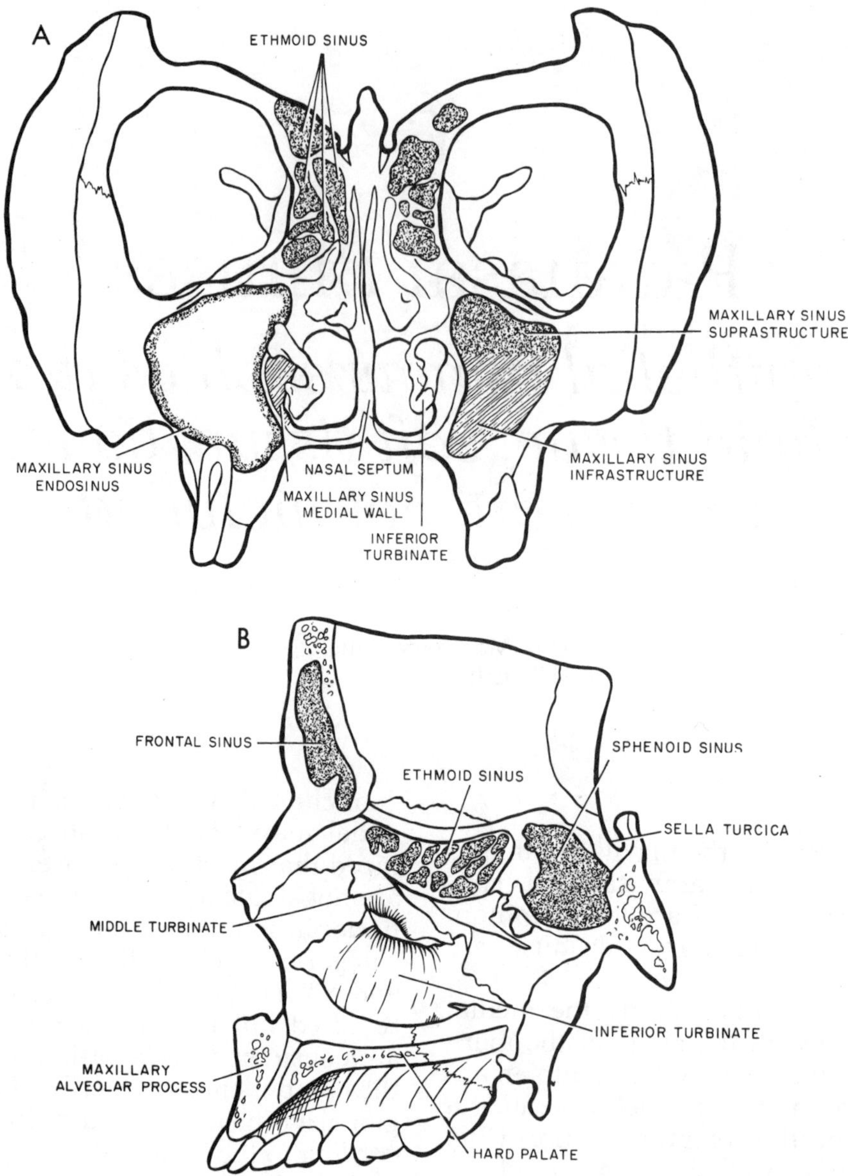

FIG. 6-1. A, B: Sites of origin of tumors of the paranasal sinuses.

RULES FOR CLASSIFICATION

Clinical Staging. The assessment of primary maxillary antrum and ethmoid tumors is based on inspection and, palpation, including examination of the orbits, nasal and oral cavities, nasopharynx, and neurologic evaluation of the cranial nerves. Cross-sectional imaging with magnetic resonance imaging (MRI) or computed tomography (CT) is mandatory for accurate pretreatment staging of malignant tumor of the sinuses. If available, MRI more accurately depicts skull base and intracranial involvement and differentiation of fluid from solid tumor. Neck nodes are assessed by palpation ± imaging. Imaging for possible nodal metastases is probably unnecessary in the presence of a clinically-negative neck. Examinations for distant metastases include appropriate radiographs, blood chemistries, blood count, and other routine studies as indicated.

Pathologic Staging. Complete resection of primary sites and major nodal dissections allow the use of this designation. Specimens that are resected after radiation or chemotherapy need to be so designated.

DEFINITION OF TNM

Maxillary Sinus

Primary Tumor (T)

TX Primary tumor cannot be assessed
T0 No evidence of primary tumor
Tis Carcinoma *in situ*
T1 Tumor limited to the antral mucosa with no erosion or destruction of bone
T2 Tumor causing bone erosion or destruction, except for the posterior antral wall, including extension into the hard palate and/or the middle nasal meatus
T3 Tumor invades any of the following: bone of the posterior wall of maxillary sinus, subcutaneous tissues, skin of cheek, floor or medial wall of orbit, infratemporal fossa, pterygoid plates, ethmoid sinuses
T4 Tumor invades orbital contents beyond the floor or medial wall including any of the following: the orbital apex, cribriform plate, base of skull, nasopharynx, sphenoid, frontal sinuses

Ethmoid Sinus

Primary Tumor (T)

T1 Tumor confined to the ethmoid with or without bone erosion
T2 Tumor extends into the nasal cavity
T3 Tumor extends to the anterior orbit, and/or maxillary sinus
T4 Tumor with intracranial extension, orbital extension including apex, involving sphenoid, and/or frontal sinus and/or skin of external nose

Regional Lymph Nodes (N)

NX Regional lymph nodes cannot be assessed
N0 No regional lymph node metastasis
N1 Metastasis in a single ipsilateral lymph node, 3 cm or less in greatest dimension
N2 Metastasis in a single ipsilateral lymph node, more than 3 cm but not more than 6 cm in greatest dimension dimension, or in multiple ipsilateral lymph nodes, none more than 6 cm in greatest dimension, or in bilateral or contralateral lymph nodes, none more than 6 cm in greatest dimension
N2a Metastasis in a single ipsilateral lymph node more than 3 cm but not more than 6 cm in greatest dimension
N2b Metastasis in multiple ipsilateral lymph nodes, none more than 6 cm in greatest dimension
N2c Metastasis in bilateral or contralateral lymph nodes, none more than 6 cm in greatest dimension
N3 Metastasis in a lymph node more than 6 cm in greatest dimension

Distant Metastasis (M)

MX Distant metastasis cannot be assessed
M0 No distant metastasis
M1 Distant metastasis

STAGE GROUPING

Stage 0	Tis	N0	M0
Stage I	T1	N0	M0
Stage II	T2	N0	M0
Stage III	T3	N0	M0
	T1	N1	M0
	T2	N1	M0
	T3	N1	M0
Stage IVA	T4	N0	M0
	T4	N1	M0
Stage IVB	Any T	N2	M0
	Any T	N3	M0
Stage IVC	Any T	Any N	M1

HISTOPATHOLOGIC TYPE

The predominant cancer is squamous cell carcinoma. Nonepithelial tumors such as those of lymphoid tissue, soft tissue, bone, and cartilage are not included. Histologic diagnosis is required to use this classification. Histopathologic grading of squamous carcinoma is recommended. The grade is subjective and uses a descriptive as well as a numerical form; i.e., well, moderately well, and poorly differentiated depending upon the degree of closeness to, or deviation from, squamous epithelium in mucosal sites. Also recommended where feasible is a quantitative evaluation of the depth of infiltration of the primary tumor and the presence of endovascular/perineural invasion. The pathologic description of any lymphadenectomy specimen should describe the size, number, and level of involved lymph node(s).

HISTOPATHOLOGIC GRADE (G)

GX Grade cannot be assessed
G1 Well differentiated
G2 Moderately differentiated
G3 Poorly differentiated

BIBLIOGRAPHY

Bridger GP, Mendelsohn MS, Baldwinn M, et al: Paranasal sinus cancer. Aust N Z J Surg 61:290–294, 1991

Jiang GL, Ang KA, Peters LJ, et al: Maxillary sinus carcinomas: natural history and results of postoperative radiotherapy. Radiother Oncol 21:193–200, 1991

Kondo M, Horiuchi M, Shiga H, et al: CT of malignant tumors of the nasal cavity and paranasal sinuses. Cancer 50:226–231, 1982

Sisson GA, Toriumi DM, Stiyah RH: Paranasal sinus malignancy: a comprehensive update. Laryngoscope 99:143–150, 1989

Som PM, Dillon WP, Sze G, et al: Benign and malignant sinonasal lesions with intracranial extension: differentiation with MR imaging. Radiology 172:763–766, 1989

Som PM, Shapiro MD, Biller HF, et al: Sinonasal tumors and inflammatory tissues: differentiation with MR imaging. Radiology 167:803–808, 1988

Som PM, Shugar JMA, Biller HF: The early detection of antral malignancy in the postmaxillectomy patient. Radiology 143:509–512, 1982

Van Tassel P, Lee YY: Gd-DTPA enhanced MR for detecting intracranial extension of sinonasal malignancies. JCAT 15:387–392, 1991

PARANASAL SINUSES

Data Form for Cancer Staging

Patient identification
Name ______
Address ______
Hospital or clinic number ______
Age ____ Sex ____ Race ______

Institution identification
Hospital or clinic ______
Address ______

Oncology Record

Anatomic site of cancer ______
Histologic type ______
Grade (G) ______
Date of classification ______

Clin	Path	DEFINITIONS	
		Primary Tumor (T)	
[ ]	[ ]	TX	Primary tumor cannot be assessed
[ ]	[ ]	T0	No evidence of primary tumor
[ ]	[ ]	Tis	Carcinoma *in situ*
		Maxillary Sinus	
[ ]	[ ]	T1	Tumor limited to the antral mucosa with no erosion or destruction of bone
[ ]	[ ]	T2	Tumor causing bone erosion or destruction, except for the posterior antral wall, including extension into the hard palate and/or the middle nasal meatus
[ ]	[ ]	T3	Tumor invades any of the following: bone of the posterior wall of maxillary sinus, subcutaneous tissues, skin of cheek, floor or medial wall of orbit, infratemporal fossa, pterygoid plates, ethmoid sinuses
[ ]	[ ]	T4	Tumor invades orbital contents beyond the floor or medial wall including any of the following: the orbital apex, cribiform plate, base of skull, nasopharynx, sphenoid, frontal sinuses
		Ethmoid Sinus	
[ ]	[ ]	T1	Tumor confined to the ethmoid with or without bone erosion
[ ]	[ ]	T2	Tumor extends into the nasal cavity
[ ]	[ ]	T3	Tumor extends to the anterior orbit and/or maxillary sinus
[ ]	[ ]	T4	Tumor with intracranial extension, orbital extension including apex, involving sphenoid and/or frontal sinus and/or skin of external nose
		Regional Lymph Nodes (N)	
[ ]	[ ]	NX	Regional lymph nodes cannot be assessed
[ ]	[ ]	N0	No regional lymph node metastasis
[ ]	[ ]	N1	Metastasis in a single ipsilateral lymph node, 3 cm or less in greatest dimension
[ ]	[ ]	N2	Metastasis in a single ipsilateral lymph node, more than 3 but not more than 6 cm in greatest dimension, or in multiple ipsilateral lymph nodes, none more than 6 cm in greatest dimension, or in bilateral or contralateral lymph nodes, none more than 6 cm in greatest dimension
[ ]	[ ]	N2a	Metastasis in a single ipsilateral lymph node more than 3 cm but not more than 6 cm in greatest dimension
[ ]	[ ]	N2b	Metastasis in multiple ipsilateral lymph nodes, none more than 6 cm in greatest dimension
[ ]	[ ]	N2c	Metastasis in bilateral or contralateral lymph nodes, none more than 6 cm in greatest dimension
[ ]	[ ]	N3	Metastasis in a lymph node more than 6 cm in greatest dimension
		Distant Metastasis (M)	
[ ]	[ ]	MX	Distant metastasis cannot be assessed
[ ]	[ ]	M0	No distant metastasis
[ ]	[ ]	M1	Distant metastasis

(continued on next page)

Stage Grouping

Clin	Path	Stage	T	N	M
[ ]	[ ]	0	Tis	N0	M0
[ ]	[ ]	I	T1	N0	M0
[ ]	[ ]	II	T2	N0	M0
[ ]	[ ]	III	T3	N0	M0
			T1	N1	M0
			T2	N1	M0
			T3	N1	M0
[ ]	[ ]	IVA	T4	N0	M0
			T4	N1	M0
[ ]	[ ]	IVB	Any T	N2	M0
			Any T	N3	M0
[ ]	[ ]	IVC	Any T	Any N	M1

Staged by ____________________ M.D.

____________________ Registrar

Date ____________________

Location of Tumor

[ ] Antrum
- [ ] Infrastructure
- [ ] Suprastructure
- [ ] Both

[ ] Nasal Cavity
- [ ] Septum
- [ ] Root
- [ ] Lateral wall
- [ ] Floor

[ ] Ethmoid
- [ ] Anterior
- [ ] Posterior

[ ] Sphenoid

[ ] Frontal

Histopathologic Type

The predominant cancer is squamous cell carcinoma. Nonepithelial tumors such as those of lymphoid tissue, soft tissue, bone and cartilage are not included in this system.

Histopathologic Grade (G)

[ ] GX Grade cannot be assessed
[ ] G1 Well differentiated
[ ] G2 Moderately differentiated
[ ] G3 Poorly differentiated

Illustrations

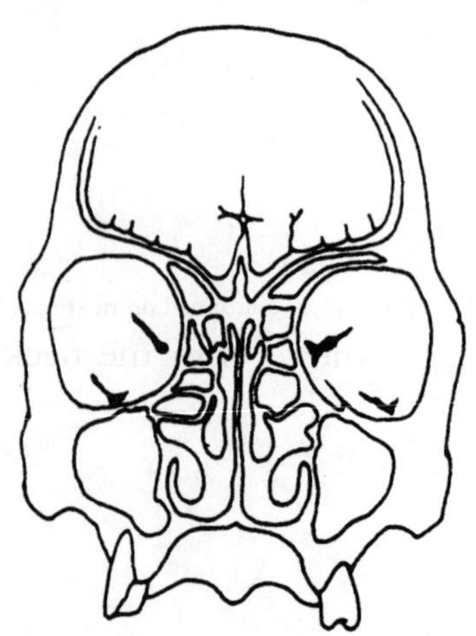

Indicate on diagram primary tumor.

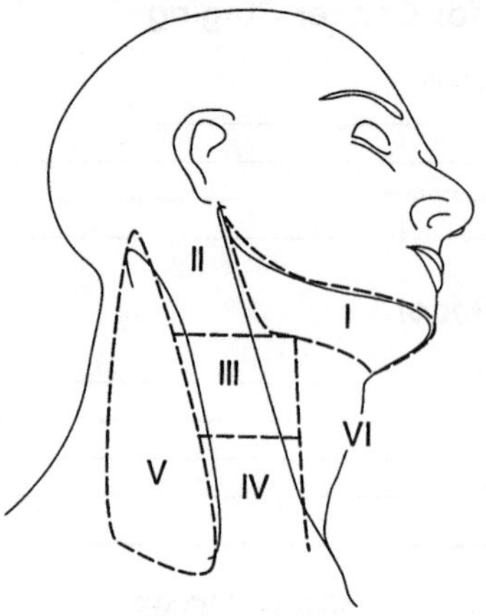

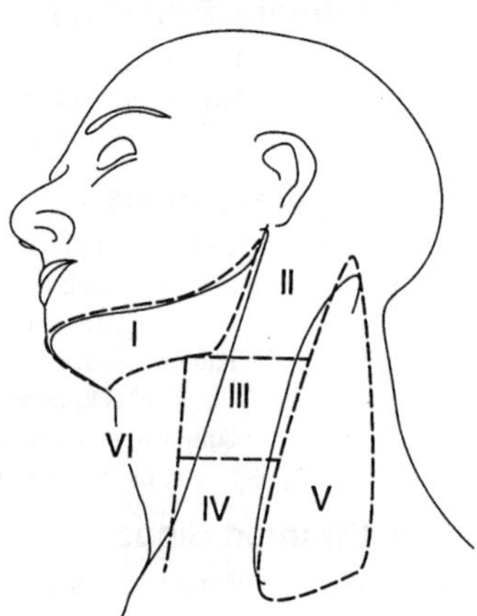

Indicate on diagram regional nodes involved.

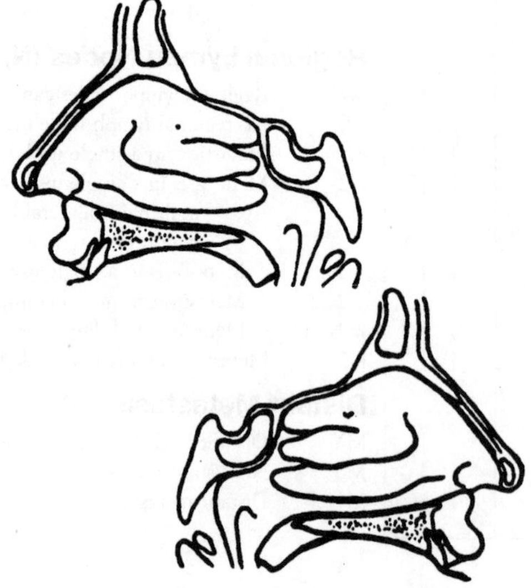

7

Major Salivary Glands (Parotid, Submandibular, and Sublingual)

C07.9 Parotid gland

C08.0 Submandibular gland
C08.1 Sublingual gland (submental)
C08.8 Overlapping lesion
C08.9 Major salivary gland, NOS

This staging system is based on an extensive retrospective study of malignant tumors of the major salivary glands collected from eleven participating United States and Canadian institutions. Statistical analysis of the data revealed that numerous factors affected patient survival, including the histologic diagnosis, cellular differentiation of the tumor, site, size, degree of fixation, or local extension, and nerve involvement. The status of regional lymph nodes and of distant metastases were also of major importance. The classification here proposed involves only four clinical variables: tumor size, local extension of the tumor, the palpability and appearance of nodes, and the presence or absence of distant metastasis. It offers a simple but effective and accurate method of evaluating the stage of salivary gland cancer.

ANATOMY

Primary Site. The major salivary glands include the parotid, submandibular and submental (sublingual) glands. Tumors arising in minor salivary glands (mucous-secreting glands in the lining membrane of the upper aerodigestive tract) are included at the anatomic site of origin (e.g., lip). Primary tumors of the parotid comprise the largest proportion of salivary gland tumors. Sublingual primary cancers are rare and may be difficult to distinguish with certainty from minor salivary gland primary tumors of the anterior floor of mouth. Extraparenchymal extension is clinical or macroscopic evidence of invasion of skin, soft tissues, bone, or nerve. Microscopic extension alone is not extraparenchymal extension for classification purposes.

Regional Lymph Nodes. Regional lymphatic spread from salivary gland cancer is less common than from head and neck mucosal cancers and relates to the histology and size of the primary tumor. Most nodal metastases will be clinically apparent on initial evaluation. Low grade tumors rarely metastasize to regional nodes, while the risk of regional spread is substantially higher from the high grade cancers. Regional dissemination tends to be orderly, to adjacent intra-periparotid, submandibular nodes, then to upper and midjugular, and occasionally retropharyngeal nodes. Bilateral lymphatic dissemination is rare. In addition to the components to describe the N-category, regional lymph nodes should also be described according to the level of the neck that is involved. Extra-facial/cervical nodal deposits are considered distant metastases.

For pN, histologic examination of a selected neck dissection will ordinarily include 6 or more lymph nodes or histological examination of a radical or modified radical neck dissection will ordinarily include 10 or more lymph nodes.

Metastatic Sites. Distant spread is most frequently to the lungs.

RULES FOR CLASSIFICATION

Clinical Staging. The assessment of primary salivary gland tumors includes inspection, palpation and neurologic evaluation of the cranial nerves. Radiologic studies may add valuable information for staging. When staging parotid malignancy, magnetic resonance imaging (MRI) best delineates the deep tissue and perineural extent of the tumor. The soft tissues of the neck from the skull base to the hyoid bone must be studied with the lower neck included whenever lymph node metastases are suspected. Images of the intratemporal facial nerve are critical to the identification of perineural tumor in this area. Cancers of the submandibular and sublingual salivary glands merit cross-sectional imaging. Computed tomography (CT) or MRI may be useful in assessing extent of deep extraglandular tumor, bone invasion, deep tissue extent (extrinsic tongue muscle, and/or soft tissues of neck). Radiologic nodal staging should be done simultaneously.

Pathologic Staging. The surgical pathology report and all other available data should be used to assign a pathologic classification to those patients who have resection of the cancer.

DEFINITION OF TNM

Primary Tumor (T)

TX Primary tumor cannot be assessed
T0 No evidence of primary tumor
T1 Tumor 2 cm or less in greatest dimension without extraparenchymal extension
T2 Tumor more than 2 cm but not more than 4 cm in greatest dimension without extraparenchymal extension
T3 Tumor having extraparenchymal extension without seventh nerve involvement and/or more than 4 cm but not more than 6 cm in greatest dimension
T4 Tumor invades base of skull, seventh nerve, and/or exceeds 6 cm in greatest dimension

Regional Lymph Nodes (N)

NX Regional lymph nodes cannot be assessed
N0 No regional lymph node metastasis
N1 Metastasis in a single ipsilateral lymph node, 3 cm or less in greatest dimension
N2 Metastasis in a single ipsilateral lymph node, more than 3 cm but not more than 6 cm in greatest dimension, or in multiple ipsilateral lymph nodes, none more than 6 cm in greatest dimension, or in bilateral or contralateral lymph nodes, none more than 6 cm in greatest dimension
  N2a Metastasis in a single ipsilateral lymph node more than 3 cm but not more than 6 cm in greatest dimension
  N2b Metastasis in multiple ipsilateral lymph nodes, none more than 6 cm in greatest dimension
  N2c Metastasis in bilateral or contralateral lymph nodes, none more than 6 cm in greatest dimension
N3 Metastasis in a lymph node more than 6 cm in greatest dimension

Distant Metastasis (M)

MX Distant metastasis cannot be assessed
M0 No distant metastases
M1 Distant metastasis

STAGE GROUPING

Stage I	T1	N0	M0
	T2	N0	M0
Stage II	T3	N0	M0
Stage III	T1	N1	M0
	T2	N1	M0
Stage IV	T4	N0	M0
	T3	N1	M0
	T4	N1	M0
	Any T	N2	M0
	Any T	N3	M0
	Any T	Any N	M1

HISTOPATHOLOGIC TYPE

The suggested histopathologic typing is that proposed by the World Health Organization. Other more rare entities also exist and are classified in the World Health Organization fascicle.

Acinic cell carcinoma
Adenoid cystic carcinoma
Salivary duct carcinoma
Carcinoma ex pleomorphic adenoma

Adenocarcinoma
Mucoepidermoid carcinoma
Polymorphous low-grade adenocarcinoma (terminal duct adenocarcinoma)

HISTOPATHOLOGIC GRADE (G)

Histologic grading is applicable only to some types of salivary gland cancer: mucoepidermoid, adenoid cystic and acinic cell carcinomas. In other instances the histologic type defines the grade (i.e., salivary duct carcinoma, whether arising from a pleomorphic adenoma or *de novo*, is high grade; terminal duct adenocarcinoma is low grade). Data indicate there is univariate significance to a three-tiered grading system for mucoepidermoid, adenoid cystic, and acinic cell carcinomas, based upon a combination of architectural growth patterns and cytologic differentiation.

BIBLIOGRAPHY

Batsakis JG, Luna MA: Histopatholgoic grading of salivary gland neoplasms: I. Mucoepidermoid carcinomas. Ann Otol Rhinol Laryngol 99:835–838, 1990

Calearo C and Pastore A: Parotid carinoma. In Hermanek P, Gospodarowicz MK, Henson DE, Hutter RVP, Sobin LH (Eds.), Prognostic factors in cancer, UICC, Geneva. Berlin-New York: Springer-Verlag; 23–27, 1995

Goepfert H, Luna MA, Lindberg RH, et al: Malignant salivary gland tumors of the paranasal sinuses and nasal cavity. Arch Otolaryngol 109:662–668, 1983

McNaney D, McNeese MD, Guillamondegui OM, et al: Postoperative irradiation in malignant epithelial tumors of the parotid. Int J Radiation Oncology Biol Phys 9:1289–1295, 1983

Seifert G, Sobin LH: Histological typing of salivary gland tumours. WHO international histological classification of tumours, 2nd ed. Berlin-Heidelberg-New York: Springer-Verlag, 1991

Spiro RH: Salivary neoplasms: overview of a 35-year experience with 2807 patients. Head Neck Surg 8:177–184, 1986

Spiro RH, Hajdu SI, Strong EW: Tumors of the submaxillary gland. Am J Surg 132:463–468, 1976

Szanto PA, Luna MA, Tortoledo ME, et al: Histologic grading of adenoid cystic carcinoma of the salivary glands. Cancer 54:1062–1069, 1984

Data Form for Cancer Staging

Patient identification
Name ______
Address ______
Hospital or clinic number ______
Age ____ Sex ____ Race ______

Institution identification
Hospital or clinic ______
Address ______

Oncology Record

Anatomic site of cancer ______
Histologic type ______
Grade (G) ______
Date of classification ______

Clin	Path	DEFINITIONS	
		Primary Tumor (T)	
[ ]	[ ]	TX	Primary tumor cannot be assessed
[ ]	[ ]	T0	No evidence of primary tumor
[ ]	[ ]	T1	Tumor 2 cm or less in greatest dimension without extraparenchymal extension
[ ]	[ ]	T2	Tumor more than 2 cm but not more than 4 cm in greatest dimension without extraparenchymal extension
[ ]	[ ]	T3	Tumor having extraparenchymal extension without seventh nerve involvement and/or more than 4 cm but not more than 6 cm in greatest dimension
[ ]	[ ]	T4	Tumor invades base of skull, seventh nerve, and/or exceeds 6 cm in greatest dimension
		Regional Lymph Nodes (N)	
[ ]	[ ]	NX	Regional lymph nodes cannot be assessed
[ ]	[ ]	N0	No regional lymph node metastasis
[ ]	[ ]	N1	Metastasis in a single ipsilateral lymph node, 3 cm or less in greatest dimension
[ ]	[ ]	N2	Metastasis in a single ipsilateral lymph node, more than 3 cm but not more than 6 cm in greatest dimension, or in multiple ipsilateral lymph nodes, none more than 6 cm in greatest dimension or in bilateral or in contralateral lymph nodes, none more than 6 cm in greatest dimension
[ ]	[ ]	N2a	Metastasis in a single ipsilateral lymph node more than 3 cm but not more than 6 cm in greatest dimension
[ ]	[ ]	N2b	Metastasis in multiple ipsilateral lymph nodes, none more than 6 cm in greatest dimension
[ ]	[ ]	N2c	Metastasis in bilateral or contralateral lymph nodes, none more than 6 cm in greatest dimension
[ ]	[ ]	N3	Metastasis in a lymph node more than 6 cm in greatest dimension
		Distant Metastasis (M)	
[ ]	[ ]	MX	Distant metastasis cannot be assessed
[ ]	[ ]	M0	No distant metastasis
[ ]	[ ]	M1	Distant metastasis

Clin	Path	Stage Grouping			
[ ]	[ ]	I	T1	N0	M0
			T2	N0	M0
[ ]	[ ]	II	T3	N0	M0
[ ]	[ ]	III	T1	N1	M0
			T2	N1	M0
[ ]	[ ]	IV	T4	N0	M0
			T3	N1	M0
			T4	N1	M0
			Any T	N2	M0
			Any T	N3	M0
			Any T	Any N	M1

Staged by ______ M.D.
______ Registrar
Date ______

(continued on next page)

Histopathologic Grade (G)

Histologic grading is applicable only to some types of salivary gland cancer: mucoepidermoid, adenoid cystic and acinic cell carcinomas. In other instances the histologic type defines the grade.

Histopathologic Type

The suggested histopathologic typing is that proposed by the World Health Organization. Other more rare entities also exist and are classified in the WHO fascicle.

Acinic cell carcinoma
Adenoid cystic carcinoma
Salivary duct carcinoma
Carcinoma ex pleomorphic adenoma
Adenocarcinoma
Mucoepidermoid carcinoma
Polymorphous low-grade adenocarcinoma (terminal duct adenocarcinoma).

Other data that might be pertinent to the biologic behavior of the tumor.

____
____
____
____

Illustrations

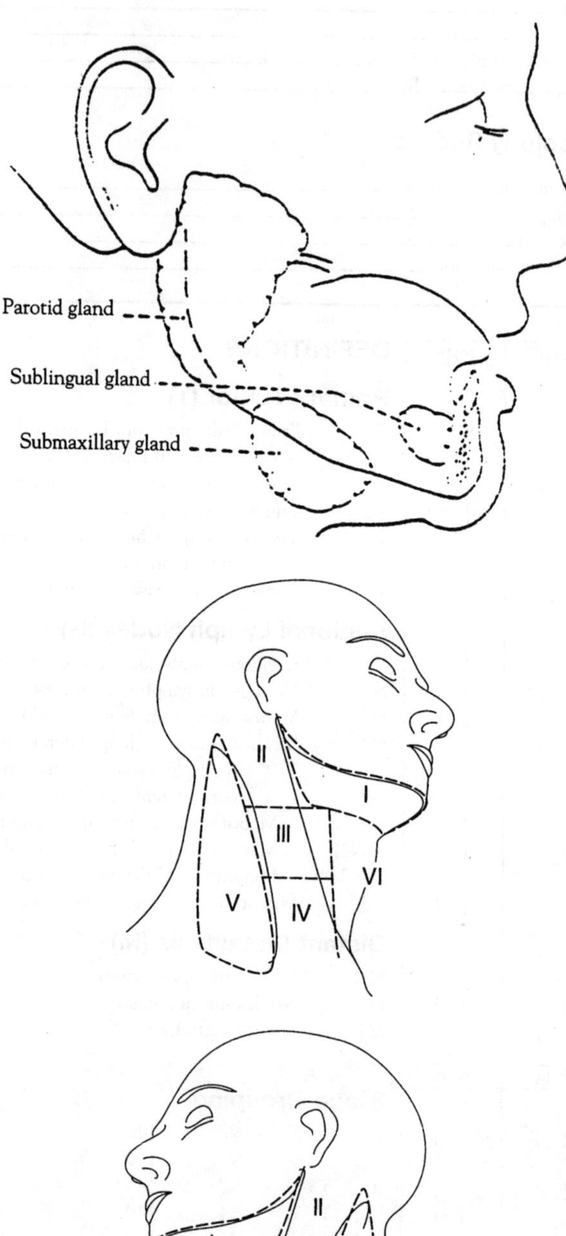

Indicate on diagram primary tumor and regional nodes involved.

8

Thyroid Gland

C73.9 Thyroid gland

Although staging for cancers in other head and neck sites is based entirely on the anatomic extent of disease, it is not possible to follow this pattern for the unique group of malignant tumors that arise in the thyroid. Both the histologic diagnosis and the age of the patient are of such importance in the behavior and prognosis of thyroid cancer that these factors are included in this staging system.

ANATOMY

Primary Site. The thyroid gland ordinarily is composed of a right and a left lobe lying adjacent and lateral to the upper trachea and esophagus. An isthmus connects the two lobes and in some cases a pyramidal lobe is present extending upward anterior to the thyroid cartilage.

Regional Lymph Nodes. Regional lymph node spread from thyroid cancer is common but of less prognostic significance in the generally well-differentiated tumors (papillary, follicular) than in medullary cancers. The first echelon of nodal metastasis is the paralaryngeal and paratracheal, prelaryngeal (Delphian) nodes adjacent to the thyroid, but involvement of these nodal stations is not prognostic and, therefore, not part of the staging system. Metastases secondarily involve mid- and lower jugular, supraclavicular nodes, and, much less commonly, submental, submandibular, spinal accessory nodes. Upper mediastinal nodal spread occurs frequently, both anteriorly and posteriorly. Retropharyngeal nodal metastases may be seen, usually in the presence of extensive cervical metastases. Bilateral nodal spread is common. In addition to the components to describe the N-category, regional lymph nodes should also be described according to the level of the neck that is involved. Nodal metastases from medullary thyroid cancer carry a much more ominous prognosis although they follow a similar pattern of spread.

For pN, histologic examination of a selected neck dissection will ordinarily include 6 or more lymph nodes or histological examination of a radical or modified radical neck dissection will ordinarily include 10 or more lymph nodes.

Metastatic Sites. Distant spread occurs by hematogenous routes, for example, to lungs and bones, but many other sites may be involved.

RULES FOR CLASSIFICATION

Clinical Staging. The assessment of a thyroid tumor depends on inspection and palpation of the thyroid gland and regional lymph nodes. Indirect laryngoscopy to evaluate vocal cord motion is important. A variety of imaging procedures can provide additional useful information. These include radioisotope thyroid scans, computed tomography (CT) scans, magnetic resonance imaging (MRI) scans, and ultrasound examinations. When cross-sectional imaging is utilized MRI is recommended so as to avoid contamination of the body with the iodinated contrast medium generally used with CT. Iodinated contrast media will delay the possibility of administering radioactive Iodine^{131} postoperatively. The diagnosis of thyroid cancer must be confirmed by needle biopsy or open biopsy of the tumor. Further information for clinical staging may be obtained by biopsy of lymph nodes or other areas of suspected local or distant spread. All information available prior to first treatment should be used.

Pathologic Staging. All available clinical data are combined with pathologic study of the surgically resected specimen for pathologic staging. The surgeon's evaluation of gross unresected residual tumor must be included.

DEFINITION OF TNM

Primary Tumor (T)

Note: All categories may be subdivided: (a) solitary tumor, (b) multifocal tumor (the largest determines the classification).

TX Primary tumor cannot be assessed
T0 No evidence of primary tumor
T1 Tumor 1 cm or less in greatest dimension limited to the thyroid
T2 Tumor more than 1 cm but not more than 4 cm in greatest dimension limited to the thyroid
T3 Tumor more than 4 cm in greatest dimension limited to the thyroid
T4 Tumor of any size extending beyond the thyroid capsule

Regional Lymph Nodes (N)

Regional lymph nodes are the cervical and upper mediastinal lymph nodes.

NX Regional lymph nodes cannot be assessed
N0 No regional lymph node metastasis
N1 Regional lymph node metastasis
 N1a Metastasis in ipsilateral cervical lymph node(s)
 N1b Metastasis in bilateral, midline, or contralateral cervical or mediastinal lymph node(s)

Distant Metastasis (M)

MX Distant metastasis cannot be assessed
M0 No distant metastasis
M1 Distant metastasis

HISTOPATHOLOGIC TYPE

There are four major histopathologic types:

Papillary carcinoma (including those with follicular foci)
Follicular carcinoma
Medullary carcinoma
Undifferentiated (anaplastic) carcinoma

STAGE GROUPING

Separate stage groupings are recommended for papillary, follicular, medullary, or undifferentiated (anaplastic).

Papillary or Follicular

	UNDER 45 YEARS	45 YEARS AND OLDER
Stage I	Any T, Any N, M0	T1, N0, M0
Stage II	Any T, Any N, M1	T2, N0, M0
		T3, N0, M0
Stage III		T4, N0, M0
		Any T, N1, M0
Stage IV		Any T, Any N, M1

Medullary

Stage I	T1	N0	M0
Stage II	T2	N0	M0
	T3	N0	M0
	T4	N0	M0
Stage III	Any T	N1	M0
Stage IV	Any T	Any N	M1

Undifferentiated (anaplastic)

All cases are stage IV.

Stage IV	Any T	Any N	Any M

BIBLIOGRAPHY

Ain KB: Papillary thyroid carcinoma: etiology, assessment, and therapy. Endocrinol Metab Clin North Am 24:711–760, 1995

Antonaci A, Brierley G, Bacchi F, Consorti C, et al: Thyroid cancer. In Hermanek P, Gospodarowicz MK, Henson DE, et al (Eds.), Prognostic factors in cancer. Berlin: Springer-Verlag; 28–36, 1995

Brierly JD, Panzarella T, Tsang RW, et al: Comparing staging classifications using thyroid cancer as an example. Cancer 79:2414–2423, 1997

Brierley J, Tsang R, Panzarella T, Simpson WJ: Medullary thyroid cancer—analyses of survival and prognostic factors and the role of radiation therapy in local control. Thyroid 6:305, 1996

Cady B, Rossi R, Silverman M, et al: Further evidence of the validity of risk group definition in differentiated thyroid carcinoma. Surgery 98:1171–1178, 1985

Cohn K, Blackdahl M, Forsslund G, et al: Prognostic value of nuclear DNA content in papillary thyroid carcinoma. World J Surg 8:474–480, 1984

Hay ID, Grant CS, Taylor WF, et al: Ipsilateral lobectomy versus bilateral lobar resection in papillary thyroid carcinoma: a retrospective analysis of surgical outcome using a novel prognostic scoring system. Surgery 102:1088–1095, 1987

Hedinger Chr: Histological typing of thyroid tumours. WHO international histological classification of tumours, 2nd ed. Berlin-Heidelberg-New York: Springer-Verlag, 1988

LiVolsi VA: Surgical pathology of the thyroid. Philadelphia: WB Saunders Company, 1990

Mazzaferri EL, Jhiang S: Longterm impact of initial surgical and medical therapy on papillary and follicular thyroid cancer. Am J Med 97:418–428, 1994

McConahey WM, Hay ID, Woolner LB, et al: Papillary thyroid cancer treated at the Mayo Clinic 1946–1970: initial manifestations, pathologic findings, therapy and outcome. Mayo Clinic Proc 61:978–996, 1986

Rosai J, Carcangiu ML, DeLellis RA: Tumors of the thyroid gland, 3rd series. Washington, DC: Armed Forces Institute of Pathology, 1992

Rossi R: Prognosis of undifferentiated carcinoma and lymphoma of the thyroid. Am J Surg 135:589–596, 1978

Saad MF, Ordonez NG, Rashid RK, et al: Medullary carcinoma of the thyroid: a study of the clinical features and prognostic factors in 161 patients. Medicine 63:319–342, 1984

Shah JP, Loree TR, Dharker D, et al: Prognostic factors in differentiated carcinoma of the thyroid gland. Am J Surg 164:658–661, 1992

Simpson WL, Panzarella T, Carruthers JS, et al: Papillary and follicular thyroid cancer: impact of treatment in 1578 patients. Int J Radiation Oncol Biol Phys 14:1063–1075, 1988

Young RL, Mazzaferri EL, Rahea J, et al: Pure follicular thyroid carcinoma: impact of therapy in 214 patients. J Nucl Med 21:733–737, 1980

Data Form for Cancer Staging

Patient identification
Name ______
Address ______
Hospital or clinic number ______
Age ____ Sex ____ Race ______

Institution identification
Hospital or clinic ______
Address ______

Oncology Record

Anatomic site of cancer ______
Histologic type ______
Grade (G) ______
Date of classification ______

DEFINITIONS

Primary Tumor (T)

All categories may be subdivided: (a) solitary tumor; (b) multifocal tumor (the largest determines the classification)

Clin	Path		
[ ]	[ ]	TX	Primary tumor cannot be assessed
[ ]	[ ]	T0	No evidence of primary tumor
[ ]	[ ]	T1	Tumor 1 cm or less in greatest dimension limited to the thyroid
[ ]	[ ]	T2	Tumor more than 1 cm but not more than 4 cm in greatest dimension limited to the thyroid
[ ]	[ ]	T3	Tumor more than 4 cm in greatest dimension limited to the thyroid
[ ]	[ ]	T4	Tumor of any size extending beyond the thyroid capsule

Regional Lymph Nodes (N)

Regional nodes are the cervical and upper mediastinal lymph nodes

Clin	Path		
[ ]	[ ]	NX	Regional lymph nodes cannot be assessed
[ ]	[ ]	N0	No regional lymph node metastasis
[ ]	[ ]	N1	Regional lymph node metastasis
[ ]	[ ]	N1a	Metastasis in ipsilateral cervical lymph node(s)
[ ]	[ ]	N1b	Metastasis in bilateral, midline, or contralateral cervical or mediastinal lymph node(s)

Distant Metastasis (M)

Clin	Path		
[ ]	[ ]	MX	Distant metastasis cannot be assessed
[ ]	[ ]	M0	No distant metastasis
[ ]	[ ]	M1	Distant metastasis

Stage Grouping

Separate stage groupings are recommended for papillary, follicular, medullary, or undifferentiated (anaplastic)

Papillary or Follicular

Under 45 Years

Clin	Path	Stage	
[ ]	[ ]	Stage I	Any T, Any N, M0
[ ]	[ ]	Stage II	Any T, Any N, M1

45 Years and Over

Clin	Path	Stage	
[ ]	[ ]	Stage I	T1, N0, M0
[ ]	[ ]	Stage II	T2, N0, M0
			T3, N0, M0
[ ]	[ ]	Stage III	T4, N0, M0
			Any T, N1, M0
[ ]	[ ]	Stage IV	Any T, Any N, M1

Medullary

Clin	Path	Stage	T	N	M
[ ]	[ ]	Stage I	T1	N0	M0
[ ]	[ ]	Stage II	T2	N0	M0
			T3	N0	M0
			T4	N0	M0
[ ]	[ ]	Stage III	Any T	N1	M0
[ ]	[ ]	Stage IV	Any T	Any N	M1

Undifferentiated (anaplastic)

All cases are Stage IV

Clin	Path	Stage	T	N	M
[ ]	[ ]	Stage IV	Any T	Any N	Any M

Staged by ______ M.D.
______ Registrar

Date ______

(continued on next page)

Nodal Involvement

Cervical unilateral ______
Cervical bilateral ______
Delphian ______
Mediastinal ______

Indicate on diagram primary tumor and regional nodes involved.

Histopathologic Type

There are four major histopathologic types:
Papillary carcinoma (including those with follicular foci)
Follicular carcinoma
Medullary carcinoma
Undifferentiated (anaplastic) carcinoma

Illustrations

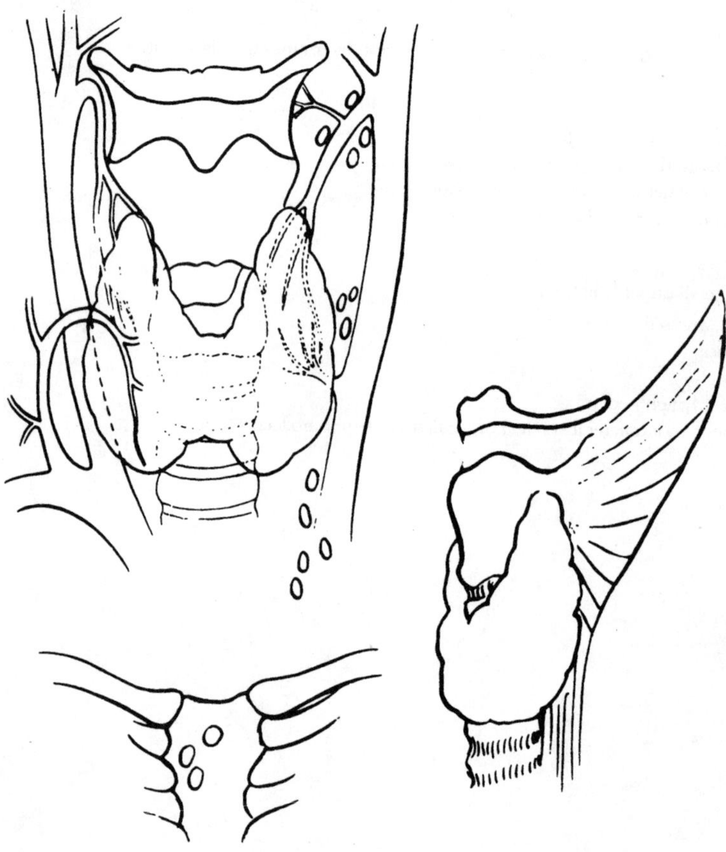

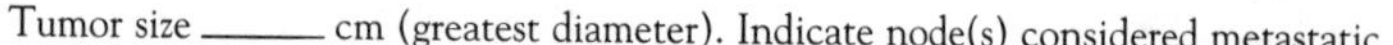

Tumor size ______ cm (greatest diameter). Indicate node(s) considered metastatic.

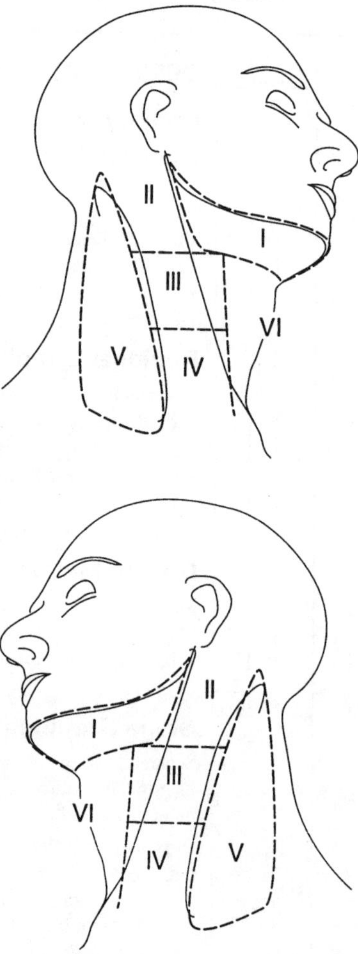

Indicate on diagram regional nodes involved.

DIGESTIVE SYSTEM

9

Esophagus

(Sarcomas are not included.)

C15.0 Cervical
C15.1 Thoracic
C15.2 Abdominal
C15.3 Upper third
C15.4 Middle third
C15.5 Lower third
C15.8 Overlapping lesion
C15.9 Esophagus, NOS

Occurring more often in males, cancer of the esophagus accounts for 5.5% of all malignant tumors of the gastrointestinal tract and less than 1% of all cancers in the United States. Predisposing factors include a high alcohol intake and heavy use of tobacco. The disease may be difficult to diagnose in its early stages. Most cancers arise in the middle or lower third of the thoracic esophagus. Squamous cell carcinomas are the most common, although the frequency of adenocarcinomas has increased in recent years. Esophageal cancers, regardless of the histologic type, may extend over wide areas of the mucosal surface. Only the depth of penetration is considered in staging, however. Squamous cell carcinomas may arise from either the cervical or thoracic esophagus while adenocarcinomas are usually found in the distal esophagus. Dysphagia is the most common clinical symptom for all lesions.

ANATOMY

Primary Site. Beginning at the hypopharynx, the esophagus lies posterior to the trachea and the heart, passing through the posterior mediastinum and entering the stomach through an opening in the diaphragm called the hiatus.

Histologically, the esophagus has four layers—mucosa, submucosa, muscle coat or muscularis propria, and adventitia. There is no serosa.

For classification, staging, and reporting of cancer, the esophagus is divided into four regions. Because the behavior of esophageal cancer and its treatment vary with the anatomic divisions, these regions should be recorded and reported separately. The location of the esophageal cancer at the time of endoscopy is often measured from the incisors (front teeth).

Cervical esophagus:

The cervical esophagus begins at the lower border of the cricoid cartilage and ends at the thoracic inlet (the suprasternal notch), approximately 18 cm from the upper incisor teeth.

Intrathoracic esophagus:

Upper thoracic portion: The upper thoracic portion extends from the thoracic inlet to the level of the tracheal bifurcation, approximately 24 cm from the upper incisor teeth.

Midthoracic portion: This is the portion of the esophagus between the tracheal bifurcation and the distal esophagus just above the esophago-gastric junction. The lower level of this portion is approximately 32 cm from the upper incisor teeth.

Lower thoracic portion: Approximately 8 cm in length, the lower thoracic esophagus includes the intra-abdominal portion of the esophagus and the esophago-gastric junction. The latter is approximately 40 cm from the upper incisor teeth.

Regional Lymph Nodes. For pN, a mediastinal lymphadenectomy specimen will ordinarily include 6 or more lymph nodes. Specific regional lymph nodes are listed as follows:

Cervical esophagus:
- Scalene
- Internal jugular
- Upper cervical
- Peri-esophageal
- Supraclavicular
- Cervical, NOS

Intrathoracic esophagus—upper, middle, and lower:
- Tracheobronchial
- Superior mediastinal
- Peritracheal
- Carinal
- Hilar (pulmonary roots)
- Peri-esophageal
- Perigastric
- Paracardial
- Mediastinal, NOS

Involvement of more distant nodes (e.g., cervical or celiac axis nodes) is considered distant metastasis for intrathoracic lesions.

The listing of specific lymph nodes for each region includes those lying within the defined boundaries for that region. For example, the supraclavicular and peri-esophageal nodes superior to the thoracic inlet would be considered regional for tumors located in the cervical esophagus, but distant metastasis for tumors originating in the thoracic esophagus.

Metastatic Sites. The liver, lungs, pleura, and kidneys are the most common sites of distant metastases. Occasionally, the tumor may extend directly into mediastinal structures before distant metastasis is evident.

RULES FOR CLASSIFICATION

Clinical Staging. Clinical staging depends on the anatomic extent of the primary tumor that can be ascertained by examination before treatment. Such an examination may include medical history, physical examination, biopsy, routine laboratory studies, endoscopic examination, and imaging. Endoscopic ultrasound and computed tomography (CT) are useful for identifying tumor location, depth of invasion, and lymph node metastasis. The anatomic location of the primary tumor (cervical, upper thoracic, midthoracic or lower thoracic) should be recorded since prognosis will vary, depending on the site of origin.

Pathologic Staging. Pathologic staging is based on surgical exploration and on the examination of the surgically resected esophagus and associated lymph nodes. Involvement of the adjacent structures depends on the location of the primary tumor. This extension and the presence of distant metastases should be specifically documented. A single classification serves all regions of the esophagus. It serves both clinical and pathologic staging.

DEFINITION OF TNM

Primary Tumor (T)

- TX Primary tumor cannot be assessed
- T0 No evidence of primary tumor
- Tis Carcinoma *in situ*
- T1 Tumor invades lamina propria or submucosa
- T2 Tumor invades muscularis propria
- T3 Tumor invades adventitia
- T4 Tumor invades adjacent structures

Regional Lymph Nodes (N)

- NX Regional lymph nodes cannot be assessed
- N0 No regional lymph node metastasis
- N1 Regional lymph node metastasis

Distant Metastasis (M)

- MX Distant metastasis cannot be assessed
- M0 No distant metastasis
- M1 Distant metastasis
  - Tumors of the lower thoracic esophagus:
    - M1a Metastasis in celiac lymph nodes
    - M1b Other distant metastasis
  - Tumors of the midthoracic esophagus:
    - M1a Not applicable
    - M1b Nonregional lymph nodes and/or other distant metastasis
  - Tumors of the upper thoracic esophagus:
    - M1a Metastasis in cervical nodes
    - M1b Other distant metastasis

For tumors of midthoracic esophagus use only M1b, since these tumors with metastasis in nonregional lymph nodes have an equally poor prognosis as those with metastasis in other distant sites.

STAGE GROUPING

Stage 0	Tis	N0	M0
Stage I	T1	N0	M0
Stage IIA	T2	N0	M0
	T3	N0	M0
Stage IIB	T1	N1	M0
	T2	N1	M0
Stage III	T3	N1	M0
	T4	Any N	M0
Stage IV	Any T	Any N	M1
Stage IVA	Any T	Any N	M1a
Stage IVB	Any T	Any N	M1b

HISTOPATHOLOGIC TYPE

The classification applies to all carcinomas. Sarcomas are not included. Squamous cell carcinomas are the most common but the prevalence of adenocarcinoma is increasing. Adenocarcinomas arising from Barrett's esophagus are included in the classification.

HISTOLOGIC GRADE (G)

GX Grade cannot be assessed
G1 Well differentiated
G2 Moderately differentiated
G3 Poorly differentiated
G4 Undifferentiated

PROGNOSTIC FACTORS

Anatomic location is an important prognostic variable with upper- and midthoracic lesions having a less favorable outcome than other sites. Depth of invasion (T) is an independent variable while tumor length is not. This has encouraged pretreatment endoscopic ultrasound for staging, particularly in patients who may be candidates for nonoperative therapy. Lymphatic spread is a strong independent prognostic variable as are distant metastases. In the latter category, distant organ metastasis leads to a worse prognosis than distant nonregional lymph node metastasis. The histologic type (squamous cell carcinoma versus adenocarcinoma) is not a prognostic factor except for T1 lesions where adenocarcinoma appears to be more favorable than squamous carcinoma. Tumor differentiation, DNA ploidy status, various oncogenes, growth factors, and other markers are being intensively studied as prognostic indicators, but data are still insufficient for a conclusive statement regarding these potential prognostic factors.

BIBLIOGRAPHY

Akiyama H, Tsurumaru M, Udagawa H, Kajiyama Y: Radical lymph nodes dissection for cancer of the thoracic esophagus. Ann Surg 220:364–373, 1994

Baba M, Aikou T, Yoshnika H, et al: Long-term results of esophagectomy with three field lymphadenectomy for carcinoma of the thoracic esophagus. Ann Surg 219:310–316, 1994

Bergman F: Cancer of the esophagus: a histological study of development and local spread of 10 cases of squamous cell carcinoma in the lower third of oesophagus. Acta Chir Scand 117:356–365, 1959

Bottger T, Storkel S, Stockle M, et al: DNA image cytometry. A prognostic tool in squamous cell carcinoma of the esophagus? Cancer 67:2290–2294, 1991

Cancer Facts and Figures—1996. Georgia: American Cancer Society, Inc., 1996

Ellis FH Jr, Watkins E Jr, Krasna MJ, et al: Staging of the esophagus and cardia: a comparison of different staging criteria. J Surg Oncol 52:231–235, 1993

Fu-Sheng L, Ling L, Song-Liang Q: Clinical and pathological characteristics of early oesophageal cancer. Clin Oncol 1(2):539-557, 1982

Gion M, Tremolada C, Mione R, et al: Tumor markers in serum of patients with primary squamous cell carcinoma of the esophagus. Tumori 75:489–493, 1989

Harvey JC, Kagan AP, Ahn C, et al: Adenocarcinoma of the esophagus: a survival study. J Surg Oncol 45:29–32, 1990

Hermanek P, Sobin LH: UICC TNM Classification of malignant tumors. 4th ed. Berlin-Heidelberg-New York: Springer-Verlag, 1987

Holscher AH, Bollschweiler E, Schneider PM, Siewert JR: Prognosis of early esophageal cancer (comparison between adeno-and squamous cell carcinoma) Cancer 76:178–186, 1995

Iizuka T, Isono K, Kakegawa T, et al: Parameters linked to ten-year survival in Japan of resected esophageal carcinoma. Chest 96:1005–1011, 1989

Lund O, Hasenkam JM, Aagaard MT, Kimose HH: Time-related changes in characteristics of prognostic significance in carcinomas of the esophagus and cardia. Br J Surg 76:1301–1307, 1989

Petrovich Z, Lam K, Langholz B, et al: Surgical therapy and radiotherapy for carcinoma of the esophagus. Treatment results in 195 patients. J Thorac Cardiovasc Surg 98:614–617, 1989

Rice TW, Boyce GA, Sivak MV: Esophageal ultrasound and the preoperative staging of carcinoma of the esophagus. J Thorac Cardiovasc Surg 101:536–543, 1991

Siewert JR, Holscher AH, Dittler HJ: Preoperative staging and risk analysis in esophageal carcinoma. Hepatogastroenterology 37:382–387, 1990

Skinner DB, Ferguson MK, Little AG: Selection of operation for esophageal cancer based on staging. Ann Surg 204:391–400, 1986

Stephens JK, Bibbo M, Dytch H, et al: Correlation between automated karyometric measurements of squamous cell carcinoma of the esophagus and histopathologic and clinical features. Cancer 64:83–87, 1989

Tio TL, Coene PP, Hartog Jager FC, et al: Preoperative TNM classification of esophageal carcinoma by endosonography. Hepatogastroenterology 37:376–381, 1990

Vilgrain V, Mompoint D, Palazzo L, et al: Staging of esophageal carcinoma: comparison of results with endoscopic sonography and CT. Am J Roentgenol 155:277–281, 1990

Watanabe H, Jass JR, Sobin LH: Histological typing of esophageal and gastric tumors. WHO international histological classification of tumors, 2nd ed. Berlin-New York: Springer-Verlag, 1990

Data Form for Cancer Staging

Patient identification
Name ______
Address ______
Hospital or clinic number ______
Age ____ Sex ____ Race ______

Institution identification
Hospital or clinic ______
Address ______

Oncology Record

Anatomic site of cancer ______
Histologic type ______
Grade (G) ______
Date of classification ______

Clin	Path	DEFINITIONS	
		Primary Tumor (T)	
[ ]	[ ]	TX	Primary tumor cannot be assessed
[ ]	[ ]	T0	No evidence of primary tumor
[ ]	[ ]	Tis	Carcinoma *in situ*
[ ]	[ ]	T1	Tumor invades lamina propria or submucosa
[ ]	[ ]	T2	Tumor invades muscularis propria
[ ]	[ ]	T3	Tumor invades adventitia
[ ]	[ ]	T4	Tumor invades adjacent structures
		Regional Lymph Nodes (N)	
[ ]	[ ]	NX	Regional lymph nodes cannot be assessed
[ ]	[ ]	N0	No regional lymph node metastasis
[ ]	[ ]	N1	Regional lymph node metastasis
		Distant Metastasis (M)	
[ ]	[ ]	MX	Distant metastasis cannot be assessed
[ ]	[ ]	M0	No distant metastasis
[ ]	[ ]	M1	Distant metastasis
		Tumors of the lower thoracic esophagus:	
[ ]	[ ]	M1a	Metastasis in celiac lymph nodes
[ ]	[ ]	M1b	Other distant metastasis
		Tumors of the midthoracic esophagus:	
[ ]	[ ]	M1a	Not applicable
[ ]	[ ]	M1b	Nonregional lymph nodes and/or other distant metastasis
		Tumors of the upper thoracic esophagus:	
[ ]	[ ]	M1a	Metastasis in cervical nodes
[ ]	[ ]	M1b	Other distant metastasis

For tumors of midthoracic esophagus use only M1b, since these tumors with metastasis in nonregional lymph nodes and those with metastasis in other distant sites have an equally poor prognosis.

Stage Grouping

Clin	Path	Stage	T	N	M
[ ]	[ ]	0	Tis	N0	M0
[ ]	[ ]	I	T1	N0	M0
[ ]	[ ]	IIA	T2	N0	M0
			T3	N0	M0
[ ]	[ ]	IIB	T1	N1	M0
			T2	N1	M0
[ ]	[ ]	III	T3	N1	M0
			T4	Any N	M0
[ ]	[ ]	IV	Any T	Any N	M1
[ ]	[ ]	IVA	Any T	Any N	M1a
[ ]	[ ]	IVB	Any T	Any N	M1b

Staged by ______ M.D.
______ Registrar
Date ______

Histopathologic Grade (G)

[ ] GX Grade cannot be assessed
[ ] G1 Well differentiated
[ ] G2 Moderately differentiated
[ ] G3 Poorly differentiated
[ ] G4 Undifferentiated

Histopathologic Type

The classification applies to all carcinomas. Sarcomas are not included. Squamous cell carcinomas are the most common, but the prevalence of adenocarcinoma is increasing. Adenocarcinomas arising from Barrett's esophagus are included in the classification.

10

Stomach

(Lymphomas, sarcomas, and carcinoid tumors are not included.)

C16.0 Cardia, NOS
C16.1 Fundus
C16.2 Body
C16.3 Antrum
C16.4 Pylorus
C16.5 Lesser curvature
C16.6 Greater curvature
C16.8 Overlapping lesion
C16.9 Stomach, NOS

Gastric cancer is currently estimated to be the thirteenth most common cancer and the eighth most deadly in the United States. There has been a steady decline in the incidence since 1930, when it was the number one cancer killer comprising 38% of all cancer deaths. It is of interest that this reduction in incidence has not occurred in all countries, and, despite some reasonable dietary hypotheses (such as change in methods of food preservation, increasing intake of Vitamin C, and "inadvertent" antibiotic control of *Helicobacter pylori* infection) this decline has not been the result of any planned health promotion or prevention intervention. Although the etiology of gastric cancer is uncertain, chronic atrophic gastritis is considered a predisposing factor, and there is circumstantial evidence for the role of nitrosamine production from dietary nitrate ingestion. Adenomatous polyps in the stomach have an association with gastric cancer but these are too infrequent to be a common precancerous lesion. Chronic peptic ulcer is clearly not a precancerous state despite the gross presentation of some gastric cancers as "ulcero-cancers."

A trend in gastric cancer presentation over the last few decades has been a shift in the anatomic location of the primary lesion. There has been a change from predominately distal gastric cancers to a greater frequency of lesions arising in the proximal stomach. Another trend in the last few decades has been an increase in incidence of primary gastric lymphoma (non-Hodgkin's lymphoma). However, 90% of gastric cancers are still adenocarcinomas.

ANATOMY

Primary Site. The stomach is the first division of the abdominal alimentary tract. Its first part is the esophagogastric junction which is located immediately below the diaphragm and is often called the cardia. The upper or proximal part of the stomach is the fundus, and the distal part is the antrum. The pylorus is continuous with the duodenum. The shorter right border forms the lesser curvature and the longer border on the left is the greater curvature. Histologically, the wall of the stomach has five layers: mucosal, submucosal, muscular, subserosa, and serosal.

Regional Lymph Nodes. The regional lymph nodes are the perigastric nodes found along the lesser and greater curvatures and the nodes located along the left gastric, common hepatic, splenic, and celiac arteries. For pN, a regional lymphadenectomy specimen will ordinarily contain at least 15 lymph nodes.

Involvement of other intra-abdominal lymph nodes, such as the hepatoduodenal, retropancreatic, mesenteric, and para-aortic, is classified as distant metastasis. The following is a specific list of regional and distant lymph nodes.

Greater Curvature of Stomach:

Greater curvature
Greater omental
Gastroduodenal
Gastroepiploic, right, or NOS
Gastroepiploic, left
Pyloric, including subpyloric and infra pyloric
Pancreaticoduodenal (anteriorly along first part of the duodenum)

Pancreatic and Splenic Area:

Pancreaticolienal
Peripancreatic
Splenic hilum

Lesser Curvature of Stomach:

Lesser curvature
Lesser omental
Left gastric
Paracardial; cardial
Cardioesophageal
Perigastric, NOS
Common hepatic
Celiac
Hepatoduodenal

All other lymph nodes are considered distant. They include:

Retropancreatic
Para-aortic
Portal
Retroperitoneal
Mesenteric

Metastatic Sites. Distant spread to the liver, the peritoneal surfaces and nonregional lymph nodes is common, while the central nervous system and lungs are infrequent sites for metastasis. Frequently, there is direct extension to the liver, the transverse colon, the pancreas, or the undersurface of the diaphragm.

RULES FOR CLASSIFICATION

Clinical Staging. Designated as cTNM, clinical staging is based on evidence of extent of disease acquired before definitive treatment is instituted. It includes physical examination, radiologic imaging, endoscopy, biopsy, and laboratory findings. All cancers should be confirmed histologically.

Pathologic Staging. Pathologic staging depends on data acquired clinically, along with findings of subsequent surgical exploration and examination of the pathologic specimen if resection is accomplished. Pathologic assessment of the regional lymph nodes entails their removal and histologic examination to evaluate the number that contain metastatic tumor. Metastatic nodules in the fat adjacent to a gastric carcinoma, without evidence of residual lymph node tissue, are considered regional lymph node metastases, but nodules implanted on peritoneal surfaces are considered distant metastasis. If there is uncertainty concerning the appropriate T, N, or M assignment, the lower (less advanced) category should be selected. This will also be reflected in the stage grouping.

DEFINITION OF TNM

Primary Tumor (T)

TX Primary tumor cannot be assessed
T0 No evidence of primary tumor
Tis Carcinoma *in situ:* intra-epithelial tumor without invasion of the lamina propria
T1 Tumor invades lamina propria or submucosa
T2 Tumor invades muscularis propria or subserosa*
T3 Tumor penetrates serosa (visceral peritoneum) without invasion of adjacent structures**,***
T4 Tumor invades adjacent structures**,***

**Note:* A tumor may penetrate the muscularis propria with extension into the gastrocolic or gastrohepatic ligaments, or into the greater or lesser omentum without perforation of the visceral peritoneum covering these structures. In this case, the tumor is classified T2. If there is perforation of the visceral peritoneum covering the gastric ligaments or the omentum, the tumor should be classified T3.

***Note:* The adjacent structures of the stomach include the spleen, transverse colon, liver, diaphragm, pancreas, abdominal wall, adrenal gland, kidney, small intestine, and retroperitoneum.

****Note:* Intramural extension to the duodenum or esophagus is classified by the depth of greatest invasion in any of these sites, including stomach.

Regional Lymph Nodes (N)

NX Regional lymph node(s) cannot be assessed
N0 No regional lymph node metastasis
N1 Metastasis in 1 to 6 regional lymph nodes
N2 Metastasis in 7 to 15 regional lymph nodes
N3 Metastasis in more than 15 regional lymph nodes

Distant Metastasis (M)

MX Distant metastasis cannot be assessed
M0 No distant metastasis
M1 Distant metastasis

STAGE GROUPING

Stage 0	Tis	N0	M0
Stage IA	T1	N0	M0
Stage IB	T1	N1	M0
	T2	N0	M0
Stage II	T1	N2	M0
	T2	N1	M0
	T3	N0	M0
Stage IIIA	T2	N2	M0
	T3	N1	M0
	T4	N0	M0
Stage IIIB	T3	N2	M0
Stage IV	T4	N1	M0
	T1	N3	M0
	T2	N3	M0
	T3	N3	M0
	T4	N2	M0
	T4	N3	M0
	Any T	Any N	M1

HISTOPATHOLOGIC TYPE

The staging recommendations apply only to carcinomas. Lymphomas, sarcomas, and carcinoid tumors are not included. Adenocarcinomas may be divided into the general subtypes (listed below), intestinal, diffuse, or mixed.

The histologic subtypes are:

Adenocarcinoma
Papillary adenocarcinoma
Tubular adenocarcinoma
Mucinous adenocarcinoma
Signet ring cell carcinoma
Adenosquamous carcinoma
Squamous cell carcinoma
Small cell carcinoma
Undifferentiated carcinoma

HISTOLOGIC GRADE (G)

GX Grade cannot be assessed
G1 Well differentiated
G2 Moderately differentiated
G3 Poorly differentiated
G4 Undifferentiated

PROGNOSTIC FACTORS

Treatment is a major prognostic factor for gastric cancer. All patients who cannot be or who are not resected have a poor prognosis with survival ranging from 3 to 11 months. For those patients undergoing complete resection, factors affecting prognosis include the location of the tumor in the stomach and the gross pathologic type, as well as the T and N classification. The prognosis for proximal gastric cancer is less favorable than for distal lesions and the classic gross pathologic type, as described by Borrmann (I-polypoid, II-ulcerocancer, III-ulcerating and infiltrating, and IV-infiltrating), has prognostic impact. Polypoid and ulcerocancers (I and II) that are resected have a considerably better prognosis than Borrmann III and IV, independent of the presence or absence of regional lymph node involvement.

Depth of invasion into the gastric wall (T) correlates with reduced survival while regional lymphatic spread is probably the most powerful prognostic factor. The histologic classification of Lauren has some impact on prognosis but diffuse lesions are more often proximally located and larger than the intestinal type lesions that generally tend to be distal. Histologic grade is an important prognostic factor. High preoperative serum levels for tumor markers CEA and CA 19-9 have been associated with a less favorable outcome.

BIBLIOGRAPHY

Cancer Facts and Figures—1996. Georgia: American Cancer Society, Inc., 1996

Coller FA, Kay EB, MacIntyre RS: Regional lymphatic metastases of carcinoma of the stomach. Arch Surg 43:748–761, 1941

Cook AO, Levine BA, Sirinek KR, et al: Evaluation of gastric adenocarcinoma: abdominal computed tomography does not replace celiotomy. Arch Surg 121:603–606, 1986

Dulchavshy S, Dahn MS, Wilson RF: The preoperative staging of malignant tumors of the stomach by computed tomagraphy and liver function tests. Current Surgery 46:26–28, 1989

Dupont JB Jr, Lee JR, Burton GR, et al: Adenocarcinoma of the stomach: review of 1,497 cases. Cancer 41:941–947, 1978

Kennedy BJ: TNM classification of stomach cancer. Cancer 26:971–983, 1970

Kennedy BJ: The unified international gastric cancer staging classification system. Scand J Gastroenterol 22(Suppl 133):11–13, 1987

Lauren P: The two histological main types of gastric carcinoma. Acta Pathol Microbiol Scand 64:31–49, 1965

Lawrence W, Menck HR, Steele GD, Winchester DP: The National Cancer Data Base report on gastric cancer. Cancer 75:1734–1744, 1995

Lewin K, Appelman HD: Tumors of the esophagus and stomach. Atlas of tumor pathology, Third Series, Fascicle 18. Washington, D.C.: Armed Forces Institute of Pathology, 1996

McNeer GP, Lawrence W Jr, Ashley MP, Pack GT: End results in the treatment of gastric cancer. Surgery 43:879–896, 1958

Miller BA, Ries LAG, Hankey BF, et al: Cancer statistics review: 1973–1990. Bethesda, Maryland: National Cancer Institute. NIH Publication No. 93-2789, 1993

Noguchi M, Miyazaki I: Prognostic significance in surgical management of lymph node metastasis in gastric cancer. Br J Surg 83:156–161, 1996

Rhode H, Gebbensleben P, Bauer P, et al: Has there been any improvement in the staging of gastric cancer? Findings from the German Gastric Cancer TNM Study Group. Cancer 64:2465–2481, 1989

Saario I, Schroder T, Talppanen EM, et al: Factors influencing 5-year survival in gastric malignancies after total gastrectomy. Annales Chirurgiae et Gynaccologiae (Helsinki) 75:23–27, 1986

Salvon-Harman JC, Cady B, Nikulasson S, et al: Shifting proportions of gastric adenocarcinomas. Arch Surg 129:381–389, 1994

Serlin O, Keehn RJ, Higgins GA, et al: Factors related to survival following resection for gastric carcinoma: analysis of 903 cases. Cancer 40:1318–1329, 1977

Severson RK, Davis S: Increasing incidence of primary gastric lymphoma. Cancer 66:1283–1287, 1990

Shiu MH, Perrotti M, Brennan MF: Adenocarcinoma of the stomach: a multivariate analysis of clinical, pathologic, and treatment factors. Hepatogastroenterology 36:7–12, 1989

Wanebo HJ, Kennedy BJ, Chmiel J, et al: Cancer of the stomach: a patient care study of the American College of Surgeons. Ann Surg 218:583–593, 1993

Watanabe H, Jass JR, Sobin LH: Histological typing of esophageal and gastric tumors. WHO international histological classification of tumours, 2nd ed. Berlin: Springer-Verlag, 1990

STOMACH

Data Form for Cancer Staging

Patient identification
Name ____________
Address ____________
Hospital or clinic number ____________
Age ____ Sex ____ Race ____________

Institution identification
Hospital or clinic ____________
Address ____________

Oncology Record

Anatomic site of cancer ____________
Histologic type ____________
Grade (G) ____________
Date of classification ____________

Clin	Path	DEFINITIONS	
		Primary Tumor (T)	
[ ]	[ ]	TX	Primary tumor cannot be assessed
[ ]	[ ]	T0	No evidence of primary tumor
[ ]	[ ]	Tis	Carcinoma *in situ*: intraepithelial tumor without invasion of lamina propria
[ ]	[ ]	T1	Tumor invades lamina propria or submucosa
[ ]	[ ]	T2	Tumor invades muscularis propria or subserosa*
[ ]	[ ]	T3	Tumor penetrates serosa (visceral peritoneum) without invasion of adjacent structures**,***
[ ]	[ ]	T4	Tumor invades adjacent structures**,***

* A tumor may penetrate the muscularis propria with extension into the gastrocolic or gastrohepatic ligaments or into the greater or lesser omentum without perforation of the visceral peritoneum covering these structures. In this case, the tumor is classified T2. If there is perforation of the visceral peritoneum covering the gastric ligaments or the omentum, the tumor should be classified T3.

** The adjacent structures of the stomach include the spleen, transverse colon, liver, diaphragm, pancreas, abdominal wall, adrenal gland, kidney, small intestine, and retroperitoneum.

*** Intramural extension to the duodenum or esophagus is classified by the depth of greatest invasion in any of these sites, including stomach.

Clin	Path	**Regional Lymph Nodes (N)**	
[ ]	[ ]	NX	Regional lymph node(s) cannot be assessed
[ ]	[ ]	N0	No regional lymph node metastasis
[ ]	[ ]	N1	Metastasis in 1 to 6 regional lymph nodes
[ ]	[ ]	N2	Metastasis in 7 to 15 regional lymph nodes
[ ]	[ ]	N3	Metastasis in more than 15 regional lymph nodes

Clin	Path	**Distant Metastasis (M)**	
[ ]	[ ]	MX	Distant metastasis cannot be assessed
[ ]	[ ]	M0	No distant metastasis
[ ]	[ ]	M1	Distant metastasis

Stage Grouping

Clin	Path	Stage	T	N	M
[ ]	[ ]	0	Tis	N0	M0
[ ]	[ ]	IA	T1	N0	M0
[ ]	[ ]	IB	T1	N1	M0
			T2	N0	M0
[ ]	[ ]	II	T1	N2	M0
			T2	N1	M0
			T3	N0	M0
[ ]	[ ]	IIIA	T2	N2	M0
			T3	N1	M0
			T4	N0	M0
[ ]	[ ]	IIIB	T3	N2	M0
[ ]	[ ]	IV	T4	N1	M0
			T1	N3	M0
			T2	N3	M0
			T3	N3	M0
			T4	N2	M0
			T4	N3	M0
			Any T	Any N	M1

Staged by ____________ **M.D.**
____________ **Registrar**
Date ____________

(continued on next page)

Histopathologic Grade (G)

[ ] GX Grade cannot be assessed
[ ] G1 Well differentiated
[ ] G2 Moderately differentiated
[ ] G3 Poorly differentiated
[ ] G4 Undifferentiated

Histopathologic Type

The staging recommendations apply only to carcinomas. Lymphomas, sarcomas, and carcinoid tumors are not included. Adenocarcinomas may be divided into the general subtypes (listed below), intestinal, diffuse, or mixed. The histologic subtypes are:

Adenocarcinoma
Papillary adenocarcinoma
Tubular adenocarcinoma
Mucinous adenocarcinoma
Signet ring cell carcinoma
Adenosquamous carcinoma
Squamous cell carcinoma
Small cell carcinoma
Undifferentiated carcinoma

Illustration

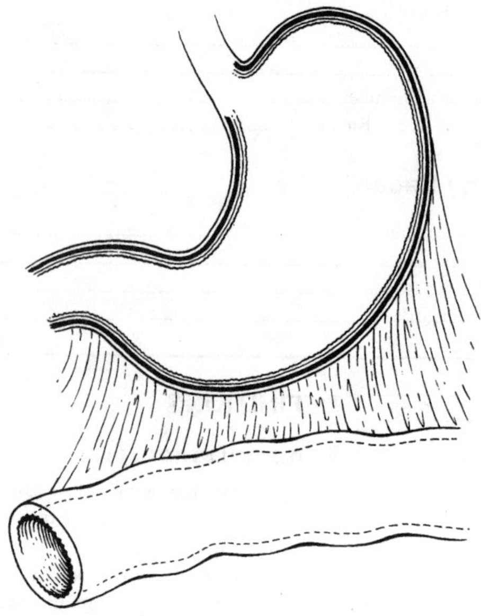

Indicate on diagram primary tumor and regional nodes involved.

11

Small Intestine

(Lymphomas, carcinoid tumors, and visceral sarcomas are not included.)

C17.0 Duodenum
C17.1 Jejunum
C17.2 Ileum
C17.8 Overlapping lesion
C17.9 Small intestine, NOS

Cancers of the small intestine account for less than 2% of all malignant tumors of the gastrointestinal tract. Most occur in the first or second part of the duodenum. Adenocarcinomas are the most frequent histologic type but they comprise less than 50% of all primary malignant tumors of the small intestine. Considered together, sarcomas, lymphomas, and malignant carcinoid tumors are more common than adenocarcinomas. Because primary cancers of the small bowel are rare, a staging system was not published by the International Union Against Cancer or by the American Joint Committee on Cancer until recently. Also, since they are uncommon, information on their method of spread and biologic behavior is incomplete. However, there is no reason to believe that any of these small bowel tumors behave much differently than similar lesions arising in other parts of the gastrointestinal tract. The classification and stage grouping described here is used for both clinical and pathologic staging of carcinomas of the small bowel and does not apply to the other types of malignant small bowel tumors.

ANATOMY

Primary Site. This classification applies to carcinomas arising in the duodenum, jejunum, and ileum. It does not apply to carcinomas arising in the ileocecal valve or to carcinomas that may arise in Meckel's diverticulum. Carcinomas arising in the ampulla of Vater are staged according to the system described in Chapter 17. Carcinomas arising in the vermiform appendix are staged according to the classification listed for the colon (see Chapter 12).

Duodenum. About 25 cm in length, the duodenum extends from the pyloric sphincter of the stomach to the jejunum. It is usually divided anatomically into four parts with the common bile duct and pancreatic duct opening into the second part at the ampulla of Vater.

Jejunum and Ileum. The jejunum and ileum extend from the junction with the duodenum proximally to the ileo cecal valve distally. The division point between the jejunum and ileum is arbitrary. As a general rule, the jejunum includes about 40% proximally and the ileum 60% distally of the small intestine, exclusive of the duodenum.

General. The jejunal and ileal portions of the small intestine are supported by a fold of the peritoneum containing the blood supply and the regional lymph nodes, the mesentery. The shortest segment, the duodenum, has no real mesentery and is only covered by peritoneum anteriorly. The wall of all parts of the small intestine has five layers: mucosal, submucosal, muscular, subserosal, and serosal. A very thin layer of smooth muscle cells, the muscularis mucosae, separates the mucosa from the submucosa. The small intestine is entirely ensheathed by peritoneum except for a narrow strip of bowel that is attached to the mesentery and that part of the duodenum that is located retroperitoneally.

Regional Lymph Nodes. For pN, histologic examination of a regional lymphadenectomy specimen will ordinarily include 6 or more regional lymph nodes.

Duodenum:
- Duodenal
- Hepatic
- Pancreaticoduodenal
- Infrapyloric
- Gastroduodenal
- Pyloric
- Superior mesenteric
- Pericholedochal
- Regional lymph nodes, NOS

Ileum and Jejunum:
- Posterior cecal (terminal ileum only)
- Ileocolic (terminal ileum only)
- Superior mesenteric
- Mesenteric, NOS
- Regional lymph nodes, NOS

Metastatic Sites. Cancers of the small intestine can metastasize to most organs, especially the liver, or to the peritoneal surfaces. Involvement of regional lymph nodes and invasion of adjacent structures is most common.

RULES FOR CLASSIFICATION

The primary tumor is staged according to its depth of penetration and the involvement of adjacent structures or distant sites. Lateral spread within the duodenum, or within the jejunum or ileum, is not considered in this classification, only the depth of tumor penetration in the bowel wall.

Although similar, differences between this staging system and that of the colon should be noted. In the colon, pTis applies to intraepithelial (*in situ*) as well as to intramucosal lesions. In the small intestine, intramucosal spread is listed as pT1 instead of pTis. In this regard, the pT1 definition for the small bowel is essentially the same as the pT1 defined for stomach lesions. Invasion through the wall is staged the same as colon cancer. Discontinuous hematogenous metastases or peritoneal metastases are coded as M1. In addition there is no subdivision within the N category based on the number of nodes involved with tumor.

DEFINITION OF TNM

Primary Tumor (T)

TX Primary tumor cannot be assessed
T0 No evidence of primary tumor
Tis Carcinoma *in situ*
T1 Tumor invades lamina propria or submucosa
T2 Tumor invades muscularis propria
T3 Tumor invades through the muscularis propria into the subserosa or into the nonperitonealized perimuscular tissue (mesentery or retroperitoneum) with extension 2 cm or less.*
T4 Tumor perforates the visceral peritoneum, or directly invades other organs or structures (includes other loops of small intestine, mesentery, or retroperitoneum more than 2 cm, and abdominal wall by way of serosa; for duodenum only, invasion of pancreas).

**Note:* The nonperitonealized perimuscular tissue is, for jejunum and ileum, part of the mesentery and, for duodenum in areas where serosa is lacking, part of the retroperitoneum.

Regional Lymph Nodes (N)

NX Regional lymph nodes cannot be assessed
N0 No regional lymph node metastasis
N1 Regional lymph node metastasis

Distant Metastasis (M)

MX Distant metastasis cannot be assessed
M0 No distant metastasis
M1 Distant metastasis

STAGE GROUPING

Stage 0	Tis	N0	M0
Stage I	T1	N0	M0
	T2	N0	M0
Stage II	T3	N0	M0
	T4	N0	M0
Stage III	Any T	N1	M0
Stage IV	Any T	Any N	M1

HISTOPATHOLOGIC TYPE

This staging classification applies only to carcinomas arising in the small intestine. Lymphomas, carcinoid tumors, and visceral sarcomas are not included. The three major histopathologic types are carcinomas (e.g., adenocarcinoma), carcinoid tumors, and lymphomas (extranodal). Primary lymphomas are staged as extranodal lymphomas. Carcinoid tumors of the small intestine have no staging system but size, depth of invasion, regional lymph node status, and distant metastasis are considered significant prognostic factors. Less common malignant tumors include leiomyosarcoma although leiomyomas are plentiful.

HISTOLOGIC GRADE (G)

GX Grade cannot be assessed
G1 Well differentiated
G2 Moderately differentiated
G3 Poorly differentiated
G4 Undifferentiated

PROGNOSTIC FACTORS

Small bowel carcinoma is rare, so various clinical prognostic factors, such as age, gender, and ethnic origin are impossible to assess. The anatomic extent of the tumor is the strongest indicator of outcome when the tumor can be resected. Prognosis after incomplete removal is poor.

The pathologic extent of tumor, in terms of the depth of invasion through the bowel wall, is a significant prognostic factor as is regional lymphatic spread. Prognosis is also influenced by histologic grade. There are insufficient data to assess the impact of other more sophisticated pathologic factors and serum tumor markers, but it is logical to believe the effect of those factors would be similar to that observed with colorectal cancer.

BIBLIOGRAPHY

Brookes VS, Waterhouse JAH, Powell DJ: Malignant lesions of the small intestine: a ten-year survey. Brit J Surg 55:405–410, 1968

Cohen A, McNeill D, Terz JJ, et al: Neoplasms of the small intestine. Am J Dig Dis 16:815–824, 1971

Dudiak KM, Johnson CD, Stephens DH: Primary tumors of the small intestine: CT evaluation. Am J Roentgenol 152:995–998, 1989

Hancock RJ: An 11-year review of primary tumours of the small bowel including the duodenum. Can Med Assoc J 103:1177–1179, 1970

Jass JR, Sobin LH: Histological typing of intestinal tumours. WHO international histological classification of tumours, 2nd ed. Berlin-New York: Springer-Verlag, 1989

Lien GS, Mori M, Enjoji M: Primary carcinoma of the small intestine. A clinicopathologic and immunohistochemical study. Cancer 61:316–322, 1988

Maglinte DD, O'Connor K, Bessette J, et al: The role of the physician in the late diagnosis of primary malignant tumors of the small intestine. Am J Gastroenterol 86:304–308, 1991

Mittal VK, Bodzin JH: Primary malignant tumors of the small bowel. Am J Surg 140:396–399, 1980

Sindelar WF: Cancer of the small intestine. In DeVita VT, Hellman S, Rosenberg, SA (Eds.), Cancer: principles and practice of oncology, 2nd ed. Philadelphia: Lippincott, 1985

Data Form for Cancer Staging

Patient identification
Name ______
Address ______
Hospital or clinic number ______
Age ____ Sex ____ Race ______

Institution identification
Hospital or clinic ______
Address ______

Oncology Record

Anatomic site of cancer ______
Histologic type ______
Grade (G) ______
Date of classification ______

DEFINITIONS

Primary Tumor (T)

Clin	Path		
[ ]	[ ]	TX	Primary tumor cannot be assessed
[ ]	[ ]	T0	No evidence of primary tumor
[ ]	[ ]	Tis	Carcinoma *in situ*
[ ]	[ ]	T1	Tumor invades lamina propria or submucosa
[ ]	[ ]	T2	Tumor invades muscularis propria
[ ]	[ ]	T3	Tumor invades through the muscularis propria into the subserosa or into the nonperitonealized perimuscular tissue (mesentery or retroperitoneum) with extension 2 cm or less*
[ ]	[ ]	T4	Tumor perforates the visceral peritoneum, or directly invades other organs and structures, (includes other loops of small intestine, mesentery, or retroperitoneum more than 2 cm, and the abdominal wall by way of the serosa; for the duodenum only includes invasion of the pancreas)

* *Note:* The nonperitonealized perimuscular tissue is, for jejunum and ileum, part of the mesentery and, for duodenum in areas where serosa is lacking, part of the retroperitoneum.

Regional Lymph Nodes (N)

Clin	Path		
[ ]	[ ]	NX	Regional lymph nodes cannot be assessed
[ ]	[ ]	N0	No regional lymph node metastasis
[ ]	[ ]	N1	Regional lymph node metastasis

Distant Metastasis (M)

Clin	Path		
[ ]	[ ]	MX	Distant metastasis cannot be assessed
[ ]	[ ]	M0	No distant metastasis
[ ]	[ ]	M1	Distant metastasis

Stage Grouping

Clin	Path				
[ ]	[ ]	0	Tis	N0	M0
[ ]	[ ]	I	T1	N0	M0
			T2	N0	M0
[ ]	[ ]	II	T3	N0	M0
			T4	N0	M0
[ ]	[ ]	III	Any T	N1	M0
[ ]	[ ]	IV	Any T	Any N	M1

Staged by ______ M.D.
______ Registrar

Date ______

Histopathologic Type

This staging classification applies only to *carcinomas* arising in the small intestine. Lymphomas, carcinoid tumors, and visceral sarcomas are not included. The three major histopathologic types are carcinomas (e.g., adenocarcinoma), carcinoid tumors, and lymphomas (extranodal). Primary lymphomas are staged as extranodal lymphomas. Carcinoid tumors of the small intestine have no staging system, but size, depth of invasion, regional lymph node status, and distant metastasis are considered significant prognostic factors. Less common malignant tumors include leiomyosarcomas although leiomyomas are plentiful.

Histopathologic Grade (G)

[ ]	GX	Grade cannot be assessed
[ ]	G1	Well differentiated
[ ]	G2	Moderately differentiated
[ ]	G3	Poorly differentiated
[ ]	G4	Undifferentiated

12

Colon and Rectum

(Sarcomas, lymphomas, and carcinoid tumors of the large intestine or appendix are not included.)

C18.0 Cecum
C18.1 Appendix
C18.2 Ascending
C18.3 Hepatic flexure
C18.4 Transverse
C18.5 Splenic flexure
C18.6 Descending
C18.7 Sigmoid
C18.8 Overlapping lesion
C18.9 Colon, NOS

C19.9 Rectosigmoid junction

C20.9 Rectum

The TNM classification for carcinomas of the colon and rectum provides more detail than other staging systems. Compatible with Dukes, the TNM adds greater precision in the identification of prognostic subgroups. The TNM is based on the depth of tumor invasion into the wall of the intestine, extension to adjacent structures, the number of regional lymph nodes involved, and the presence or absence of distant metastasis. The TNM classification applies to both clinical and pathologic staging. Most cancers of the colon or rectum, however, are staged after pathologic examination of the resected specimen. This staging system applies to all carcinomas arising in the colon, rectum, or in the vermiform appendix.

ANATOMY

Divisions of the Colon and Rectum:
Cecum
Ascending colon
Hepatic flexure
Transverse colon
Splenic flexure
Descending colon
Sigmoid colon
Rectosigmoid junction
Rectum

Cancers that occur in the anal canal are staged according to the classification used for the anus (see Chapter 13).

Primary Site. The large intestine (colorectum) extends from the terminal ileum to the anal canal. Excluding the rectum and vermiform appendix, the colon is divided into four parts: the right or ascending colon, the middle or transverse colon, the left or descending colon, and the sigmoid colon. The sigmoid is continuous with the rectum which terminates at the anal canal.

The cecum is a large pouch that forms the proximal segment of the right colon. It usually measures 6 cm by 9 cm and is covered with peritoneum. The ascending colon measures 15 to 20 cm in length and is located retroperitoneally. Connecting the ascending colon to the transverse colon is the hepatic flexure which lies under the right lobe of the liver near the duodenum.

The transverse colon lies more anteriorly than the other divisions of the colon. It is supported by the transverse mesocolon which is attached to the pancreas. Anteriorly, its serosa is continuous with the gastrocolic ligament. The transverse colon is connected to the descending colon by the splenic flexure which is located near the spleen and tail of the pancreas. The descending colon, which measures 10 to 15 cm in length, is also located retroperitoneally. The descending colon becomes the sigmoid at the origin of the mesosigmoid. The sigmoid loop extends from the medial border of the left posterior major psoas muscle to the rectum, which begins at the termination of the mesosigmoid.

Approximately 12 cm in length, the rectum extends from the third sacral vertebra to the apex of the prostate gland in the male and to the apex of the perineal body in the female; that is, to a point 4 cm anterior to the tip of the coccyx. It is often defined as the distal 10 cm of the large intestine as measured from the anal verge with a sigmoidoscope. The rectosigmoid segment is usually 10 to 15 cm from the anal mucocutaneous junction. The rectum is covered by peritoneum in front and on both sides in its upper third and only on the anterior wall in its middle third. The peritoneum is reflected laterally from the rectum to form the perirectal fossa and anteriorly the uterine or rectovesical fold. There is no peritoneal covering in the lower third, which is often known as the rectal ampulla. The anal canal, which measures 4 to 5 cm in length, courses downward and backward from the apex of the prostate gland or from the perineal body to the anal verge. (See Figs. 12-1A and 12-1B.)

Regional Lymph Nodes. Regional nodes are located: (1) along the course of the major vessels supplying the colon and rectum; (2) along the vascular arcades of the marginal artery; and (3) adjacent to the colon; that is, located along the mesocolic border of the colon. Specifically, the regional lymph nodes are the pericolic and perirectal nodes and those found along the ileocolic, right colic, middle colic, left colic, inferior mesenteric artery, superior rectal (hemorrhoidal), and internal iliac arteries.

For pN, the number of lymph nodes sampled should be recorded. It is desirable to obtain at least 12 lymph nodes in radical colon resections; however, in cases in which tumor is resected for palliation or in patients who have received pre-operative radiation, only a few lymph nodes may be present.

The regional lymph nodes for each segment of the colon are:

SEGMENT	REGIONAL LYMPH NODES
Cecum and appendix	Anterior cecal, posterior cecal, ileocolic, right colic
Ascending colon	Ileocolic, right colic, middle colic
Hepatic flexure	Middle colic, right colic
Transverse colon	Middle colic
Splenic flexure	Middle colic, left colic, inferior mesenteric
Descending colon	Left colic, inferior mesenteric, sigmoid
Sigmoid colon	Inferior mesenteric, superior rectal, (hemorrhoidal), sigmoidal, sigmoid mesenteric
Rectosigmoid	Perirectal, left colic, sigmoid mesenteric, sigmoidal, inferior mesenteric, superior rectal (hemorrhoidal), middle rectal (hemorrhoidal)
Rectum	Perirectal, sigmoid mesenteric, inferior mesenteric, lateral sacral presacral, internal iliac, sacral promontory (Gerota's), superior rectal (hemorrhoidal), middle rectal (hemorrhoidal), inferior rectal (hemorrhoidal)

Metastatic Sites. Although carcinomas of the colon and rectum can metastasize to almost any organ, the liver and lungs are the most common sites. Seeding of other segments of the colon or small intestine can also occur.

RULES FOR CLASSIFICATION

Clinical Staging. Clinical assessment is based on medical history, physical examination, routine and special imaging procedures, sigmoidoscopy, colonoscopy with biopsy, and special examinations designed to demonstrate the presence of extracolonic metastasis, for example, chest films, liver function tests, and liver scans.

Pathologic Staging. Colorectal cancers are usually staged after pathologic examination of

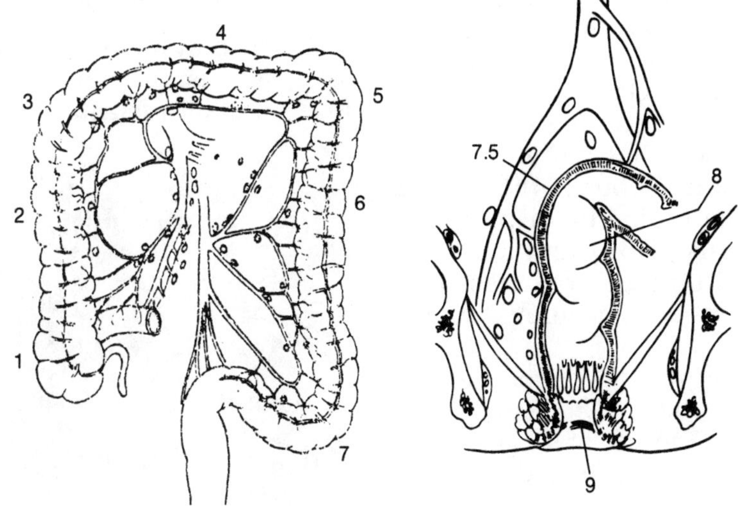

A

	MEASUREMENT FROM ANAL VERGE	AVERAGE SEGMENT LENGTH	
		GRAY'S	TNM
Anus	0–4 cm	4 cm	4–5 cm
Rectum	4–16 cm	12 cm	12 cm
* Rectosigmoid	(at 15–17 cm)		
Sigmoid	17–57 cm	40 cm	n/a
Descending	57–82 cm	25 cm	10–15 cm
Transverse	82–132 cm	50 cm	n/a
Ascending	132–147 cm	15 cm	15–20 cm
Cecum	at 150 cm	6 cm	6 cm

(Total length of large intestine approximately 150 cm).
* The rectosigmoid is of anatomic and surgical importance because of the blood supply and the disappearance of the mesosigmoid. While the rectosigmoid is truly a junction, some authors include 1 inch of the sigmoid above and 1 inch of rectum below and refer to it as the rectosigmoid region.
These measurements are APPROXIMATIONS ONLY. Each person is different and these measurements should be used as GUIDELINES ONLY.

B

FIG. 12-1. The anatomic areas of the colon and rectum are: cecum *(1);* ascending colon *(2);* hepatic flexure *(3);* transverse colon *(4);* splenic flexure *(5);* descending colon *(6);* sigmoid *(7);* rectosigmoid *(7.5);* rectum *(8);* anal canal *(9).*

the resected specimen and surgical exploration of the abdomen. The definition of *in situ* carcinoma—pTis—includes cancer cells confined within the glandular basement membrane (intraepithelial) or lamina propria (intramucosal) with no extension through the muscularis mucosae into the submucosa. This definition of pTis is different from that used for the other divisions of the gastrointestinal tract. Neither intraepithelial nor intramucosal carcinomas of the large intestine have a significant potential for metastasis.

Tumor that invades the stalk of a polyp is classified according to the pT definitions adopted for colorectal carcinomas. For instance, tumor that is limited to the lamina propria is listed as pTis, whereas tumor that has invaded the muscularis mucosae and entered the submucosa of the stalk is classified T1.

Lymph nodes are classified N1 or N2 according to the number involved with metastatic tumor. Involvement of 1 to 3 nodes is N1.

Patients with tumor located on the serosal surface as a result of direct extension through the colon are assigned T4. Seeding of abdominal organs, for instance, the distal ileum from a carcinoma of the transverse colon, is considered discontinuous metastasis and should be recorded as M1. Metastatic nodules or foci found in the pericolic or perirectal fat or in adjacent mesentery (mesocolic fat) without evidence of residual lymph node tissue are equivalent to regional lymph node metastasis. Multiple metastatic foci seen microscopically only in the pericolic fat should be considered as metastasis in a single lymph node for classification. A tumor nodule greater than 3 mm in diameter in the perirectal or pericolic fat without histologic evidence of a residual node in the nodule is classified as regional perirectal or pericolic lymph node metastasis. However, a tumor nodule 3 mm or less in diameter is classified in the T category as a discontinuous extension, that is T3.

Metastasis in the external iliac or common iliac lymph nodes is classified M1.

If the tumor recurs at the site of surgery, it is anatomically assigned to the proximal segment of the anastomosis.

DEFINITION OF TNM

The same classification is used for both clinical and pathologic staging.

Primary Tumor (T)

- TX Primary tumor cannot be assessed
- T0 No evidence of primary tumor
- Tis Carcinoma *in situ:* intraepithelial or invasion of lamina propria*
- T1 Tumor invades submucosa
- T2 Tumor invades muscularis propria
- T3 Tumor invades through the muscularis propria into the subserosa, or into nonperitonealized pericolic or perirectal tissues
- T4 Tumor directly invades other organs or structures, and/or perforates visceral peritoneum**

**Note:* Tis includes cancer cells confined within the glandular basement membrane (intraepithelial) or lamina propria (intramucosal) with no extension through the muscularis mucosae into the submucosa.

***Note:* Direct invasion in T4 includes invasion of other segments of the colorectum by way of the serosa; for example, invasion of the sigmoid colon by a carcinoma of the cecum.

Regional Lymph Nodes (N)

- NX Regional lymph nodes cannot be assessed
- N0 No regional lymph node metastasis
- N1 Metastasis in 1 to 3 regional lymph nodes
- N2 Metastasis in 4 or more regional lymph nodes

Distant Metastasis (M)

- MX Distant metastasis cannot be assessed
- M0 No distant metastasis
- M1 Distant metastasis

STAGE GROUPING

AJCC/UICC				Dukes*
Stage 0	Tis	N0	M0	–
Stage I	T1	N0	M0	A
	T2	N0	M0	–
Stage II	T3	N0	M0	B
	T4	N0	M0	–
Stage III	Any T	N1	M0	C
	Any T	N2	M0	–
Stage IV	Any T	Any N	M1	–

*Dukes B is a composite of better (T3 N0 M0) and worse (T4 N0 M0) prognostic groups, as is Dukes C (Any TN1 M0 and Any T N2 M0)

HISTOPATHOLOGIC TYPE

This staging classification applies to carcinomas that arise in the colon, rectum, or appendix. The classification does not apply to sarcomas, lymphomas, or to carcinoid tumors of the large intestine or appendix. The histologic types include:

Adenocarcinoma *in situ**
Adenocarcinoma
Mucinous carcinoma, (colloid type) (greater than 50% mucinous carcinoma)
Signet ring cell carcinoma (greater than 50% signet ring cell)
Squamous cell (epidermoid) carcinoma
Adenosquamous carcinoma
Small cell carcinoma
Undifferentiated carcinoma
Carcinoma, NOS

*The terms "high grade dysplasia" or "severe dysplasia" may be used as synonyms for *in situ* adenocarcinoma or *in situ* carcinoma. These cases should be assigned pTis.

HISTOLOGIC GRADE (G)

- GX Grade cannot be assessed
- G1 Well differentiated
- G2 Moderately differentiated
- G3 Poorly differentiated
- G4 Undifferentiated

PROGNOSTIC FACTORS

In addition to the TNM, independent prognostic factors that are generally used in patient management and well-supported in the literature include histologic type, histologic grade, serum carcinoembryonic antigen level, extramural venous invasion, and submucosal vascular invasion by carcinomas arising in adenomas. Small cell carcinomas, signet ring cell carcinomas, and undifferentiated carcinomas have a less favorable outcome that other histologic types. Submucosal vascular invasion by carcinomas arising in adenomas is associated with a greater risk of regional lymph node involvement.

BIBLIOGRAPHY

Astler VB, Coller FA: The prognostic significance of direct extension of carcinoma of the colon and rectum. Ann Surg 139:846–852, 1954

Bauer K, Bagwell C, Giaretti W, et al: Consensus review of the clinical utility of DNA flow cytometry in colorectal cancer. Cytometry 14:486–491, 1993

Butch RJ, Stark DD, Wittenberg J, et al: Staging rectal cancer by MR and CT. AJR Am J Roentgenol 146:1155–1160, 1986

Chapuis PH, Fisher R, Dent DF, et al: The relationship between different staging methods and survival in colorectal carcinoma. Dis Colon Rectum 28:158–161, 1985

Dukes CE: Cancer of the rectum: an analysis of 1000 cases. J Pathol Bacteriol 50:527–539, 1940

Fenoglio-Preiser CM, Hutter RVP: Colorectal polyps: pathologic diagnosis and clinical significance. Cancer J Clin 35:322–344, 1985

Fielding LP: Clinicopathological staging for colorectal cancer: an International Documentation System (IDS) and an International Comprehensive Anatomical Terminology (ICAT). J Gastroenterol Hepatol, 1991

Fielding LP, Ballantyne GH: Classification systems for staging colorectal cancer. Problems Gen Surg 4:39–53, 1987

Fielding LP, Pettigrew N: College of American Pathologists Conference XXVI on clinical relevance of prognostic markers in solid tumors: report of the Colorectal Working Group. Arch Pathol Lab Med 119:1115–1121, 1995

Fielding LP, Phillips RK, Frey JS, et al: The prediction of outcome after curative resection for large bowel cancer. Lancet 2:904–907, 1986

Fielding LP, Phillips RK, Hittinger R: Factors influencing mortality after curative resection for large bowel cancer in elderly patients. Lancet 1:595–597, 1989

Griffin MR, Bergstralh EJ, Coffey RJ, et al: Predictors of survival after curative resection of carcinoma of the colon and rectum. Cancer 60:2318–2324, 1987

Harrison JC, Dean PJ, El-Zeky F, et al: From Dukes through Jass: pathological prognostic indicators in rectal cancer. Hum Pathol 25:498–505, 1994

Henson DE, Hutter RVP, Sobin LH, et al: Protocol of the examination of specimens removed from patients with colorectal carcinoma. Arch Pathol Lab Med 118:122–125, 1994

Hermanek P: Colorectal carcinoma. Histopathological diagnosis and staging. Baillieres Clin Gastroenterol 3:511–529, 1989

Hermanek P: Problems of pTNM classification of carcinoma of the stomach, colorectum and anal margin. Pathol Res Pract 181:296–300, 1986

Hermanek P, Gall FP: Early (microinvasive) colorectal carcinoma: pathology, diagnosis, surgical treatment. Int J Colorectal Dis 1:79–84, 1986

Hermanek P, Giedl J, Dworak O: Two programs for examination of regional lymph nodes in colorectal carcinoma with regard to the new pN classification. Pathol Res Pract 185:867–873, 1989

Hermanek P, Guggenmoos-Holzmann I, Gall FP: Prognostic factors in rectal carcinoma. A contribution to the further development of tumor classification. Dis Colon Rectum 32:593–599, 1989

Hermanek P, Henson DE, Hutter RVP, Sobin LH: TNM Supplement 1993: a commentary on uniform use. Berlin: Springer-Verlag, 1993

Hermanek P, Sobin LH: Colorectal carcinoma. In Hermanek P, Gospodarowicz MK, Henson DE, et al (Eds.), Prognostic factors in cancer. Berlin: Springer-Verlag, 1995

Herrera-Ornelas L, Justiniano J, Castillo, N, et al: Metastases in small lymph nodes from colon cancer. Arch Surg 122:1253–1256, 1987

Jass JR, Atkin WS, Cuzick J, et al: The grading of rectal cancer: historical perspectives and a multivariate analysis of 447 cases. Histopathology 10:437–459, 1986

Jass JR, Love SB, Northover JMA: A new prognostic classification of rectal cancer. Lancet i:1303–1306, 1987

Jass JR, Mukawa K, Goh HS, et al: Clinical importance of DNA content in rectal cancer measured by flow cytometry. J Clin Pathol 42:254–259, 1989

Jass JR, Sobin LH: Histological typing of intestinal tumours. WHO International Histological Classification of Tumours, 2nd ed. Berlin-New York: Springer-Verlag, 1989

Kokal W, Sheibani K, Terz J, et al: Tumor DNA content in the prognosis of colorectal carcinoma. JAMA 255:3123–3127, 1986

Kotanagi H, Fukuoka T, Shibata Y, et al: Blood-vessel invasions in metastatic nodes for development of liver metastasis in colorectal cancer. Hepato-Gastroenterol 42:771–774, 1995

Lindmark G, Gerdin B, Sundberg C, et al: Prognostic significance of the microvascular count in colorectal cancer. J Clin Oncol 14:461–466, 1996

Lipper S, Kahn LB, Ackerman LV: The significance of microscopic invasive cancer in endoscopically removed polyps of the large bowel: a clinicopathologic study of 51 cases. Cancer 52:1691, 1983

Minsky BD, Mies C, Rich TA, et al: Lymphatic vessel invasion is an independent prognostic factor for survival in colorectal cancer. Int J Radiat Oncol 17:311–318, 1989

Newland RC, Chapuis PH, Pheils MT, et al: The relationship of survival to staging and grading of colorectal carcinoma: a prospective study of 503 cases. Cancer 47:1424–1429, 1981

Ondero H, Maetani S, Nishikawa T, et al: The reappraisal of prognostic classifications for colorectal cancer. Dis Colon Rectum 32:609–614, 1989

Phillips RKS, Hittinger R, Blesovsky L, et al: Large bowel cancer: surgical pathology and its relationship to survival. Br J Surg 71:604–610, 1984

Qizilbash AH: Pathologic studies in colorectal cancer: a guide to the surgical pathology examination of colorectal specimens and review of features of prognostic significance. Pathol Annu 17(1): 1–46, 1982

Scott KWM, Grace RH: Detection of lymph node metastases in colorectal carcinoma before and after fat clearance. Br J Surg 76:1165–1167, 1989

Scott NA, Rainwater LM, Wieland HS, et al: The relative prognostic value of flow cytometric DNA analysis and conventional clinicopathologic criteria in patients with operative rectal carcinoma. Dis Colon Rectum 30:513–520, 1987

Shepherd NA, Saraga EP, Love SB, et al: Prognostic factors in colonic cancer. Histopathology 14:613–620, 1989

Steinberg SM, Barkin JS, Kaplan RS, et al: Prognostic indicators of colon tumors: the gastrointestinal tumor study group experience. Cancer 57: 1866–1870, 1986

Talbot IC, Ritchie S, Leighton MH, et al: The clinical significance of invasion of veins by rectal cancer. Br J Surg 67:439–442, 1980

Talbot IC, Ritchie S, Leighton MH, et al: Spread of rectal cancer within veins: histologic features and clinical significance. Am J Surg 141:15–17, 1981

Williams NS, Durdey P, Qwihe P, et al: Pre-operative staging of rectal neoplasm and its impact on clinical management. Br J Surg 72:868–874, 1985

Wolmark N, Fisher B, Wieand HS: The prognostic value of the modifications of the Dukes' C class of colorectal cancer: an analysis of the NSABP clinical trials. Ann Surg 203:115–122, 1986

Wolmark N, Fisher ER, Wieand HS, et al: The relationship of depth of penetration and tumor size to the number of positive nodes in Dukes' C colorectal cancer. Cancer 53:2707–2712, 1984

Data Form for Cancer Staging

Patient identification
Name ______
Address ______
Hospital or clinic number ______
Age ____ Sex ____ Race ______

Institution identification
Hospital or clinic ______
Address ______

Oncology Record

Anatomic site of cancer ______
Histologic type ______
Grade (G) ______
Date of classification ______

DEFINITIONS

Primary Tumor (T)

Clin	Path		
[ ]	[ ]	TX	Primary tumor cannot be assessed
[ ]	[ ]	T0	No evidence of primary tumor
[ ]	[ ]	Tis	Carcinoma *in situ:* intraepithelial or invasion of lamina propria*
[ ]	[ ]	T1	Tumor invades submucosa
[ ]	[ ]	T2	Tumor invades muscularis propria
[ ]	[ ]	T3	Tumor invades through muscularis propria into subserosa, or into nonperitonealized pericolic or perirectal tissues
[ ]	[ ]	T4	Tumor directly invades other organs or structures, and/or perforates visceral peritoneum**

** Tis includes cancer cells confined within the glandular basement membrane (intraepithelial) or lamina propria (intramucosal) with no extension through the muscularis mucosae into the submucosa.*

*** Direct invasion in T4 includes invasion of other segments of the colorectum by way of the serosa, for example, invasion of the sigmoid colon by a carcinoma of the cecum.*

Regional Lymph Nodes (N)

Clin	Path		
[ ]	[ ]	NX	Regional lymph nodes cannot be assessed
[ ]	[ ]	N0	No regional lymph node metastasis
[ ]	[ ]	N1	Metastasis in 1 to 3 regional lymph nodes
[ ]	[ ]	N2	Metastasis in 4 or more regional lymph nodes

Distant metastasis (M)

Clin	Path		
[ ]	[ ]	MX	Distant metastasis cannot be assessed
[ ]	[ ]	M0	No distant metastasis
[ ]	[ ]	M1	Distant metastasis

Stage Grouping

Clin	Path	Stage	T	N	M	Dukes*
[ ]	[ ]	0	Tis	N0	M0	
[ ]	[ ]	I	T1	N0	M0	A
			T2	N0	M0	
[ ]	[ ]	II	T3	N0	M0	B
			T4	N0	M0	
[ ]	[ ]	III	Any T	N1	M0	C
			Any T	N2	M0	
[ ]	[ ]	IV	Any T	Any N	M1	

* Dukes B is a composite of better (T3 N0 M0) and worse (T4 N0 M0) prognostic groups, as is Dukes C (Any T N1 M0 and Any T N2 M0).

Histopathologic Grade (G)

[ ] GX Grade cannot be assessed
[ ] G1 Well differentiated
[ ] G2 Moderately differentiated
[ ] G3 Poorly differentiated
[ ] G4 Undifferentiated

Histopathologic Type

This staging classification applies to carcinomas that arise in the colon, rectum, or appendix. The classification does not apply to sarcomas, lymphomas, or to carcinoid tumors of the large intestine or appendix. The histologic types include:

Adenocarcinoma *in situ**
Adenocarcinoma
Mucinous carcinoma (colloid type) (greater than 50% mucinous carcinoma)
Signet ring cell carcinoma (greater than 50% signet ring cell)
Squamous cell (epidermoid) carcinoma
Adenosquamous carcinoma
Small cell carcinoma
Undifferentiated carcinoma
Carcinoma, NOS

** The terms high grade dysplasia or severe dysplasia may be used as synonyms for in situ adenocarcinoma or in situ carcinoma. These cases should be assigned pTis.*

Staged by ______ M.D.
______ Registrar

Date ______

(continued on next page)

Illustrations

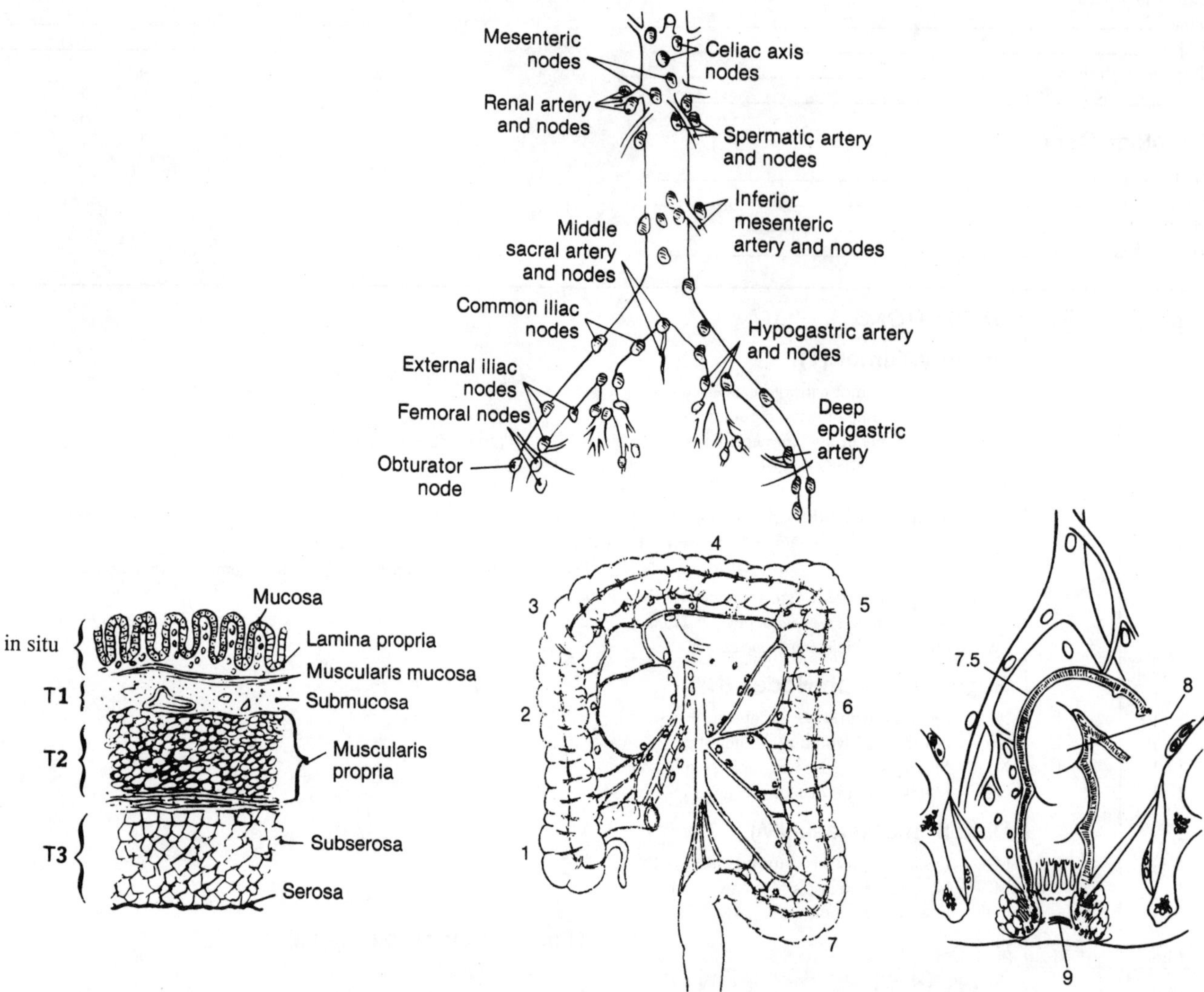

For anatomic areas corresponding to numbers, see list below.
Indicate on diagram primary and regional nodes involved.

Anatomic Areas of Colon and Rectum

1. Cecum
2. Ascending colon
3. Hepatic flexure
4. Transverse colon
5. Splenic flexure
6. Descending colon
7. Sigmoid

7.5 Rectosigmoid

8. Rectum
9. Anal canal

13

Anal Canal

(Melanomas are not included.)

C21.0 Anus, NOS
C21.1 Anal canal
C21.2 Cloacogenic zone
C21.8 Overlapping lesion of rectum, anus and anal canal

Two different staging systems are needed for carcinomas that arise in the anal canal, one for carcinomas arising in the anal canal proper and the other for carcinomas arising at the anal margin. The two systems are needed because carcinomas that arise in these sites have different modes of spread and treatment options.

Carcinomas of the anal canal are staged clinically according to the size and extent of the primary tumor. Thus, patients with cancer of the canal can be classified at presentation by inspection of the lesion and palpation of adjacent structures, including the regional lymph nodes. Although additional information concerning depth of penetration is often provided by the pathologist after resection, in many cases, especially those initially treated with radiation and chemotherapy, the depth of invasion cannot always be assessed. Radiation and chemotherapy not only destroy tumor cells but also cause inflammatory changes and edema, which often makes it difficult for the pathologist to assess the extent of disease. The most important indicator of outcome is spread of tumor outside the pelvis. Lymph nodes should be specifically identified.

Cancers that arise at the anal margin, that is, the junction of the hair-bearing skin and the mucous membrane of the anal canal, or more distal, are staged according to the system used for cancers of the skin (see Chapters 23 and 24).

ANATOMY

Primary Site. The anal canal extends from the rectum to the perianal skin and is lined by a mucous membrane that covers the internal sphincter. The mucous membrane extends to the junction of the hair-bearing skin.

Regional Lymph Nodes. For pN, histologic examination of a regional perirectal-peripelvic lymphadenectomy specimen will ordinarily include 12 or more regional lymph nodes; or histologic examination of an inguinal lymphadenectomy specimen will ordinarily include 6 or more lymph nodes. The regional lymph nodes are as follows:

Perirectal:
- Anorectal
- Perirectal
- Lateral sacral

Internal iliac (hypogastric)

Inguinal:
- Superficial
- Deep femoral

All other nodal groups represent sites of distant metastasis. The sites of regional node involvement are governed by the lymphatic drainage, above to the rectal ampulla and below to the perineum. Tumors that arise in the anal canal usually spread initially to the anorectal and perirectal nodes, and those that arise at the anal margin spread to the superficial inguinal nodes.

Metastatic Sites. Cancers of the anus can metastasize to most organs, especially to the liver and lungs. Involvement of the abdominal cavity is not unusual.

RULES FOR CLASSIFICATION

The TNM classification for tumors of the anal canal depends largely on clinical observations. The primary tumor is staged according to its size and local extent as determined by clinical or pathologic examination. For most of the histologic types, the diameter of the tumor correlates with its depth of penetration. Extension to the anorectal, perirectal, superficial inguinal, or femoral nodes, as well as to adjacent structures, can usually be assessed by palpation. Tumor can extend to the rectal mucosa or submucosa, subcutaneous perianal tissue, perianal skin, ischiorectal fat, and/or local skeletal muscles, such as the external anal sphincter, levator ani, and coccygeus muscles. Tumor can also invade the perineum, vulva, prostate gland, urinary bladder, urethra, vagina, cervix uteri, corpus uteri, pelvic peritoneum, and broad ligaments. Organs invaded by tumor should be specified.

The staging system does not preclude the surgeon from recording the depth of penetration or extension of tumor based on information provided by the pathologist or radiologist. This information, however, is not included in the staging classification.

Metastasis to other nodal groups, such as the inferior mesenteric, can often be suspected by computed tomography (CT) or magnetic resonance imaging (MRI).

Clinical Staging. Anal cancers are staged primarily by inspection and palpation. Imaging may help to define the extent of tumor. In rare cases of rectal excision, tumors of the anal canal may be staged pathologically. Direct invasion of the rectal wall, perirectal skin, or subcutaneous tissue is not considered T4. The tumor is classified by size.

DEFINITION OF TNM

The following is the TNM classification for the staging of cancers that arise in the anal canal only. Cancers that arise at the anal margin are staged according to the classification for cancers of the skin.

Primary Tumor (T)

TX Primary tumor cannot be assessed
T0 No evidence of primary tumor
Tis Carcinoma *in situ*
T1 Tumor 2 cm or less in greatest dimension
T2 Tumor more than 2 cm but not more than 5 cm in greatest dimension
T3 Tumor more than 5 cm in greatest dimension
T4 Tumor of any size invades adjacent organ(s), e.g., vagina, urethra, bladder (involvement of the sphincter muscle[s] alone is not classified as T4)

Regional Lymph Nodes (N)

NX Regional lymph nodes cannot be assessed
N0 No regional lymph node metastasis
N1 Metastasis in perirectal lymph node(s)
N2 Metastasis in unilateral internal iliac and/or inguinal lymph node(s)
N3 Metastasis in perirectal and inguinal lymph nodes and/or bilateral internal iliac and/or inguinal lymph nodes

Distant Metastasis (M)

MX Distant metastasis cannot be assessed
M0 No distant metastasis
M1 Distant metastasis

STAGE GROUPING

Stage 0	Tis	N0	M0
Stage I	T1	N0	M0
Stage II	T2	N0	M0
	T3	N0	M0
Stage IIIA	T1	N1	M0
	T2	N1	M0
	T3	N1	M0
	T4	N0	M0
Stage IIIB	T4	N1	M0
	Any T	N2	M0
	Any T	N3	M0
Stage IV	Any T	Any N	M1

HISTOPATHOLOGIC TYPE

The staging system applies to all carcinomas arising in the anal canal, including carcinomas that arise within anorectal fistulas. The classification also includes cloacogenic carcinomas. Melanomas are excluded.

HISTOLOGIC GRADE (G)

GX Grade cannot be assessed
G1 Well differentiated
G2 Moderately differentiated
G3 Poorly differentiated
G4 Undifferentiated

PROGNOSTIC FACTORS

Because of the infrequent occurrence of carcinomas of the anal canal, the evaluation of prognostic factors is difficult. However, poor histologic grade is associated with a less favorable outcome than cases that are well differentiated.

BIBLIOGRAPHY

Boman BM, Moertel CG, O'Connell MJ, et al: Carcinoma of the anal canal: a clinical and pathologic study of 188 cases. Cancer 54:114–125, 1984

Cummings BJ: Anal canal carcinoma. In Hermanek P, Gospodarowicz MK, Henson DE, et al (Eds.), Prognostic factors in cancer. Berlin: Springer-Verlag, 1995

Flam MS, John M, Lovalvo LJ, et al: Definitive nonsurgical therapy of epithelial malignancies of the anal canal. Cancer 51:1378–1387, 1983

Greenall MJ, Quan SHQ, Stearns MW, et al: Epidermoid cancer of the anal margin. Am J Surg 149:95–101, 1985

Longo WE, Vernava AM 3rd, Wade TP, et al: Recurrent squamous cell carcinoma of the anal canal: predictors of initial treatment failure and results of salvage therapy. Ann Surg 220:40–49, 1994

Nigro ND: An evaluation of combined therapy for squamous cell cancer of the anal canal. Dis Colon Rectum 27:763–766, 1984

Nigro ND: Treatment of squamous cell cancer of the anus. Cancer Treat Res 18:221–242, 1984

Nigro ND, Vaitkeviceus VK, Herskovic AM: Preservation of function in the treatment of cancer of the anus. Important Adv Oncol 161–177, 1989

Paradis P, Douglass HO Jr, Holyoke ED: The clinical implications of a staging system for carcinoma of the anus. Surg Gynecol Obstet 141:411–416, 1975

Pintor MP, Northover JM, Nicholls RJ: Squamous cell carcinoma of the anus at one hospital from 1948. Br J Surg 76:806–810, 1989

Roseau G, Palazzo L, Colardelle P, et al: Endoscopic ultrasonography in the staging and follow-up of epidermoid carcinoma of the anal canal. Gastrointest Endosc 40:447–450, 1994

Salmon RJ, Fenton J, Asselain B, et al: Treatment of epidermoid anal canal cancer. Am J Surg 147:43–47, 1984

Salmon RJ, Zafrani B, Labib A, et al: Prognosis of cloacogenic and squamous cancers of the anal canal. Dis Colon Rectum 29:336–340, 1986

Schraut WH, Wang CH, Dawson PJ, et al: Depth of invasion, location, and size of cancer of the anus dictate operative treatment. Cancer 51:1291–1296, 1983

Scott NA, Beart RW Jr, Weiland LH, et al: Carcinoma of the anal canal and flow cytometric DNA analysis. Br J Cancer 60:56–58, 1989

Shank B: Treatment of anal canal carcinoma. Cancer 55(Suppl):2156–2162, 1985

Shepherd NA, Scholefield JH, Love SB, et al: Prognostic factors in anal squamous carcinoma: A multivariate analysis of clinical, pathological and flow cytometric parameters in 235 cases. Histopathology 16:545–555, 1990

Spratt JS (Ed.): Neoplasms of the colon, rectum, and anus. Philadelphia, WB Saunders, 1984

Data Form for Cancer Staging

Patient identification
Name ______
Address ______
Hospital or clinic number ______
Age ____ Sex ____ Race ______

Institution identification
Hospital or clinic ______
Address ______

Oncology Record

Anatomic site of cancer ______
Histologic type ______
Grade (G) ______
Date of classification ______

DEFINITIONS

The following is the TNM classification for the staging of cancers that arise in the anal canal only. Cancers that arise in the anal margin are staged according to the classification for cancers of the skin.

Primary Tumor (T)

Clin	Path		
[ ]	[ ]	TX	Primary tumor cannot be assessed
[ ]	[ ]	T0	No evidence of primary tumor
[ ]	[ ]	Tis	Carcinoma *in situ*
[ ]	[ ]	T1	Tumor 2 cm or less in greatest dimension
[ ]	[ ]	T2	Tumor more than 2 cm but not more than 5 cm in greatest dimension
[ ]	[ ]	T3	Tumor more than 5 cm in greatest dimension
[ ]	[ ]	T4	Tumor of any size invades adjacent organ(s): e.g., vagina, urethra, bladder (involvement of sphincter muscle[s] *alone* is not classified as T4)

Regional Lymph Nodes (N)

Clin	Path		
[ ]	[ ]	NX	Regional lymph nodes cannot be assessed
[ ]	[ ]	N0	No regional lymph node metastasis
[ ]	[ ]	N1	Metastasis in perirectal lymph node(s)
[ ]	[ ]	N2	Metastasis in unilateral internal iliac and/or inguinal lymph node(s)
[ ]	[ ]	N3	Metastasis in perirectal and inguinal lymph nodes and/or bilateral internal iliac and/or inguinal lymph nodes

Distant Metastasis (M)

Clin	Path		
[ ]	[ ]	MX	Distant metastasis cannot be assessed
[ ]	[ ]	M0	No distant metastasis
[ ]	[ ]	M1	Distant metastasis

Stage Grouping

Clin	Path	Stage	T	N	M
[ ]	[ ]	0	Tis	N0	M0
[ ]	[ ]	I	T1	N0	M0
[ ]	[ ]	II	T2	N0	M0
			T3	N0	M0
[ ]	[ ]	IIIA	T1	N1	M0
			T2	N1	M0
			T3	N1	M0
			T4	N0	M0
[ ]	[ ]	IIIB	T4	N1	M0
			Any T	N2	M0
			Any T	N3	M0
[ ]	[ ]	IV	Any T	Any N	M1

Histopathologic Type

The staging system applies to all carcinomas arising in the anal canal, including carcinomas that arise within anorectal fistulas. The classification also includes cloacogenic carcinomas. Melanomas are excluded.

Histopathologic Grade (G)

[ ] GX Grade cannot be assessed
[ ] G1 Well differentiated
[ ] G2 Moderately differentiated
[ ] G3 Poorly differentiated
[ ] G4 Undifferentiated

Illustration

7.5
8
9

Indicate on diagram primary tumor and regional nodes involved.

Staged by ______ M.D.
______ Registrar
Date ______

14

Liver (Including Intrahepatic Bile Ducts)

(Sarcomas and tumors metastatic to the liver are not included.)

C22.0 Liver
C22.1 Intrahepatic bile duct

The largest parenchymatous organ in the body, the liver is often the site of metastatic cancer, especially from carcinomas that arise in abdominal viscera. Primary cancers of the liver are uncommon in the United States, although common in many other countries. Several distinctive malignant tumors are found in the liver. These include hepatocellular carcinomas that originate from hepatocytes, cholangiocarcinomas or intrahepatic bile duct carcinomas that arise from bile ducts, and sarcomas that arise from mesenchymal elements. Hepatocellular carcinomas are often associated with pre-existing liver disease, usually cirrhosis, which may dominate the clinical picture. The liver has a dual blood supply: the hepatic artery which branches from the celiac artery and the portal vein which drains the intestine. Blood from the liver passes through the hepatic vein and enters the inferior vena cava. Hepatocellular carcinomas have a proclivity to invade blood vessels, a fact that is considered in the TNM classification. Invasion of adjacent structures such as the diaphragm, adrenal gland, inferior vena cava, or hilar vessels often makes resection of the tumor difficult or impossible. The most important indicators of outcome are resectability for cure and extent of disease.

ANATOMY

Primary Site. The liver is located in the right upper abdominal cavity immediately below the right leaf of the diaphragm. It extends from the fifth rib and midclavicular line on the left side to the inferior costal margin and midaxillary line on the right side. Covered by a smooth, reddish-brown capsule, the organ is divided into right and left lobes, the former being much larger. Two small lobes—the quadrate and the caudate—are subdivisions of the undersurface of the liver. They are located on the left side of a plane projecting between the bed of the gallbladder and the inferior vena cava. For classification, the quadrate lobe is considered part of the left lobe. The quadrate lobe is inferior and the caudate superior to the porta hepatis, through which the hepatic artery passes.

Histologically, the liver is divided into lobules. Between the lobules are the portal areas that contain the intrahepatic bile ducts and small arteries and veins.

Regional Lymph Nodes. The regional lymph nodes are the hilar (i.e., those in the hepatoduodenal ligament), the hepatic, and the periportal nodes. Specifically, regional nodes include those along the hepatic artery, portal vein, and inferior vena cava. Histologic examination of a regional lymphadenectomy specimen will ordinarily include a minimum of 3 lymph nodes.

Involvement beyond these lymph nodes is considered distant metastasis and should be coded as M1. Involvement of the inferior phrenic lymph nodes should also be considered M1.

Metastatic Sites. Carcinomas of the liver can spread to most organs in the body. The most common sites are the lungs and bone. Tumors may extend through the capsule to the diaphragm.

RULES FOR CLASSIFICATION

The T classification is based on the number of tumor nodules, the size of the largest nodule (2 cm is the discriminating limit), and the presence of vascular invasion. The TNM classification does not consider etiologic mechanisms such as whether multiple nodules represent independent primary tumors or intra-hepatic metastasis from a single primary hepatic carcinoma. For pathologic classification, vascular invasion includes either the macroscopic or the histologic involvement of vessels.

Because of the tendency for hepatomas to invade blood vessels, imaging of the liver is important for staging, unless distant metastasis (M1) is present at the time of diagnosis.

Clinical Staging. Staging depends on imaging procedures designed to demonstrate the size of the primary tumor and vascular invasion. Surgical exploration is usually not carried out because the possibility for complete resection is minimal, especially for larger tumors.

Pathologic Staging. If surgical exploration is carried out and there is resection then Pathologic Staging should be recorded.

Note: For classification, the plane projecting between the bed of the gallbladder and the inferior vena cava divides the liver into two lobes.

DEFINITION OF TNM

Primary Tumor (T)

TX Primary tumor cannot be assessed
T0 No evidence of primary tumor
T1 Solitary tumor 2 cm or less in greatest dimension without vascular invasion
T2 Solitary tumor 2 cm or less in greatest dimension with vascular invasion, or multiple tumors limited to one lobe, none more than 2 cm in greatest dimension without vascular invasion, or a solitary tumor more than 2 cm in greatest dimension without vascular invasion
T3 Solitary tumor more than 2 cm in greatest dimension with vascular invasion, or multiple tumors limited to one lobe, none more than 2 cm in greatest dimension, with vascular invasion, or multiple tumors limited to one lobe, any more than 2 cm in greatest dimension, with or without vascular invasion
T4 Multiple tumors in more than one lobe or tumor(s) involve(s) a major branch of the portal or hepatic vein(s) or invasion of adjacent organs other than the gallbladder or perforation of the visceral peritoneum

Regional Lymph Nodes (N)

NX Regional lymph nodes cannot be assessed
N0 No regional lymph node metastasis
N1 Regional lymph node metastasis

Distant Metastasis (M)

MX Distant metastasis cannot be assessed
M0 No distant metastasis
M1 Distant metastasis

STAGE GROUPING

Stage I	T1	N0	M0
Stage II	T2	N0	M0
Stage IIIA	T3	N0	M0
Stage IIIB	T1	N1	M0
	T2	N1	M0
	T3	N1	M0
Stage IVA	T4	Any N	M0
Stage IVB	Any T	Any N	M1

HISTOPATHOLOGIC TYPE

The staging system applies only to primary carcinomas of the liver. These include hepatomas or hepatocellular carcinomas and intrahepatic bile duct carcinomas or cholangiocarcinomas, bile duct cystadenocarcinomas, and mixed types. Hepatomas are by far the most common. The classification does not apply to sarcomas or to metastatic tumors. The histologic type should be recorded, since it may contain prognostic information.

HISTOLOGIC GRADE (G)

The grading scheme of Edmondson and Steiner is recommended. The system employs four grades.

GX Grade cannot be assessed
G1 Well differentiated
G2 Moderately differentiated
G3 Poorly differentiated
G4 Undifferentiated

PROGNOSTIC FACTORS

This includes preceding liver disease, such as cirrhosis, and invasion of the portal vein. Positive surgical margins is another adverse prognostic factor in resected cases. Long-term outcome indicators include portal involvement, number of tumors in the liver, and serum alphafetoprotein level.

BIBLIOGRAPHY

Akashi Y, Koreeda C, Enomoto S, et al: Prognosis of unresectable hepatocellular carcinoma: an evaluation based on multivariate analysis of 90 cases. Hepatology 14:262–268, 1991

Asemia R, Shimizu K, Ii T, Yagi M, et al: Prognostic factors of hepatocellular carcinoma in patients undergoing hepatic resection. Gastroenterology 106:720–727, 1994

Bartok I, Remenar E, Toth J, et al: Clinicopathological studies of liver cirrhosis and hepatocellular carcinoma in a general hospital. Hum Pathol 12:794–803, 1981

Chuong JJ, Livstone EM, Barwick KW: The histopathologic and clinical indicators of prognosis in hepatoma. J Clin Gastroenterol 4:547–552, 1982

Craig JR, Peters RL, Edmondson HA: Tumors of liver and intrahepatic bile ducts, Fascicle 26, Second Series. Washington D.C.: Armed Forces Institute of Pathology, 1989

Edmondson HA, Steiner PE: Primary carcinoma of the liver. Cancer 7:462–503, 1954

Haratake J, Takeda S, Kasai T, et al: Predictable factors for estimating prognosis of patients after resection of hepatocellular carcinoma. Cancer 72: 1178–1183, 1993

Ishak KG, Anthony PP, Sobin LH: Histological typing of tumours of the liver. WHO international classification of tumours. Geneva: World Health Organization, 1994

Kenmochi K, Sugihara S, Kojiro M: Relationship of histologic grade of hepatocellular carcinoma (HCC) to tumor size, and demonstration of tumor cells of multiple different grades in single small HCC. Liver 7:18–26, 1987

Liver Cancer Study Group of Japan: Predictive factors for long-term prognosis after partial hepatectomy for patients with hepatocellular carcinoma in Japan. Cancer 74:2772–2780, 1994

Okuda K, Peters RL (Eds): Hepatocellular carcinoma. New York: Wiley Publications, 1976

Schaff Z, Lapis K, Henson DE: Liver. In Henson DE, Albores-Saavedra J (Eds.), The pathology of incipient neoplasia, 2nd ed. Philadelphia: WB Saunders, 1993

Sutton FM, Russell NC, Guinee VF, et al: Factors affecting the prognosis of primary liver carcinoma. J Clin Oncol 6:321–328, 1988

Wittekind C: Hepatocellular carcinoma. In Hermanek P, Gospodarowicz MK, Henson DE, et al (Eds.), Prognostic factors in cancer. Berlin: Springer-Verlag, 1995

Yamanaka N, Okamoto E, Oriyama T, et al: A prediction scoring system to select the surgical treatment of liver cancer. Further refinement based on 10 years of use. Ann Surg 219:342–346, 1994

Data Form for Cancer Staging

Patient identification
Name ____
Address ____
Hospital or clinic number ____
Age ____ Sex ____ Race ____

Institution identification
Hospital or clinic ____
Address ____

Oncology Record

Anatomic site of cancer ____
Histologic type ____
Grade (G) ____
Date of classification ____

DEFINITIONS

Primary Tumor (T)

Clin	Path		
[ ]	[ ]	TX	Primary tumor cannot be assessed
[ ]	[ ]	T0	No evidence of primary tumor
[ ]	[ ]	T1	Solitary tumor 2 cm or less in greatest dimension without vascular invasion
[ ]	[ ]	T2	Solitary tumor 2 cm or less in greatest dimension with vascular invasion, or multiple tumors limited to one lobe none more than 2 cm in greatest dimension without vascular invasion, or a solitary tumor more than 2 cm in greatest dimension without vascular invasion
[ ]	[ ]	T3	Solitary tumor more than 2 cm in greatest dimension with vascular invasion, or multiple tumors limited to one lobe, none more than 2 cm in greatest dimension, with vascular invasion, or multiple tumors limited to one lobe, any more than 2 cm in greatest dimension, with or without vascular invasion
[ ]	[ ]	T4	Multiple tumors in more than one lobe or tumor(s) involve(s) a major branch of portal or hepatic vein(s) or invasion of adjacent organs other than the gallbladder or perforation of the visceral peritoneum

Regional Lymph Nodes (N)

Clin	Path		
[ ]	[ ]	NX	Regional lymph nodes cannot be assessed
[ ]	[ ]	N0	No regional lymph node metastasis
[ ]	[ ]	N1	Regional lymph node metastasis

Distant Metastasis (M)

Clin	Path		
[ ]	[ ]	MX	Distant metastasis cannot be assessed
[ ]	[ ]	M0	No distant metastasis
[ ]	[ ]	M1	Distant metastasis

Stage Grouping

Clin	Path	Stage	T	N	M
[ ]	[ ]	I	T1	N0	M0
[ ]	[ ]	II	T2	N0	M0
[ ]	[ ]	IIIA	T3	N0	M0
[ ]	[ ]	IIIB	T1	N1	M0
			T2	N1	M0
			T3	N1	M0
[ ]	[ ]	IVA	T4	Any N	M0
[ ]	[ ]	IVB	Any T	Any N	M1

Histopathologic Grade (G)

[ ]	GX	Grade cannot be assessed
[ ]	G1	Well differentiated
[ ]	G2	Moderately differentiated
[ ]	G3	Poorly differentiated
[ ]	G4	Undifferentiated

Illustration

Indicate on diagram primary tumor and regional nodes involved.

Histopathologic Type

The staging system applies only to primary carcinomas of the liver. These include hepatomas or hepatocellular carcinomas and intrahepatic bile duct carcinomas or cholangiocarcinomas, bile duct cystadenocarcinomas, and mixed types. Hepatomas are by far the most common. The classification does not apply to sarcomas or to metastatic tumors. The histologic type should be recorded, since it may contain prognostic information.

Staged by ____ M.D.
____ Registrar

Date ____

15

Gallbladder

(Carcinoid tumors and sarcomas are not included.)

C23.9 Gallbladder

ANATOMY

Cancers of the gallbladder are staged according to their depth of penetration and extent of spread. These cancers frequently spread to the liver, which is involved in 70% of patients at the time of surgical evaluation. Malignant tumors of the gallbladder are insidious in their growth, often metastasizing early before a diagnosis is made. This proclivity for early spread before the appearance of signs and symptoms includes all carcinomas known to occur in the gallbladder. Tumors can also perforate the wall of the gallbladder eventually causing intra-abdominal metastases, carcinomatosis, and ascites. Because gallbladder cancer is uncommon and usually diagnosed late, physicians have tended to ignore anatomic staging, even though its importance for survival, management, and prognosis has been emphasized. Many cases are not suspected clinically and are first discovered at laparotomy or incidentally by the pathologist. More than 75% of carcinomas of the gallbladder are associated with cholelithiasis. Survival correlates with the extent of tumor.

Primary Site. The gallbladder is a pear-shaped saccular organ located under the liver in the gallbladder fossa. It has three parts: a fundus, a body, and a neck that tapers into the cystic duct. The wall of the gallbladder is much thinner than that of the intestine, lacking a circular and transverse muscle layer. The wall has a mucosa, that is, an epithelial lining and lamina propria, a smooth muscle layer analogous to the muscularis mucosae of the small intestine, perimuscular connective tissue, and serosa. In contrast to the intestine, there is no submucosa. Along the attachment to the liver, no serosa exists, and the perimuscular connective tissue is continuous with the interlobular connective tissue of the liver. Tumors that arise in the cystic duct are classified according to the scheme for the extrahepatic bile ducts.

Regional Lymph Nodes. The regional lymph nodes include the following:

Cystic duct
Pericholedochal
Hilar
Celiac
Periduodenal
Periportal
Peripancreatic
Superior mesenteric

The hilar nodes include those along the inferior vena cava, hepatic artery, portal vein, and hepatic pedicle. For pN, histologic examination of a regional lymphadenectomy specimen will ordinarily include 3 or more lymph nodes.

Peripancreatic nodes located along the body and tail of the pancreas are sites of distant metastasis.

Metastatic Sites. Cancers of the gallbladder usually metastasize to the lungs, pleura, diaphragm, and intra-abdominally. Any site can be involved.

RULES FOR CLASSIFICATION

Gallbladder cancers are staged primarily on the basis of surgical exploration or resection. Many *in situ* and early stage carcinomas are not recognized grossly. They are usually staged pathologically after histologic examination of the resected specimen.

The T classification depends on the depth of tumor penetration into the wall of the gallbladder, extent of invasion into the liver, and the number of adjacent organs involved. The liver is not considered a metastatic (M) site. Tumor confined to the gallbladder is classified either T1 or T2 depending on the depth of invasion.

To separate N1 from N2, the lymph nodes must be specifically identified.

Clinical Staging. Clinical evaluation usually depends on the results of ultrasound and computed tomography. It may also be the result of surgical exploration.

Pathologic Staging. Staging is based on examination of the resected specimen.

DEFINITION OF TNM

Primary Tumor (T)

TX Primary tumor cannot be assessed
T0 No evidence of primary tumor
Tis Carcinoma *in situ*
T1 Tumor invades lamina propria or muscle layer
  T1a Tumor invades lamina propria
  T1b Tumor invades muscle layer
T2 Tumor invades perimuscular connective tissue; no extension beyond serosa or into liver
T3 Tumor perforates the serosa (visceral peritoneum) or directly invades one adjacent organ, or both (extension 2 cm or less into liver)
T4 Tumor extends more than 2 cm into liver, and/or into two or more adjacent organs (stomach, duodenum, colon, pancreas, omentum, extrahepatic bile ducts, any involvement of liver)

Regional Lymph Nodes (N)

NX Regional lymph nodes cannot be assessed
N0 No regional lymph node metastasis
N1 Metastasis in cystic duct, pericholedochal, and/or hilar lymph nodes (i.e., in the hepatoduodenal ligament)
N2 Metastasis in peripancreatic (head only), periduodenal, periportal, celiac, and/or superior mesenteric lymph nodes

Distant Metastasis (M)

MX Distant metastasis cannot be assessed
M0 No distant metastasis
M1 Distant metastasis

STAGE GROUPING

Stage 0	Tis	N0	M0
Stage I	T1	N0	M0
Stage II	T2	N0	M0
Stage III	T1	N1	M0
	T2	N1	M0
	T3	N0	M0
	T3	N1	M0
Stage IVA	T4	N0	M0
	T4	N1	M0
Stage IVB	Any T	N2	M0
	Any T	Any N	M1

HISTOPATHOLOGIC TYPE

The staging system applies only to primary carcinomas of the gallbladder. It does not apply to carcinoid tumors or to sarcomas. Adenocarcinomas are the most common histologic type. More than 98% of gallbladder cancers are carcinomas. The carcinomas are listed below.

Carcinoma *in situ*
Adenocarcinoma, NOS
Papillary carcinoma
Adenocarcinoma, intestinal type
Clear cell adenocarcinoma
Mucinous carcinoma
Signet ring cell carcinoma
Squamous cell carcinoma
Adenosquamous carcinoma
Small cell carcinoma*
Undifferentiated carcinoma*
  Spindle and giant cell type
  Small cell type
Carcinoma, NOS
Carcinosarcoma
Other (specify)

*Grade 4 by definition

HISTOLOGIC GRADE (G)

GX Grade cannot be assessed
G1 Well differentiated
G2 Moderately differentiated
G3 Poorly differentiated
G4 Undifferentiated

PROGNOSTIC FACTORS

The prognostic factors include histologic type, histologic grade, and vascular invasion. Papillary carcinomas have the most favorable prognosis. Unfavorable histologic types include small cell carcinomas and undifferentiated carcinomas. Lymphatic and/or blood vessel invasion indicates a less favorable outcome. Histologic grade correlates with outcome.

BIBLIOGRAPHY

Albores-Saavedra J, Cruz-Ortiz H, Alcantara-Vazquez A, et al: Unusual types of gallbladder carcinoma. Arch Pathol Lab Med 105:287–293, 1981

Albores-Saavedra J, Henson DE: Tumors of the gallbladder and extrahepatic bile ducts. Atlas of tumor pathology, Fascicle 22, Second Series. Washington, D.C.: Armed Forces Institute of Pathology, 1986

Albores-Saavedra J, Henson DE, Sobin LH: Histological typing of tumours of the gallbladder and extrahepatic bile ducts. WHO international histological classification of tumours. Berlin: Springer-Verlag, 1991

Bergdahl L: Gallbladder carcinoma first diagnosed at microscopic examination of gallbladder removed for presumed benign disease. Ann Surg 191:19–22, 1980

Bivins BA, Meeker WR Jr, Griffen WO Jr: Importance of histologic classification of carcinoma of the gallbladder. Ann Surg 41:121–124, 1975

Fahim RB, McDonald JR, Richards JC, et al: Carcinoma of the gallbladder: a study of its modes of spread. Ann Surg 156:114–124, 1962

Friedman RB, Anderson RE, Gilchrest KW, Carbone PP: Prognostic factors in invasive gallbladder carcinoma. J Surg Oncol 23:189–194, 1983

Guo K-J, Yamaguchi K, Enjoji M: Undifferentiated carcinoma of the gallbladder. A clinicopathologic, histochemical, and immunohistochemical study of 21 patients with a poor prognosis. Cancer 61:1872–1879, 1988

Henson DE, Albores-Saavedra J, Corle D: Carcinoma of the gallbladder: histologic types, stage of disease, grade, and survival rates. Cancer 70:1493–1497, 1992

Hisatomi K, Haratake J, Horie A, et al: Relation of histopathological features to prognosis of gallbladder cancer. Am J Gastroenterol 85:567–572, 1990

Jones RS: Carcinoma of the gallbladder. Surg Clin N Amer 70:1419–1428, 1990

Nevin JE, Moran TJ, Day S, et al: Carcinoma of the gallbladder: staging, treatment, and prognosis. Cancer 37:141–148, 1976

Ogura Y, Mizumoto R, Isaji S, et al: Radical operations for carcinoma of the gallbladder: present status in Japan. World J Surg 15:337–343, 1991

Ohtani T, Shirai Y, Tsukada K, et al: Carcinoma of the gallbladder: CT evaluation of lymphatic spread. Radiology 189:875–880, 1993

Ouchi K, Owada Y, Matsuno S, et al: Prognostic factors in the surgical treatment of gallbladder carcinoma. Surg 101:736–737, 1987

Perpetuo MMO, Valdivieso M, Heilbrun LK, et al: Natural history study of gallbladder cancer. Cancer 42:330–335, 1978

Shirai Y, Tsukada K, Ohtani T, et al: Hepatic metastases from carcinoma of the gallbladder. Cancer 75:2063–2068, 1995

Shirai Y, Yoshida K, Tsukada K, et al: Identification of the regional lymphatic system of the gallbladder by vital staining. Br J Surg 79:659–662, 1992

Wanebo HJ, Castle WN, Fechner R: Is carcinoma of the gallbladder a curable lesion? Ann Surg 195:624–630, 1982

Yamamoto M, Nakajo S, Tahara E: Carcinoma of the gallbladder: the correlation between histogenesis and prognosis. Virchows Arch [A] 414:83–90, 1989

Data Form for Cancer Staging

Patient identification
Name ____________________
Address ____________________
Hospital or clinic number ____________________
Age ______ Sex ______ Race ____________________

Institution identification
Hospital or clinic ____________________
Address ____________________

Oncology Record

Anatomic site of cancer ____________________
Histologic type ____________________
Grade (G) ____________________
Date of classification ____________________

DEFINITIONS

Primary Tumor (T)

Clin	Path		
[ ]	[ ]	TX	Primary tumor cannot be assessed
[ ]	[ ]	T0	No evidence of primary tumor
[ ]	[ ]	Tis	Carcinoma *in situ*
[ ]	[ ]	T1	Tumor invades lamina propria or muscle layer
[ ]	[ ]	T1a	Tumor invades lamina propria
[ ]	[ ]	T1b	Tumor invades muscle layer
[ ]	[ ]	T2	Tumor invades perimuscular connective tissue; no extension beyond serosa or into liver
[ ]	[ ]	T3	Tumor perforates the serosa (visceral peritoneum) or directly invades one adjacent organ, or both (extension 2 cm or less into liver)
[ ]	[ ]	T4	Tumor extends more than 2 cm into liver, and/or into two or more adjacent organs (stomach, duodenum, colon, pancreas, omentum, extrahepatic bile ducts, any involvement of liver)

Regional Lymph Nodes (N)

Clin	Path		
[ ]	[ ]	NX	Regional lymph nodes cannot be assessed
[ ]	[ ]	N0	No regional lymph node metastasis
[ ]	[ ]	N1	Metastasis in cystic duct, pericholedochal, and/or hilar lymph nodes (i.e., in hepatoduodenal ligament)
[ ]	[ ]	N2	Metastasis in peripancreatic (head only), periduodenal, periportal, celiac, and/or superior mesenteric lymph nodes

Distant Metastasis (M)

Clin	Path		
[ ]	[ ]	MX	Distant metastasis cannot be assessed
[ ]	[ ]	M0	No distant metastasis
[ ]	[ ]	M1	Distant metastasis

Stage Grouping

Clin	Path	Stage	T	N	M
[ ]	[ ]	0	Tis	N0	M0
[ ]	[ ]	I	T1	N0	M0
[ ]	[ ]	II	T2	N0	M0
[ ]	[ ]	III	T1	N1	M0
			T2	N1	M0
			T3	N0	M0
			T3	N1	M0
[ ]	[ ]	IVA	T4	N0	M0
			T4	N1	M0
[ ]	[ ]	IVB	Any T	N2	M0
			Any T	Any N	M1

Staged by ____________________ M.D.
____________________ Registrar
Date ____________________

(continued on next page)

Histopathologic Type

The staging system applies only to primary carcinomas of the gallbladder. It does not apply to carcinoid tumors or to sarcomas. Adenocarcinomas are the most common histologic type. More than 98% of gallbladder cancers are carcinomas. The carcinomas are listed below.

Carcinoma *in situ*
Adenocarcinoma, NOS
Papillary carcinoma
Adenocarcinoma, intestinal type
Clear cell adenocarcinoma
Mucinous carcinoma
Signet ring cell carcinoma
Squamous cell carcinoma
Adenosquamous carcinoma
Small cell carcinoma*
Undifferentiated carcinoma*
  Spindle and giant cell type
  Small cell type
Carcinoma, NOS
Carcinosarcoma
Other (specify)

* *Grade 4 by definition*

Histopathologic Grade (G)

[ ] GX Grade cannot be assessed
[ ] G1 Well differentiated
[ ] G2 Moderately differentiated
[ ] G3 Poorly differentiated
[ ] G4 Undifferentiated

Illustration

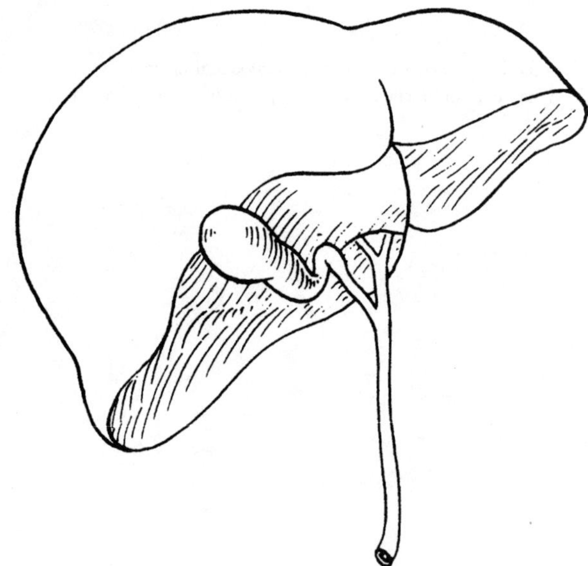

Indicate on diagram primary tumor and regional nodes involved.

16

Extrahepatic Bile Ducts

(Sarcomas and carcinoid tumors are not included.)

C24.0 Extrahepatic bile duct
C24.8 Overlapping lesion
C24.9 Biliary tract, NOS

Malignant tumors can develop anywhere along the extrahepatic bile ducts. Nearly 50% occur in the upper third, 25% in the middle third, and 20% in the lower third. In 10% of cases, the ducts are diffusely involved. Carcinomas that arise in the upper third near the hepatic hilum are associated with a worse prognosis because of direct extension to the liver. Furthermore, tumors that develop near the hilum are more difficult to resect than those arising in the lower segments of the biliary tree. Malignant tumors that originate in the right or left hepatic ducts are often described as hilar carcinomas of the liver. All malignant tumors inevitably cause partial or complete obstruction of the extrahepatic bile ducts. Because the bile ducts have a small diameter, the signs and symptoms of obstruction usually occur while the tumor is relatively small. Extrahepatic bile duct carcinomas often arise in choledochal cysts (congenital cystic dilatation).

This TNM classification applies only to cancers arising in the extrahepatic bile ducts and in the cystic duct. It does not include those arising in the ampulla of Vater or in the pancreatic ducts. It does apply to malignant tumors that develop in congenital choledochal cysts. For staging, tumors arising in the distal segment of the common bile duct should be separated from those that originate in the pancreatic duct or in the ampulla of Vater.

ANATOMY

Primary Site. Emerging from the transverse fissure of the liver are the right and left hepatic bile ducts, which join to form the common hepatic duct. The cystic duct which connects to the gallbladder joins the common hepatic duct to form the common bile duct which passes posterior to the first part of the duodenum, traverses the head of the pancreas, and then enters the second part of the duodenum through the ampulla of Vater. Histologically, the bile ducts are lined by a single layer of tall uniform columnar cells. The mucosa usually forms irregular pleats or small longitudinal folds. The wall of the bile duct has a layer of subepithelial connective tissue and surrounding muscle fibers. It should be noted that the muscle fibers are most prominent in the distal segment of the common bile duct. More proximally, the muscle fibers are sparse and the wall of the bile duct largely consists of fibrous tissue.

Regional Lymph Nodes. The regional nodes are the same as listed for the gallbladder, but also include those located near the duodenum and head of the pancreas. They include the following:

Cystic
Hilar

Superior mesenteric
Periduodenal
Posterior pancreaticoduodenal
Peripancreatic
Periportal
Pericholedochal
Celiac

Hilar nodes include those along the inferior vena cava, hepatic artery, portal vein, and hepatic pedicle. For pN, histologic examination of a regional lymphadenectomy specimen will ordinarily include 3 or more lymph nodes.

Involvement of other lymph nodes is considered distant metastasis and should be coded M1. Parapancreatic nodes located along the body and tail of the pancreas are also considered sites of distant metastasis.

Metastatic Sites. Carcinomas can extend to the liver, pancreas, ampulla of Vater, duodenum, colon, omentum, stomach, or gallbladder. Tumors arising in the right or left hepatic ducts usually extend proximally into the liver or distal to the common hepatic duct. Neoplasms from the cystic duct invade the gallbladder or the common bile duct, or both. Carcinomas that arise in the distal segment of the common duct can spread to the pancreas, duodenum, stomach, colon, or omentum. Distant metastases usually occur late in the course of the disease, most often to the lungs.

RULES FOR CLASSIFICATION

Most patients are staged following surgery and pathologic examination of the resected specimen. Evaluation of the extent of disease is most important for staging and for prognosis. The same rules apply to carcinomas arising in choledochal cysts. Invasion of perifibromuscular tissue, that is, tissue beyond the confines of the bile duct is classified T2. Invasion of the hepatic artery or portal vein is classified T3.

Clinical Staging. Evaluating the extent of disease depends on imaging, which often defines the limits of the tumor.

Pathologic Staging. Pathologic staging is based on surgical exploration with pathologic examination of the resected specimen. In some cases, it may be difficult for the surgeon to completely resect the tumor.

DEFINITION OF TNM

Primary Tumor (T)

TX Primary tumor cannot be assessed
T0 No evidence of primary tumor
Tis Carcinoma *in situ*
T1 Tumor invades subepithelial connective tissue or fibromuscular layer
 T1a Tumor invades subepithelial connective tissue
 T1b Tumor invades fibromusclar layer
T2 Tumor invades perifibromuscular connective tissue
T3 Tumor invades adjacent structures: liver, pancreas, duodenum, gallbladder, colon, stomach

Regional Lymph Nodes (N)

NX Regional lymph nodes cannot be assessed
N0 No regional lymph node metastasis
N1 Metastasis in cystic duct, pericholedochal and/or hilar lymph nodes (i.e., in the hepatoduodenal ligament)
N2 Metastasis in peripancreatic (head only), periduodenal, periportal, celiac, and/or superior mesenteric and/or posterior pancreaticoduodenal lymph nodes

Distant Metastasis (M)

MX Distant metastasis cannot be assessed
M0 No distant metastasis
M1 Distant metastasis

STAGE GROUPING

Stage 0	Tis	N0	M0
Stage I	T1	N0	M0
Stage II	T2	N0	M0
Stage III	T1	N1	M0
	T1	N2	M0
	T2	N1	M0
	T2	N2	M0
Stage IVA	T3	Any N	M0
Stage IVB	Any T	Any N	M1

HISTOPATHOLOGIC TYPE

The staging system applies to all carcinomas that arise in the extrahepatic bile ducts or in the cystic duct. Sarcomas and carcinoid tumors are excluded. Adenocarcinoma, NOS is the most common histologic type. Carcinomas account for more than 98% of cancers of the extrahepatic bile ducts. The histologic types include:

Carcinoma *in situ*
Adenocarcinoma, NOS
Adenocarcinoma, intestinal type

Clear cell adenocarcinoma
Mucinous carcinoma
Signet ring cell carcinoma
Squamous cell carcinoma
Adenosquamous carcinoma
Small cell carcinoma*
Undifferentiated carcinoma*
  Spindle and giant cell type
  Small cell type
Papillomatosis
Papillary carcinoma, noninvasive
Papillary carcinoma, invasive
Carcinoma, NOS
Other (specify)

*Grade 4 by definition

HISTOLOGIC GRADE (G)

GX Grade cannot be assessed
G1 Well differentiated
G2 Moderately differentiated
G3 Poorly differentiated
G4 Undifferentiated

PROGNOSTIC FACTORS

Several prognostic factors based on the pathologic characteristics of the primary tumor have been reported for carcinomas of the extrahepatic bile ducts. These include histologic type, histologic grade, blood vessel or lymphatic vessel invasion, and perineural invasion. Papillary carcinomas have a more favorable outcome than other types of carcinoma. Histologic grade is associated with outcome. High grade tumors (grades 3-4) have a less favorable outcome than low grade tumors (grades 1-2). Involvement of the surgical margins should also be considered an important prognostic factor. Residual tumor (R) classification should be reported if the margins are involved.

BIBLIOGRAPHY

Albores-Saavedra J, Henson DE: Tumors of the gallbladder and extrahepatic bile ducts. Atlas of tumor pathology, Fascicle 22, Second Series. Washington, D.C.: Armed Forces Institute of Pathology, 1986

Albores-Saavedra J, Henson DE, Sobin LH: Histological typing of tumours of the gallbladder and extrahepatic bile ducts. WHO international histological classification of tumours. Berlin: Springer-Verlag, 1991

Bhuiya MMR, Nimura Y, Kamiya J, et al: Clinicopathologic factors influencing survival of patients with bile duct carcinoma: multivariate statistical analysis. World J Surg 17:653–657, 1993

Bhuiya MMR, Nimura Y, Kamiya J, et al. Clinicopathologic studies on perineural invasion of bile duct carcinoma. Ann Surg 215:344–349, 1992

Braasch JW, Warren KW, Kune GA: Malignant neoplasms of the bile ducts. Surg Clin North Am 47:627–638, 1967

Hayashi S, Miyazaki M, Kondo Y, et al: Invasive growth patterns of hepatic hilar ductal carcinoma. A histologic analysis of 18 surgical cases. Cancer 73:2922–2929, 1994

Henson DE, Albores-Saavedra J, Corle D: Carcinoma of the extrahepatic bile ducts: histologic types, stage of disease, grade, and survival. Cancer 70:1498–1501, 1992

Kayahara M, Nagakawa T, Tsukioka Y, et al: Neural invasion and nodal involvement in distal bile duct cancer. Hepatogastroenterology 41:190–194, 1994

Kayahara M, Nagakawa T, Ueno K, et al: Lymphatic flow in carcinoma of the distal bile duct based on a clinicopathologic study. Cancer 72:2112–2117, 1993

Longmire WP Jr, McArthur MS, Bastounis EA, et al: Carcinoma of the extrahepatic biliary tract. Ann Surg 178:333–345, 1973

Ogura Y, Takahashi K, Tabata M, et al: Clinicopathological study on carcinoma of the extrahepatic bile-duct with special focus on cancer invasion on the surgical margins. World J Surg 18:778–784, 1994

Ouchi K, Suzuki M, Hashimoto L, Sato T. Histologic findings and prognostic factors in carcinoma of the upper bile duct. Am J Surg 157:552–556, 1989

Suzuki M, Takahashi T, Ouchi K, et al: The development and extension of hepatohilar bile duct carcinoma. A three-dimensional tumor mapping in the intrahepatic biliary tree visualized with the aid of a graphics computer system. Cancer 64:658–666, 1989

Tamada K, Ido K, Ueno N, et al: Preoperative staging of extrahepatic bile duct cancer with intraductal ultrasonography. Am J Gastroenterol 90:239–246, 1995

Tio TL, Cheng J, Wijers OB, et al: Endosonographic TNM staging of extrahepatic bile duct cancer: comparison with pathological staging. Gastroenterology 100(Pt 1):1351–1361, 1991

Tio TL, Wijers OB, Sars PR, et al: Preoperative TNM classification of proximal extrahepatic bile duct carcinoma by endosonography. Semin Liver Dis 10:114–120, 1990

Tompkins RK, Saunders K, Roslyn JJ, et al: Changing patterns in diagnosis and management of bile duct cancer. Ann Surg 211:614–620, 1990

Tompkins RK, Thomas D, Wile A, et al: Prognostic factors in bile duct carcinoma. Ann Surg 194:447–455, 1981

Tsunoda T, Eto T, Koga M, et al: Early carcinoma of the extrahepatic bile duct. Jpn J Surg 19:691–698, 1989

Yamaguchi K. Early bile duct carcinoma. Aust N Z J Surg 62:525–529, 1992

Data Form for Cancer Staging

Patient identification
Name ______
Address ______
Hospital or clinic number ______
Age ____ Sex ____ Race ______

Institution identification
Hospital or clinic ______
Address ______

Oncology Record

Anatomic site of cancer ______
Histologic type ______
Grade (G) ______
Date of classification ______

DEFINITIONS

Primary Tumor (T)

Clin	Path		
[ ]	[ ]	TX	Primary tumor cannot be assessed
[ ]	[ ]	T0	No evidence of primary tumor
[ ]	[ ]	Tis	Carcinoma *in situ*
[ ]	[ ]	T1	Tumor invades subepithelial connective tissue or fibromuscular layer
[ ]	[ ]	T1a	Tumor invades subepithelial connective tissue
[ ]	[ ]	T1b	Tumor invades fibromuscular layer
[ ]	[ ]	T2	Tumor invades perifibromuscular connective tissue
[ ]	[ ]	T3	Tumor invades adjacent structure(s), liver, pancreas, duodenum, gallbladder, colon, stomach

Regional Lymph Nodes (N)

Clin	Path		
[ ]	[ ]	NX	Regional lymph nodes cannot be assessed
[ ]	[ ]	N0	No regional lymph node metastasis
[ ]	[ ]	N1	Metastasis in cystic duct, pericholedochal and/or hilar lymph nodes (i.e., in the hepatoduodenal ligament)
[ ]	[ ]	N2	Metastasis in peripancreatic (head only), periduodenal, periportal, celiac, and/or superior mesenteric and/or posterior pancreatic duodenal lymph nodes

Distant Metastasis (M)

Clin	Path		
[ ]	[ ]	MX	Distant metastasis cannot be assessed
[ ]	[ ]	M0	No distant metastasis
[ ]	[ ]	M1	Distant metastasis

Stage Grouping

Clin	Path	Stage	T	N	M
[ ]	[ ]	0	Tis	N0	M0
[ ]	[ ]	I	T1	N0	M0
[ ]	[ ]	II	T2	N0	M0
[ ]	[ ]	III	T1	N1	M0
			T1	N2	M0
			T2	N1	M0
			T2	N2	M0
[ ]	[ ]	IVA	T3	Any N	M0
[ ]	[ ]	IVB	Any T	Any N	M1

Staged by ______ M.D.
______ Registrar
Date ______

Histopathologic Grade (G)

[ ] GX Grade cannot be assessed
[ ] G1 Well differentiated
[ ] G2 Moderately differentiated
[ ] G3 Poorly differentiated
[ ] G4 Undifferentiated

Illustration

Upper third
Middle third
Lower third
Diffuse

Indicate on diagram primary tumor and regional nodes involved.

Histopathologic Types

The staging system applies to all carcinomas that arise in the extrahepatic bile ducts or in the cystic duct. Sarcomas and carcinoid tumors are excluded. Adenocarcinoma, NOS is the most common histologic type. Carcinomas account for more than 98% of cancers of the extrahepatic bile ducts. The histologic types include:

Carcinoma *in situ*
Adenocarcinoma, NOS
Adenocarcinoma, intestinal type
Clear cell adenocarcinoma
Mucinous carcinoma
Signet ring cell carcinoma
Squamous cell carcinoma
Adenosquamous carcinoma
Small cell carcinoma*
Undifferentiated carcinoma*
  Spindle and giant cell type
  Small cell type
  Papillomatosis
  Papillary carcinoma, noninvasive
  Papillary carcinoma, invasive
  Carcinoma, NOS
  Other (specify)

* *Grade 4 by definition*

17

Ampulla of Vater

(Carcinoid tumors and other neuroendocrine tumors are not included.)

C24.1 Ampulla of Vater

The ampulla of Vater is strategically located at the confluence of the pancreatic and common bile ducts. Most tumors that arise in this small structure will obstruct the common bile duct, causing jaundice, abdominal pain, and occasionally pancreatitis. Clinically and pathologically, carcinomas of the ampulla may be difficult to differentiate from those arising in the head of the pancreas or in the distal segment of the common bile duct. Primary cancers of the ampulla are not common, although they comprise a high proportion of malignant tumors occurring in the duodenum. Tumors of the ampulla must be differentiated from those arising in the second part of the duodenum and invading the ampulla. Carcinomas of the ampulla and the periampullary region are often associated with the multiple polyposis syndrome.

ANATOMY

Primary Site. A small dilated duct, less than 1.5 cm in length, the ampulla is formed in most individuals by the union of the terminal segments of the pancreatic and common bile ducts. In 42% of individuals, however, the ampulla is the termination of the common duct only, the pancreatic duct having its own entrance into the duodenum adjacent to the ampulla. In these individuals, the ampulla may be difficult to locate or even nonexistent. The ampulla opens into the duodenum, usually on the posterior-medial wall, through a small mucosal elevation—the duodenal papilla, which is also called the papilla of Vater. Although carcinomas can arise in either the ampulla or on the papilla, they most commonly arise near the junction of the mucosa of the ampulla with that of the papilla. Nearly all cancers that arise in this area are well-differentiated adenocarcinomas. They have a variety of designations, for example: carcinoma of the ampulla of Vater; carcinoma of the periampullary portion of the duodenum; or carcinoma of the peripapillary portion of the duodenum. It may not be possible to determine the exact site of origin for large tumors.

Regional Lymph Nodes. The regional lymph nodes of the ampulla of Vater include:

Superior: Lymph nodes superior to the head and body of the pancreas
Inferior: Lymph nodes inferior to the head and body of the pancreas
Anterior: Anterior pancreaticoduodenal, pyloric and proximal mesenteric
Posterior: Posterior pancreaticoduodenal, common bile duct, and proximal mesenteric.

Other Regional Lymph Nodes:

Pancreaticoduodenal NOS
Peripancreatic
Infrapyloric
Hepatic
Subpyloric
Celiac

Superior mesenteric
Retroperitoneal
Lateral aortic

Regional metastases are most commonly found in the peripancreatic lymph nodes. For pN, histologic examination of a regional lymphadenectomy specimen will ordinarily include 10 or more regional lymph nodes. The splenic lymph nodes and those located at the tail of the pancreas are not considered regional; metastases in these nodes should be designated M1.

Metastatic Sites. Tumors of the ampulla can spread to almost every site. However, they usually infiltrate adjacent structures, such as the wall of the duodenum, head of the pancreas, and the extrahepatic bile ducts. Metastatic deposits are generally found in the liver, peritoneum, lungs, and pleura. Spread to distant sites usually occurs late in the course of the disease.

RULES FOR CLASSIFICATION

Most patients are staged pathologically after examination of the resected specimen. Classification is based primarily on local extension. The T classification depends on extension of the primary tumor through the ampulla or sphincter of Oddi into the duodenal wall or beyond into the head of the pancreas or contiguous soft tissue. If pancreatic invasion is present, the extent of invasion in centimeters must be known to separate T3 from T4. For T4, adjacent organs include the extrahepatic bile ducts and soft tissue.

Clinical Staging. Endoscopic ultrasonography and computed tomography are effective in the pre-operative staging and in evaluating resectability of ampullary carcinomas. Preoperative laparoscopy has been used to search for evidence of nonresectability.

Pathologic Staging. Staging depends on surgical resection and pathologic examination of the specimen and associated lymph nodes.

DEFINITION OF TNM

Primary Tumor (T)

TX Primary tumor cannot be assessed
T0 No evidence of primary tumor
Tis Carcinoma *in situ*
T1 Tumor limited to the ampulla of Vater or sphincter of Oddi
T2 Tumor invades duodenal wall
T3 Tumor invades 2 cm or less into the pancreas
T4 Tumor invades more than 2 cm into pancreas and/or into other adjacent organs

Regional Lymph Nodes (N)

NX Regional lymph nodes cannot be assessed
N0 No regional lymph node metastasis
N1 Regional lymph node metastasis

Distant Metastasis (M)

MX Distant metastasis cannot be assessed
M0 No distant metastasis
M1 Distant metastasis

STAGE GROUPING

Stage 0	Tis	N0	M0
Stage I	T1	N0	M0
Stage II	T2	N0	M0
	T3	N0	M0
Stage III	T1	N1	M0
	T2	N1	M0
	T3	N1	M0
Stage IV	T4	Any N	M0
	Any T	Any N	M1

HISTOPATHOLOGIC TYPE

The staging system applies to all primary carcinomas that arise in the ampulla or on the duodenal papilla. Adenocarcinomas are the most common histologic type. The classification does not apply to carcinoid tumors or to other neuroendocrine tumors.

Carcinoma *in situ*
Adenocarcinoma, NOS
Adenocarcinoma, intestinal type
Clear cell adenocarcinoma
Mucinous carcinoma
Signet ring cell carcinoma
Squamous cell carcinoma
Adenosquamous carcinoma
Small cell carcinoma*
Undifferentiated carcinoma*
  Spindle and giant cell type
  Small cell type
Papillomatosis
Papillary carcinoma, noninvasive
Papillary carcinoma, invasive
Carcinoma, NOS
Other (specify)

*Grade 4 by definition

HISTOLOGIC GRADE (G)

GX Grade cannot be assessed
G1 Well differentiated
G2 Moderately differentiated
G3 Poorly differentiated
G4 Undifferentiated

PROGNOSTIC FACTORS

Although tumor size is not part of the TNM classification, it has prognostic significance. Perineural invasion, ulceration, local extension, and histologic grade are also adverse prognostic factors. Papillary tumors have a better outcome than nonpapillary tumors.

BIBLIOGRAPHY

Allema JH, Reinders ME, van Gulik TM, et al: Prognostic factors for survival after pancreaticoduodenectomy for patients with carcinoma of the pancreatic head region. Cancer 75:2069–2076, 1995

Bakkevold KE, Kambestad B: Long-term survival following radical and palliative treatment of patients with carcinoma of the pancreas and papilla of Vater—the prognostic factors influencing the long-term results. A prospective mulitcentre study. Eur J Surg Oncol 19:147–161, 1993

Bakkevold KE, Kambestad B: Staging of carcinoma of the pancreas and ampulla of Vater. Tumor (T), lymph node (N), and distant metastasis (M) as prognostic factors. Int J Pancreatol 17:249–259, 1995

Cubilla AL, Fitzgerald PJ: Tumors of the exocrine pancreas. Atlas of tumor pathology, Second Series, Fascicle 19. Washington, D.C.: Armed Forces Institute of Pathology, 1984

Delcore R Jr, Connor CS, Thomas JH, et al: Significance of tumor spread in adenocarcinoma of the ampulla of Vater. Am J Surg 158:593–596, 1989

Griffanti-Bartoli F, Arnone GB, Ceppa P, et al: Malignant tumors in the head of the pancreas and the periampullary region, diagnostic and prognostic aspects. Anticancer Res 14:657–666, 1994

Klempnauer J, Ridder GJ, Bektas H, et al: Surgery for exocrine pancreatic cancer—who are the 5- and 10-year survivors? Oncology 52:353–359, 1995

Knox RA, Kingston RD: Carcinoma of the ampulla of Vater. Br J Surg 73:72–73, 1986

Makipour H, Cooperman A, Danzi JT, et al: Carcinoma of the ampulla of Vater. Ann Surg 183:341–344, 1976

Martin MF, Rossi RL, Dorucci V, et al: Clinical and pathologic correlations in patients with periampullary tumors. Arch Surg 125:723–726, 1990

Monson JRT, Donohue JH, McEntee GP, et al: Radical resection for carcinoma of the ampulla of Vater. Arch Surg 126:353–357, 1991

Mori K, Ikei S, Yamane T, et al: Pathological factors influencing survival of carcinoma of the ampulla of Vater. Eur J Surg Oncol 16:183–188, 1990

Neoptolemos JP, Talbot IC, Shaw DC, et al: Long-term survival after resection of ampullary carcinoma is associated independently with tumor grade and a new staging classification that assesses local invasiveness. Cancer 61:1403–1407, 1988

Shirai Y, Tsukada K, Ohtani T, et al: Carcinoma of the ampulla of Vater: histopathologic analysis to tumor spread in Whipple pancreatoduodenectomy specimens. World J Surg 19:102–107, 1995

Wise L, Pizzimbono C, Dehner IP: Periampullary cancer. Am J Surg 131:141–148, 1976

Yamaguchi K, Enjoji M: Carcinoma of the ampulla of Vater: a clinicopathologic study and pathologic staging of 109 cases of carcinoma and 5 cases of adenoma. Cancer 59:506–515, 1987

Yasuda K, Mukai H, Cho E, et al: The use of endoscopic ultrasonography in the diagnosis and staging of carcinoma of the papilla of Vater. Endoscopy 20(Suppl):218–222, 1988

Data Form for Cancer Staging

Patient identification
Name ______
Address ______
Hospital or clinic number ______
Age ______ Sex ______ Race ______

Institution identification
Hospital or clinic ______
Address ______

Oncology Record

Anatomic site of cancer ______
Histologic type ______
Grade (G) ______
Date of classification ______

DEFINITIONS

Primary Tumor (T)

Clin	Path		
[ ]	[ ]	TX	Primary tumor cannot be assessed
[ ]	[ ]	T0	No evidence of primary tumor
[ ]	[ ]	Tis	Carcinoma *in situ*
[ ]	[ ]	T1	Tumor limited to ampulla of Vater or sphincter of Oddi
[ ]	[ ]	T2	Tumor invades duodenal wall
[ ]	[ ]	T3	Tumor invades 2 cm or less into pancreas
[ ]	[ ]	T4	Tumor invades more than 2 cm into pancreas and/or into other adjacent organs

Regional Lymph Nodes (N)

Clin	Path		
[ ]	[ ]	NX	Regional lymph nodes cannot be assessed
[ ]	[ ]	N0	No regional lymph node metastasis
[ ]	[ ]	N1	Regional lymph node metastasis

Distant Metastasis (M)

Clin	Path		
[ ]	[ ]	MX	Distant metastasis cannot be assessed
[ ]	[ ]	M0	No distant metastasis
[ ]	[ ]	M1	Distant metastasis

Stage Grouping

Clin	Path	Stage	T	N	M
[ ]	[ ]	0	Tis	N0	M0
[ ]	[ ]	I	T1	N0	M0
[ ]	[ ]	II	T2	N0	M0
			T3	N0	M0
[ ]	[ ]	III	T1	N1	M0
			T2	N1	M0
			T3	N1	M0
[ ]	[ ]	IV	T4	Any N	M0
			Any T	Any N	M1

Staged by ______ M.D.
______ Registrar
Date ______

Histopathologic Grade (G)

[ ]	GX	Grade cannot be assessed
[ ]	G1	Well differentiated
[ ]	G2	Moderately differentiated
[ ]	G3	Poorly differentiated
[ ]	G4	Undifferentiated

Histopathologic Type

The staging system applies to all primary carcinomas that arise in the ampulla or on the duodenal papilla. Adenocarcinomas are the most common histologic type. The classification does not apply to carcinoid tumors or to other neuroendocrine tumors.

Carcinoma *in situ*
Adenocarcinoma, NOS
Adenocarcinoma, intestinal type
Clear cell adenocarcinoma
Mucinous carcinoma
Signet ring cell carcinoma
Squamous cell carcinoma
Adenosquamous carcinoma
Small cell carcinoma*
Undifferentiated carcinoma*
  Spindle and giant cell type
  Small cell type
Papillomatosis
Papillary carcinoma, noninvasive
Papillary carcinoma, invasive
Carcinoma, NOS
Other (specify)

** Grade 4 by definition*

18

Exocrine Pancreas

(Endocrine tumors arising from the islets of Langerhans and carcinoid tumors are not included.)

C25.0 Head
C25.1 Body
C25.2 Tail
C25.3 Pancreatic duct
C25.7 Other specified parts
C25.8 Overlapping lesion
C25.9 Pancreas, NOS

In the United States, pancreatic cancer is the third most common malignant tumor of the gastrointestinal tract and the fifth leading cause of cancer related mortality. The disease is often difficult to diagnose, especially in its early stages. Cancers of the exocrine pancreas are almost always fatal; nearly all patients die within 2 years following diagnosis. Most cancers arise in the head of the pancreas, eventually causing bile duct obstruction, pain, and clinical jaundice. Cancers arising in either the body or tail of the pancreas are insidious in their development and often far advanced when first detected. Most cancers are adenocarcinomas that usually originate from the pancreatic ducts. Surgical resection remains the only potentially curative approach. The TNM classification does not apply to endocrine tumors. Staging depends on the size and extent of the primary tumor.

ANATOMY

Primary Site. The pancreas is a long, coarsely lobulated gland that lies transversely across the posterior abdomen. It is located retroperitoneally lying in the concavity of the duodenum on its right and touching the spleen with its tail on the left. The shape of the pancreas is often compared to the letter "J" turned sideways. The organ is divided into a head with a small uncinate process, a neck, body, and tail. Anteriorly the body is in direct relation with the stomach and posteriorly with the aorta, splenic veins, and left kidney. The tail is usually in contact with the spleen.

Regional Lymph Nodes. A rich lymphatic network surrounds the pancreas with left splenic and superior and inferior right side truncal drainage. For pN, histologic examination of a regional lymphadenectomy specimen will ordinarily include 10 or more regional lymph nodes. The regional lymph nodes are the peripancreatic which are divided as follows:

Superior: Lymph nodes superior to the head and body of the pancreas
Inferior: Lymph nodes inferior to the head and body of the pancreas
Anterior: Anterior pancreaticoduodenal, pyloric, and proximal mesenteric lymph nodes

Posterior: Posterior pancreaticoduodenal, common bile duct or pericholedochal, and proximal mesenteric nodes
Splenic: Hilum of the spleen and tail of the pancreas (for tumors in the body and tail only)

The following lymph nodes are considered regional:

Peripancreatic (superior, inferior, anterior, posterior)
Hepatic artery
Infrapyloric (for tumors in the head only)
Subpyloric (for tumors in the head only)
Celiac (for tumors in the head only)
Superior mesenteric
Pancreaticolienal (for tumors in the body and tail only)
Splenic (for tumors in the body and tail only)
Retroperitoneal
Lateral aortic

Involvement of other nodal groups is considered distant metastasis.

Metastatic Sites. Distant spread occurs primarily to the liver and to the lungs. Other sites can also be involved including bones.

DEFINITION OF LOCATION

Tumors of the head of the pancreas are those arising to the right of the left border of the superior mesenteric vein. The uncinate process is part of the head.

Tumors of the body of the pancreas are those arising between the left border of the superior mesenteric vein and the left border of the aorta.

Tumors of the tail of the pancreas are those arising between the left border of the aorta and the hilum of the spleen.

RULES FOR CLASSIFICATION

Clinical Staging. Imaging procedures such as ultrasonic scanning and computed tomography along with cytology and endoscopic retrograde cholangiopancreatography (ERCP) are available. Laparotomy and surgical exploration of the pancreas with biopsy is an accurate means of assessing the extent of the tumor and staging the patient.

Pathologic Staging. Complete or subtotal resection of the pancreas along with the tumor and associated regional lymph nodes provides the information necessary for staging. Pathologic staging is often based on a Whipple procedure. A single TNM classification serves both clinical and pathologic staging.

Direct extension to an organ or structure not listed in T1-T3 should be coded as M1. For example, extension to the liver is M1. Seeding of the peritoneum is also considered M1.

For T3, the peripancreatic tissues include the soft tissues adjacent to the pancreas in addition to the common bile duct and duodenum. Specifically, peripancreatic tissues include the surrounding retroperitoneal fat, (retroperitoneal soft tissue) mesentery (mesenteric fat), mesocolon, greater and lesser omentum, and the peritoneum. Direct invasion of the ampulla of Vater should be classified as T3. For T4, the adjacent large vessels include the celiac artery, superior mesenteric artery, common hepatic artery, portal vein, superior mesenteric vein, and hepatic vein, but not the splenic vessels.

DEFINITION OF TNM

Primary Tumor (T)

TX Primary tumor cannot be assessed
T0 No evidence of primary tumor
Tis *In situ* carcinoma
T1 Tumor limited to the pancreas 2 cm or less in greatest dimension
T2 Tumor limited to the pancreas more than 2 cm in greatest dimension
T3 Tumor extends directly into any of the following: duodenum, bile duct, peripancreatic tissues
T4 Tumor extends directly into any of the following: stomach, spleen, colon, adjacent large vessels

Regional Lymph Nodes (N)

NX Regional lymph nodes cannot be assessed
N0 No regional lymph node metastasis
N1 Regional lymph node metastasis
 pN1a Metastasis in a single regional lymph node
 pN1b Metastasis in multiple regional lymph nodes

Distant Metastasis (M)

MX Distant metastasis cannot be assessed
M0 No distant metastasis
M1 Distant metastasis

STAGE GROUPING

Stage 0	Tis	N0	M0
Stage I	T1	N0	M0
	T2	N0	M0
Stage II	T3	N0	M0
Stage III	T1	N1	M0
	T2	N1	M0
	T3	N1	M0
Stage IVA	T4	Any N	M0
Stage IVB	Any T	Any N	M1

HISTOPATHOLOGIC TYPE

The staging system applies to all carcinomas that arise in the pancreas. It does not apply to endocrine tumors that usually arise from the islets of Langerhans. Carcinoid tumors are also excluded. More than 90% of malignant tumors of the pancreas are exocrine carcinomas. The following carcinomas are included:

Severe ductal dysplasia/carcinoma *in situ*
Ductal adenocarcinoma
Mucinous noncystic carcinoma
Signet ring cell carcinoma
Adenosquamous carcinoma
Undifferentiated (anaplastic) carcinoma
Mixed ductal-endocrine carcinoma
Osteoclast-like giant cell tumor
Serous cystadenocarcinoma
Mucinous cystadenocarcinoma
Intraductal papillary-mucinous carcinoma
Invasive papillary-mucinous carcinoma
Acinar cell carcinoma
Acinar cell cystadenocarcinoma
Mixed acinar-endocrine carcinoma
Pancreaticoblastoma
Solid pseudopapillary carcinoma
Other

Borderline (Uncertain Malignant Potential) Tumors
- Mucinous cystic tumor with moderate dysplasia
- Intraductal papillary-mucinous tumor with moderate dysplasia
- Solid-pseudopapillary tumor

HISTOLOGIC GRADE (G)

GX Grade cannot be assessed
G1 Well differentiated
G2 Moderately differentiated
G3 Poorly differentiated
G4 Undifferentiated

PROGNOSTIC FACTORS

Histologic grade, lymphatic vessel invasion, perineural invasion, and capsular infiltration have been shown to be adverse prognostic factors.

BIBLIOGRAPHY

Albores-Saavedra J, Gould EW, Angeles-Angeles A, et al: Cystic tumors of the pancreas (Part 2). Pathol Ann 25:19–50, 1990

Allema JH, Reinders ME, van Gulik TM, et al: Prognostic factors for survival after pancreaticoduodenectomy for patients with carcinoma of the pancreatic head region. Cancer 75:2069–2076, 1995

Baisch H, Klöppel G, Reinke B: DNA ploidy and cell-cycle analysis in pancreatic and ampullary carcinoma: flow cytometric study of formalin-fixed paraffin-embedded tissue. Virchows Arch [A] 417: 145–150, 1990

Bakkevold KE, Kambestad B: Staging of carcinoma of the pancreas and ampulla of Vater: tumor (T), Lymph node (N), and distant metastasis (M) as prognostic factors. Int J Pancreatol 17:249–259, 1995

Böttger TC, Störkel S, Wellek S, et al: Factors influencing survival after resection of pancreatic cancer. A DNA analysis and a histomorphologic study. Cancer 73:63–73, 1994

Böttger TC, Zech J, Weber W, et al: Relevant factors in the prognosis of ductal pancreatic carcinoma. Acta Chir Scand 156:781–788, 1990

Cancer of the Pancreas Task Force: Staging of cancer of the pancreas. Cancer 47:1631–1637, 1981

Cubilla AL, Fitzgerald PJ: Tumors of the exocrine pancreas. Atlas of tumor pathology, Second Series, Fascicle 19. Washington, D.C.: Armed Forces Institute of Pathology, 1984

Cubilla AL, Fortner J, Fitzgerald PJ: Lymph node involvement in carcinoma of the head of the pancreas area. Cancer 41:880–887, 1978

Eskelinen M, Lipponen P: A review of prognostic factors in human pancreatic adenocarcinoma. Cancer Detect Prevent 16:287–295, 1992

Eskelinen M, Lipponen P, Marin S, et al: Prognostic factors in human pancreatic cancer, with special reference to quantitative histology. Scand J Gastroenterol 26:483–490, 1991

Freeny PC: Radiologic diagnosis and staging of pancreatic ductal adenocarcinoma. Radiol Clin North Am 27:121–128, 1989

Geer RJ, Brennan MF: Prognostic indicators for survival after resection of pancreatic adenocarcinoma. Am J Surg 165:68–73, 1993

Giulianotti PC, Boggi U, Fornaciari G, et al: Prognostic value of histological grading in ductal adenocarcinoma of the pancreas: Klöppel vs TNM grading. Int J Pancreatol 17:279–289, 1995

Griffanti-Bartoli F, Arnone GB, Ceppa P, et al: Malignant tumors in the head of the pancreas and the periampullary region, diagnostic and prognostic aspects. Anticancer Res 14:657–666, 1994

Hermanek P: Staging of exocrine pancreatic carcinoma. Eur J Surg Oncol 17:167–172, 1991

Hermanek P, Henson DE, Hutter RVP, et al: TNM supplement 1993. Berlin: Springer-Verlag, 1993

Kellokumpu-Lehtinen P, Huovinen R, Tuominen J: Pancreatic cancer: evaluation of prognostic factors and treatment results. Acta Oncologica 28: 481–484, 1989

Klöppel G, Lingenthal G, von Bülow M, et al: Histological and fine structural features of pancreatic ductal adenocarcinoma in relation to growth and prognosis: studies in xenografted tumours and clinico-histopathological correlation in a series of 75 cases. Histopathology 9:841–856, 1985

Klöppel G, Solcia E, Longnecker D, et al: Histological typing of tumours of the exocrine pancreas. WHO international histological classification of tumours, 2nd ed. Berlin-New York: Springer-Verlag, 1996

Lack EE: Primary tumors of the exocrine pancreas: classification, overview, and recent contributions by immunohistochemistry and electron microscopy. Am J Surg Pathol 13(Suppl 1):66–88, 1989

Manabe T, Ohshio G, Baba N, et al: Factors influencing prognosis and indications for curative pancreatectomy for ductal adenocarcinoma of the head of the pancreas. Int J Pancreatol 7:187–193, 1990

Nagakawa T, Mori K, Nakano T, et al: Perineural invasion of carcinoma of the pancreas and biliary tract. Br J Surg 80:619–621, 1993

Nix GA, Dubbelman C, Wilson JH, et al: Prognostic implications of tumor diameter in carcinoma of the head of the pancreas. Cancer 67:529–535, 1991

Obertop H: Prognostic factors for survival after pancreaticoduodenectomy for patients with carcinoma of the pancreatic head region. Cancer 75:2069–2076, 1995

Reber HA: Lymph node involvement as a prognostic factor in pancreatic cancer. Int J Pancreatol 7:125–127, 1990

Safi F, Roscher R, Beger HG: The clinical relevance of the tumor marker CA 19-9 in the diagnosing and monitoring of pancreatic carcinoma. Bull Cancer (Paris) 77:83–91, 1990

Satake K, Nishiwaki H, Yokomatsu H, et al: Surgical curability and prognosis for standard versus extended resection for T1 carcinoma of the pancreas. Surg Gynecol Obstet 175:259–265, 1992

Tannapfel A, Wittekind C, Junefeld G: Ductal adenocarcinoma of the pancreas. Int J Pancreatol 12:145–152, 1992

Trapnell JE: Staging of cancer of the pancreas. Int J Pancreatol 7:109–116, 1990

Tsuchiya R, Oribe T, Noda T: Size of the tumor and other factors influencing prognosis of carcinoma of the head of the pancreas. Am J Gastroenterol 80:459–462, 1985

Tsunoda T, Ura K, Eto T, et al: UICC and Japanese stage classifications for carcinoma of the pancreas. Int J Pancreatol 8:205–214, 1991

Warshaw AL: Implications of peritoneal cytology for staging of early pancreatic cancer. Am J Surg 161:26–30, 1991

Winek T, Hamre D, Mozell E, et al: Prognostic factors for survival after pancreaticoduodenectomy for malignant disease. Am J Surg 159:454–456, 1990

Yamamoto M, Saitoh Y, Hermanek P: Exocrine pancreatic carcinoma. In Hermanek P, Gospodarowicz M, Henson DE, Hutter RVP, Sobin LH (Eds.), Prognostic factors in cancer. Berlin: Springer-Verlag, 1995

Data Form for Cancer Staging

Patient identification
Name ______
Address ______
Hospital or clinic number ______
Age ____ Sex ____ Race ______

Institution identification
Hospital or clinic ______
Address ______

Oncology Record

Anatomic site of cancer ______
Histologic type ______
Grade (G) ______
Date of classification ______

DEFINITIONS

Primary Tumor (T)

Clin	Path		
[ ]	[ ]	TX	Primary tumor cannot be assessed
[ ]	[ ]	T0	No evidence of primary tumor
[ ]	[ ]	Tis	Carcinoma *in situ*
[ ]	[ ]	T1	Tumor limited to the pancreas 2 cm or less in greatest dimension
[ ]	[ ]	T2	Tumor limited to the pancreas more than 2 cm in greatest dimension
[ ]	[ ]	T3	Tumor extends directly into any of the following: duodenum, bile duct, peripancreatic tissues
[ ]	[ ]	T4	Tumor extends directly into any one of the following: stomach, spleen, colon, adjacent large vessels

Regional Lymph Nodes (N)

Clin	Path		
[ ]	[ ]	NX	Regional lymph nodes cannot be assessed
[ ]	[ ]	N0	No regional lymph node metastasis
[ ]	[ ]	N1	Regional lymph node metastasis
[ ]	[ ]	pN1a	Metastasis in a single regional lymph node
[ ]	[ ]	pN1b	Metastasis in multiple regional lymph nodes

Distant Metastasis (M)

Clin	Path		
[ ]	[ ]	MX	Distant metastasis cannot be assessed
[ ]	[ ]	M0	No distant metastasis
[ ]	[ ]	M1	Distant metastasis

Stage Grouping

Clin	Path	Stage	T	N	M
[ ]	[ ]	0	Tis	N0	M0
[ ]	[ ]	I	T1	N0	M0
			T2	N0	M0
[ ]	[ ]	II	T3	N0	M0
[ ]	[ ]	III	T1	N1	M0
			T2	N1	M0
			T3	N1	M0
[ ]	[ ]	IVA	T4	Any N	M0
[ ]	[ ]	IVB	Any T	Any N	M1

Histopathologic Grade (G)

[ ] GX Grade cannot be assessed
[ ] G1 Well differentiated
[ ] G2 Moderately differentiated
[ ] G3 Poorly differentiated
[ ] G4 Undifferentiated

Location in Pancreas

[ ] Head
[ ] Body
[ ] Tail
[ ] Diffuse
Size (largest diameter) ____ cm

Staged by ______ M.D.
______ Registrar
Date ______

Illustration

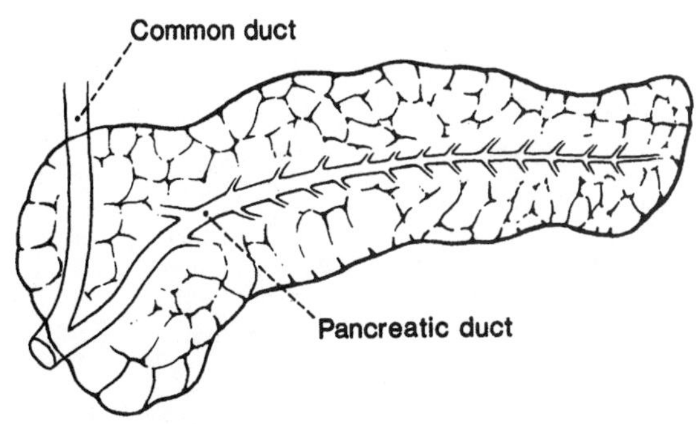

Indicate on diagram primary tumor and regional nodes involved.

(continued on next page)

Histopathologic Type

The staging system applies to all carcinomas that arise in the pancreas. It does not apply to endocrine tumors that usually arise from the islets of Langerhans. Carcinoid tumors are also excluded. More than 90% of malignant tumors of the pancreas are exocrine carcinomas. The following carcinomas are included:

Severe ductal dysplasia/carcinoma *in situ*
Ductal adenocarcinoma
Mucinous noncystic carcinoma
Signet ring cell carcinoma
Adenosquamous carcinoma
Undifferentiated (anaplastic) carcinoma
Mixed ductal-endocrine carcinoma
Osteoclast-like giant cell tumor
Serous cystadenocarcinoma
Mucinous cystadenocarcinoma
Intraductal papillary-mucinous carcinoma
Invasive papillary-mucinous carcinoma
Acinar cell carcinoma
Acinar cell cystadenocarcinoma
Mixed acinar-endocrine carcinoma
Pancreaticoblastoma
Solid pseudopapillary carcinoma
Other

Borderline (Uncertain malignant potential) Tumors
- Mucinous cystic tumor with moderate dysplasia
- Intraductal papillary-mucinous tumor with moderate dysplasia
- Solid-pseudopapillary tumor

THORAX

19

Lung

(Sarcomas and other rare tumors are not included.)

C34.0 Main bronchus
C34.1 Upper lobe
C34.2 Middle lobe
C34.3 Lower lobe
C34.8 Overlapping lesion
C34.9 Lung, NOS

Lung cancers are among the most common malignancies in the Western world and are the leading cause of cancer deaths in both men and women. It is one of the few tumors with a known carcinogen contributing to its etiology. In recent years we have come to appreciate that the initiation of lung cancer is a complex process that also involves certain biologic factors, such as the body's ability to process carcinogens. This disease is difficult to diagnose and treat, and the overall 5-year survival rate is less than 15% (Fig. 19-1). The staging of lung cancer depends on extent of disease, location of the primary tumor, and associated clinical complications. Assessment of extrapulmonary intrathoracic and extrathoracic metastasis is important for staging and patient evaluation.

ANATOMY

Primary Site. The mucosa lining the bronchus is the usual site of origin for carcinomas of the lung. The trachea, which lies in the anterior mediastinum, divides into the right and left main bronchi, which extend into the right and left lungs respectively. The bronchi then subdivide into the lobar bronchi for the upper, middle, and lower lobes on the right and the upper and lower lobes on the left. The lungs are encased in membranes called the visceral pleura. The inside of the chest cavity is lined by a similar membrane called the parietal pleura. The potential space between these two membranes is the pleural space. The mediastinum which contains the heart, thymus, great vessels, and other structures separates the lungs in the midline.

The great vessels:

Aorta
Superior caval vein
Inferior caval vein
Main pulmonary artery
Intrapericardial segments of the trunk of the right and left pulmonary artery
Intrapericardial segments of the superior or inferior right or left pulmonary veins

Regional Lymph Nodes. All regional nodes are above the diaphragm. They include the intrathoracic, scalene, and supraclavicular nodes (Fig. 19-2). For pN, a lymph node dissection will ordinarily include 6 or more lymph nodes. For purposes of staging, the intrathoracic nodes are as follows:

Mediastinal:
- Peritracheal (including those that may be designated tracheobronchial, i.e,. lower peritracheal, including azygos)
- Pre- and retrotracheal (includes precarinal)
- Aortic (includes subaortic, aorticopulmonary window, periaortic, including ascending aorta or phrenic)

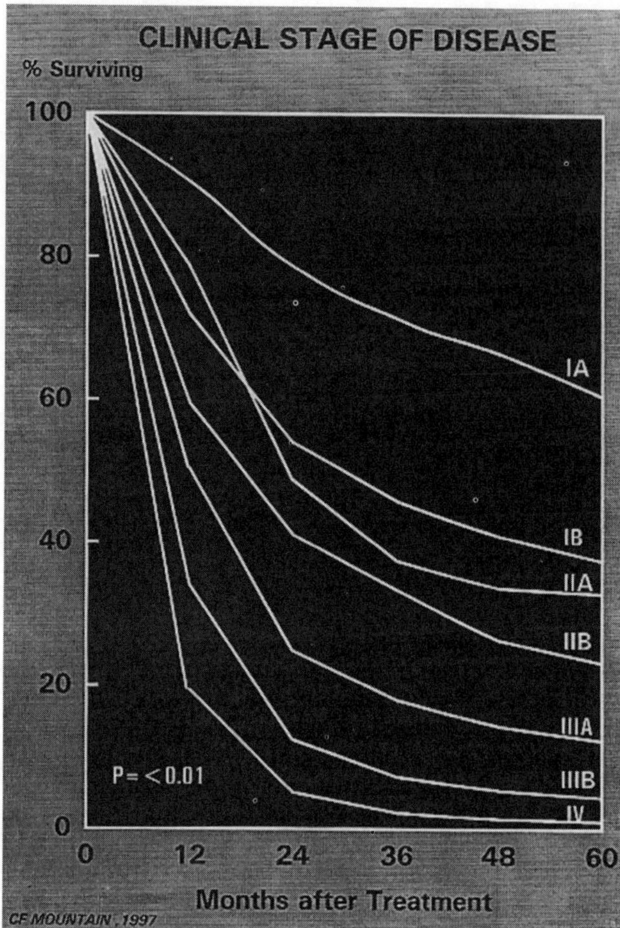

FIG. 19-1. Cumulative proportion of patients expected to survive following treatment according to clinical estimates of the stage of disease (From Mountain CF, Libshitz HI, Hermes KE: Lung cancer handbook for staging and imaging. 2nd ed. Houston: Clifton F. Mountain Foundation, 1997, with permission).

- Subcarinal
- Periesophageal
- Pulmonary ligament

Intrapulmonary:

- Hilar (proximal lobar)
- Peribronchial
- Intrapulmonary (includes interlobar, lobar, segmental)

Distant Metastatic Sites. The most common metastatic sites are the cervical lymph nodes, liver, brain, bones, adrenal glands, kidneys, and contralateral lung. No organ is safe. Synchronous separate tumor nodule(s) in a different lobe (ipsilateral or contralateral) is categorized as M1.

RULES FOR CLASSIFICATION

Clinical Staging. Clinical staging is based on the assessment of the anatomic extent of disease before definitive therapy is instituted. This includes a medical history, physical examination, various imaging procedures, and the results of selected studies (including bronchoscopy, esophagoscopy, mediastinoscopy, mediastinotomy, thoracentesis, and thoracoscopy), and other tests designed to demonstrate extrathoracic metastasis and regional extension. Information from exploratory thoracotomy is not included in the clinical classification. Patients explored and found unresectable should be pathologically staged.

If objective evidence is unavailable, clinical assignment of N2 disease may be made according to the judgment of the radiologist.

Lung cancer detected by sputum cytology but not seen radiographically or during bronchoscopy is known as "occult" carcinoma and is coded as TX. Occult cancers without evidence of regional lymph node involvement or distant metastasis are coded as TX, N0, M0. Any primary tumor that cannot be assessed, that is, no tumor mass present or evaluable, but lung cancer proven, is designated TX. In this context, bronchiolo-alveolar carcinoma presenting as a diffuse infiltrate, with no evidence of obstructive endobronchial tumor, is also designated TX.

T2 is used when there is direct extension into the visceral pleura. T3 is used if the lesion directly invades the parietal pleura covering the mediastinum and pericardium, as well as that lining the chest wall and covering the diaphragm.

Invasion of the phrenic nerve which invariably indicates direct extension of the primary tumor is classified as T3.

Peripheral tumors directly invading the chest wall and ribs are classified as T3.

Pleural tumor foci that are separate from direct pleural invasion by the primary tumor should be listed as T4. A separate lesion outside the parietal pleura, in the chest wall, or in the diaphragm should be designated as M1.

For the classification of pleural effusion, a footnote has been added to the T categories regarding the implications of pleural fluid as a staging variable. Patients with a malignant pleural effusion—that is, either cytologically positive for cancer cells or clinically related to the underlying malignancy are coded T4. Pericardial effusion is classified the same as pleural effusion.

Vocal cord paralysis (resulting from involvement of the recurrent branch of the vagus nerve), superior vena caval obstruction, or compression of the trachea or esophagus may be related to direct extension of the primary tumor or to lymph node involvement. The treatment

REGIONAL NODAL STATIONS FOR LUNG CANCER STAGING

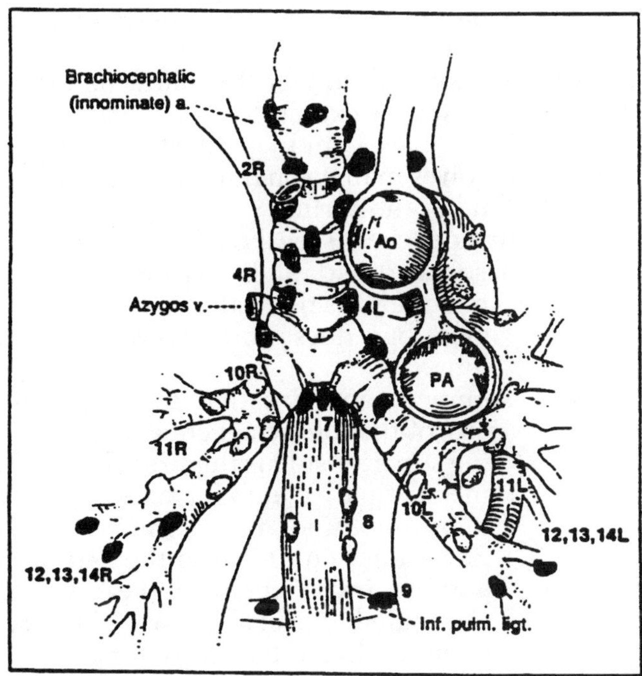

N_2 NODES
SUPERIOR MEDIASTINAL NODES

1 Highest Mediastinal

2 Upper Paratracheal

3 Pre- and Retrotracheal

4 Lower Paratracheal (including Azygos Nodes)

AORTIC NODES

5 Subaortic (A-P window)

6 Para-aortic (ascending aorta or phrenic)

INFERIOR MEDIASTINAL NODES

7 Subcarinal

8 Paraesophageal (below carina)

9 Pulmonary Ligament

N_1 NODES

10 Hilar

11 Interlobar

12 Lobar

13 Segmental

14 Subsegmental

FIG. 19-2. A revised schema for classifying regional lymph nodes, as the information relates to staging, is recommended. This classification represents a reconciliation of the prior recommendations of the American Joint Committee on Cancer and the American Thoracic Society. Nodal classifications are appropriate if lymph nodes are ipsilateral. If lymph nodes are contralateral, classify as N3. (Mountain/Dresler modifications from Naruke/ATS-LCSG Map) (© 1996 Reprints are permissible for educational use only.)

options and prognosis associated with these manifestations of disease extent fall within the T4-Stage IIIB category; therefore, a classification of T4 is recommended. If the primary tumor is peripheral and clearly unrelated to vocal cord paralysis, vena caval obstruction, or compression of the trachea and esophagus, then the nodal classification according to the established rules is appropriate.

The designation of "Pancoast" tumors relates to the symptom complex or syndrome caused by a tumor arising in the superior sulcus of the lung that involves the sympathetic nerve trunks, including the stellate ganglion. The extent of disease varies in these tumors, and they should be classified according to the established rules. If there is evidence of invasion of the vertebral body or extension into the neural foramina, the "Pancoast" tumor would be classified T4. If no criteria for T4 disease pertain, the tumor would be classified as T3.

The presence of multiple or satellite tumors (not lymph nodes) within the primary tumor lobe should be classified T4. Intrapulmonary ipsilateral metastasis in a distant, that is, nonprimary tumor lobe, is classified M1. Discontinuous tumor foci, only histologically detectable, do not affect the clinical TNM classification, but would be reflected in the pathologic staging.

Pathologic Staging. Pathologic staging is based on the information obtained from clinical staging, from thoracotomy, and from examination of the resected specimen, including lymph nodes. The same classification applies to both clinical and pathologic staging. The histologic type of cancer should be recorded because it also has a bearing on prognosis.

Multiple synchronous tumors of different histologic cell types should be considered separate primary lung cancers and each should be staged separately. For single patient data entry, the highest stage of disease should be recorded, with separate coding to identify multiple primary tumors.

DEFINITION OF TNM

Primary Tumor (T)

- TX Primary tumor cannot be assessed, or tumor proven by the presence of malignant cells in sputum or bronchial washings but not visualized by imaging or bronchoscopy
- T0 No evidence of primary tumor
- Tis Carcinoma *in situ*
- T1 Tumor 3 cm or less in greatest dimension, surrounded by lung or visceral pleura, without bronchoscopic evidence of invasion more proximal than the lobar bronchus,* (i.e., not in the main bronchus)
- T2 Tumor with any of the following features of size or extent:
  - More than 3 cm in greatest dimension
  - Involves main bronchus, 2 cm or more distal to the carina
  - Invades the visceral pleura
  - Associated with atelectasis or obstructive pneumonitis that extends to the hilar region but does not involve the entire lung.
- T3 Tumor of any size that directly invades any of the following: chest wall (including superior sulcus tumors), diaphragm, mediastinal pleura, parietal pericardium; or tumor in the main bronchus less than 2 cm distal to the carina, but without involvement of the carina; or associated atelectasis or obstructive pneumonitis of the entire lung.
- T4 Tumor of any size that invades any of the following: mediastinum, heart, great vessels, trachea, esophagus, vertebral body, carina; or separate tumor nodules in the same lobe; or tumor with a malignant pleural effusion.**

**Note:* The uncommon superficial tumor of any size with its invasive component limited to the bronchial wall, which may extend proximal to the main bronchus, is also classified T1.

***Note:* Most pleural effusions associated with lung cancer are due to tumor. However, there are a few patients in whom multiple cytopathologic examinations of pleural fluid are negative for tumor. In these cases, fluid is nonbloody and is not an exudate. When these elements and clinical judgment dictate that the effusion is not related to the tumor, the effusion should be excluded as a staging element and the patient should be staged T1, T2, or T3.

Regional Lymph Nodes (N)

- NX Regional lymph nodes cannot be assessed
- N0 No regional lymph node metastasis
- N1 Metastasis to ipsilateral peribronchial and/or ipsilateral hilar lymph nodes, and intrapulmonary nodes including involvement by direct extension of the primary tumor

N2 Metastasis to ipsilateral mediastinal and/ or subcarinal lymph node(s)

N3 Metastasis to contralateral mediastinal, contralateral hilar, ipsilateral or contralateral scalene, or supraclavicular lymph node(s)

Distant Metastasis (M)

MX Distant metastasis cannot be assessed
M0 No distant metastasis
M1 Distant metastasis present

Note: M1 includes separate tumor nodule(s) in a different lobe (ipsilateral or contralateral).

STAGE GROUPING

Stage grouping of the TNM subsets has been revised as follows:

Occult Carcinoma	TX	N0	M0
Stage 0	Tis	N0	M0
Stage IA	T1	N0	M0
Stage IB	T2	N0	M0
Stage IIA	T1	N1	M0
Stage IIB	T2	N1	M0
	T3	N0	M0
Stage IIIA	T1	N2	M0
	T2	N2	M0
	T3	N1	M0
	T3	N2	M0
Stage IIIB	Any T	N3	M0
	T4	Any N	M0
Stage IV	Any T	Any N	M1

HISTOPATHOLOGIC TYPE

There are four common types of lung cancer:

1. Squamous cell carcinoma (epidermoid carcinoma)
   Variant: Spindle cell
2. Small cell carcinoma
   Oat cell carcinoma
   Intermediate cell type
   Combined oat cell carcinoma
3. Adenocarcinoma
   Acinar adenocarcinoma
   Papillary adenocarcinoma
   Bronchiolo-alveolar carcinoma
   Solid carcinoma with mucus formation
4. Large cell carcinoma
   Variants:
   Giant cell carcinoma
   Clear cell carcinoma

This classification applies only to carcinomas, including small cell carcinoma. The classification may be applied to those tumors classified as "undifferentiated carcinomas" with no special cell types identified. Sarcomas and other rare tumors are excluded because the relationship between disease extent and prognosis has not been established or does not pertain.

HISTOPATHOLOGIC GRADE (G)

GX Grade cannot be assessed
G1 Well differentiated
G2 Moderately differentiated
G3 Poorly differentiated
G4 Undifferentiated

PROGNOSTIC FACTORS

The prognostic significance of histologic cell type and anatomic extent of disease in lung cancer is generally accepted. Small cell carcinoma, characterized by rapid growth and widespread dissemination, even in clinically "early" disease is recognized as a separate entity from the nonsmall cell histologies—adenocarcinoma, large cell carcinoma and squamous cell carcinoma. Treatment selection and survival are significantly related to the stage and histologic classifications. It must be kept in mind that the diagnostic process will affect the accuracy of clinical staging. Series of patients in whom mediastinoscopy is required for surgical selection or those in whom a complete lymph node dissection is performed at operation will have fewer errors reported than may be reported for patients in whom these procedures are not performed.

Clinical Factors

Performance status and severity of symptoms have prognostic significance in nonsmall cell carcinoma; these factors may be related either to the spread of the cancer or associated conditions that limit treatment, for example the cardiac and pulmonary complications associated with advancing age, as well as with tobacco use. Weight loss, more than 10% of body weight, has an adverse effect on prognosis and is predictive of recurrence in patients who have undergone resection. Differing studies have identified gender, age, and various physiologic components as indicators of a poor outcome; however, most are not reproduced in large scale studies of well-defined lung cancer populations.

A large number of clinical, laboratory, serologic, paraneoplastic, and immune factors have been investigated for their prognostic influence on specific groups of patients with small cell carcinoma. Lactate dehydrogenase (LDH), alkaline phosphatase, alanine, transaminase, albumin, urate, sodium, bicarbonate, hemoglobin and white blood count, and specific sites of metastasis have been identified as significant prognostic factors. A model, incorporating 21 factors, has been developed using tree classification methodology to identify four prognostic groups that are homogeneous and different from each other. These groups incorporate the influence of prognostic factors that are important for specific groups of patients. The initial branching is according to the extent of disease, followed by various factors that are significant in each category.

Anatomic Factors

Each of the staging components, the primary tumor, the regional lymph nodes, and distant metastasis has a profound effect on prognosis. The most deleterious factor is the presence of distant metastatic disease. Involvement of multiple distant sites has more serious implications than single site metastasis, which may be responsive to available treatment in a few instances: for example, surgical treatment of solitary brain lesions, or response to chemotherapy or combined regimens.

The absence of, or presence and extent of, regional lymph node metastasis has significant bearing on prognosis. When lymph node metastasis has progressed beyond the ipsilateral hemithorax, the outcome is very poor. Less than 3% of patients with clinical evidence of N3 disease are expected to survive 5 years or more. Survival rates for patients with metastasis limited to the ipsilateral mediastinal lymph nodes, N2 disease, are influenced by the number of nodes involved, the number of levels; that is, upper mediastinal, lower mediastinal, or both, and extracapsular extension. Patients with N2 disease with squamous cell carcinoma have a better outcome following resection than those with adenocarcinoma and large cell carcinoma.

The prognostic implications of intrapulmonary lymph node metastasis vary with the location of the nodes and the primary tumor status. Metastasis to hilar nodes carries a worse prognosis than disease limited to the interlobar and segmental nodes. Involvement of N1 nodes in the presence of larger more invasive tumors, T2 or T3, indicates a poorer outcome than expected for T1 tumors.

Biologic Factors

Research advances in the field of molecular biology have provided a new understanding of the genetic background of lung cancer. Knowledge of the role of genetic lesions and other biologic aberrations in tumorigenesis is the basis for many investigations of biologic markers as indicators of prognosis. In order to take marker information to clinical practice, the marker must bear a strong relationship to patient prognosis and the factor must provide additional prognostic information beyond that provided by conventional factors. Elements such as stage and histology, performance status, age, and gender must be documented and analyzed. The method of determining the factor must be reproducible within and between laboratories. Identifying the marker should bear a reasonable cost. These requirements argue for a standard format for reporting prognostic factor data. The studies of markers in the following listing report that the factor under investigation does have either independent prognostic value or correlates significantly with disease progression, and warrants large scale investigation.

Marker Studies in Lung Cancer

- Aberrant gene expression (oncogene amplification and overexpression)
  - *ras* family
  - *myc* family
  - HER-2/*neu*(p185)
  - p53
- Tumor-associated antigens
  - Blood group carbohydrate antigens
  - Antigen 43-9F
  - Serum CA125
  - Squamous cell carcinoma antigen
- Other biologic factors
  - Tumor cell DNA content
  - Growth factors
  - Tumor cell proliferation
  - Basement membrane deposition
  - Cytokeratin
  - Soluble interleukin-2 receptor
- Enzymes and Hormones
  - Neuron-specific enolase
  - Serum lactate dehydrogenase

The results of biologic marker studies available at this time are insufficient to select patients for predicted effective treatment, thus improving survival, or to withhold ineffective therapy, thus improving quality of life. Prospective clinical trials, including large patient populations, are required to validate the association/causation relationships of prognostic factors to survival. In the absence of such data, changes in present treatment policies or staging recommendations are not justified. The findings, in studies with confirmatory reports, may be taken into account as stratification variables in clinical trials.

BIBLIOGRAPHY

Angeletti CA, Macchiarini P, Mussi A, et al: Influence of T and N stages on long-term survival in resectable small cell lung cancer. Eur J Surg Oncol 15:337–340, 1989

Brundage MD, Mackillop WJ: Locally advanced nonsmall cell lung cancer: do we know the questions. Clin Epidemiol 49:183–192, 1996

Byhardt RW, Hartz A, Libnoch JA, et al: Prognostic influence of TNM staging and LDH levels in small cell carcinoma of the lung (SCCL). Int J Radiat Oncol Biol Phys 12:771–777, 1986

Capewell S, Sudlow MF: Performance and prognosis in patients with lung cancer. Thorax 45:951–956, 1990

Carr DT, Mountain CF: The staging of lung cancer. Semin Oncol 1:229–234, 1974

Costa A, Silvestrini R, Mochen C: P53 expression, DNA ploidy and s-phase cell fraction in operable locally advanced nonsmall cell lung cancer. Brit J Cancer 73:914–919, 1996

Dearing MP, Steinberg SM, Phelps R, et al: Outcome of patients with small cell lung cancer: effect of changes in staging procedures and imaging technology on prognostic factors over 14 years. J Clin Oncol 8:1042–1049, 1990

Feinstein AR, Wells CK: Lung cancer staging: a critical evaluation. Clin Chest Med 3:291–305, 1982

Feld R, Sagman U, LeBlanc M: Staging and prognostic factors: small cell carcinoma. In Pass HI, Mitchell JB, Johnson DH, Turrissi AT (Eds.), Lung cancer: principles and practice. Philadelphia: Lippincott–Raven; 495–509, 1996

Gail MH, Eagan RT, Feld R, et al: Prognostic factors in patients with resected stage I nonsmall cell lung cancer. Cancer 54:1802–1813, 1984

Ichinose Y, Yano T, Asoh H, et al: Prognostic factors obtained by a pathologic examination in completely resected nonsmall cell lung cancer. An analysis in each pathologic stage. J Thorac Cardiovasc Surg 110:601–605, 1995

Ishikawa S: Staging system on TNM classification for lung cancer. Jpn J Clin Oncol 6:19–30, 1973

Libshitz HI: Computed tomography in bronchogenic carcinoma. Semin Roentgenol 25:64–72, 1990

McKenna RJ, Libshitz HI, Mountain CF, et al: Roentgenographic evaluation of mediastinal nodes for preoperative assessment in lung cancer. Chest 88: 206–210, 1985

Mountain CF: A new international staging system for lung cancer. Chest 89(4 Suppl):25S–233S, 1986

Mountain CF: New prognostic factors in lung cancer. Prophets of cancer cell aggression. Chest 108:246–254, 1995

Mountain CF, Libshitz HI, Hermes KE: Lung cancer handbook for staging and imaging, 3rd ed. Houston: Clifton F. Mountain Foundation, 1996

Naruke T, Goya T, Tsuchiya R, et al: Prognosis and survival in resected lung carcinoma based on the new international staging system. J Thorac Cardiovasc Surg 96:440–447, 1988

Naruke T, Suemasu K, Ishikawa S: Lymph node mapping and curability at various levels of metastasis in resected lung cancer. J Thorac Cardiovas Surg 76:832–839, 1978

Nesbitt JC, Putnam JB, Walsh GL, et al: Survival in early stage nonsmall cell lung cancer. Ann Thorac Surg 60:466–472, 1995

Ogawa J, Iwazaki M, Tsurumi T, et al: Prognostic implications of DNA histogram, DNA content, and histologic changes of regional lymph nodes in patients with lung cancer. Cancer 67:1370–1376, 1991

Rawson NS, Peto J: An overview of prognostic factors in small cell lung cancer. A report from the subcommittee for the management of lung. Br J Cancer 61:597–604, 1990

Sagawa M, Saito Y, Takahashi S, et al: Clinical and prognostic assessment of patients with resected small peripheral lung cancer lesions. Cancer 66:2653–2657, 1990

Sandler HM, Curran WJ Jr, Turrisi AT III: The influence of tumor size and pretreatment staging on outcome following radiation therapy alone for stage I nonsmall cell lung cancer. Int J Radiat Oncol Biol Phys 19:9–13, 1990

Sano T, Naruke T, Kondo H, et al: Prognosis for resected lung cancer patients with tumors greater than ten centimeters in diameter. Jpn J Clin Oncol 20:369–373, 1990

Sheehan RG, Balaban EP, Cox JV, et al: The relative value of conventional staging procedures for developing prognostic models in extensive-stage small cell lung cancer. J Clin Oncol 8:2047–2053, 1990

Siu LL, Shepherd FA, Murray N, et al: Influence of age on the treatment of limited-stage small cell lung cancer. J Clin Oncol 14:821–828, 1996

Stanley KD: Prognostic factors for survival in patients with inoperable lung cancer. J Natl Cancer Inst 65:25–32, 1980

Templeton PA, Caskey CI, Zerhouni EA: Current uses of CT and MR imaging in the staging of lung cancer. Radiol Clin North Am 28:631–646, 1990

World Health Organization. Histological typing of lung tumors, 2nd ed. Geneva: World Health Organization, 1981

Zang EA, Wynder EL. Differences in lung cancer risk between men and women—examination of the evidence. J NCI 88:183–193, 1996

Data Form for Cancer Staging

Patient identification
Name ______
Address ______
Hospital or clinic number ______
Age ____ Sex ____ Race ______

Institution identification
Hospital or clinic ______
Address ______

Oncology Record

Anatomic site of cancer ______
Histologic type ______
Grade (G) ______
Date of classification ______

Clin	Path	DEFINITIONS
		Primary Tumor (T)
[ ]	[ ]	TX Primary tumor cannot be assessed, or tumor proven by presence of malignant cells in sputum or bronchial washings but not visualized by imaging or bronchoscopy
[ ]	[ ]	T0 No evidence of primary tumor
[ ]	[ ]	Tis Carcinoma *in situ*
[ ]	[ ]	T1 Tumor 3 cm or less in greatest dimension, surrounded by lung or visceral pleura, without bronchoscopic evidence of invasion more proximal than the lobar bronchus* (i.e., not in main bronchus)
[ ]	[ ]	T2 Tumor with *any* of the following features of size or extent: More than 3 cm in greatest dimension Involves main bronchus, 2 cm or more distal to the carina Invades the visceral pleura Associated with atelectasis or obstructive pneumonitis that extends to the hilar region but does not involve the entire lung
[ ]	[ ]	T3 Tumor of any size that directly invades any of the following: chest wall (including superior sulcus tumors), diaphragm, mediastinal pleura, parietal pericardium; or tumor in the main bronchus less than 2 cm distal to the carina but without involvement of the carina; or associated atelectasis or obstructive pneumonitis of the entire lung
[ ]	[ ]	T4 Tumor of any size that invades any of the following: mediastinum, heart, great vessels, trachea, esophagus, vertebral body, carina; separate tumor nodule(s) in the same lobe; or tumor with a malignant pleural effusion**
		** The uncommon superficial tumor of any size with its invasive component limited to the bronchial wall, which may extend proximal to the main bronchus, is also classified T1.*
		*** Most pleural effusions associated with lung cancer are due to tumor. However, there are a few patients in whom multiple cytopathologic examinations of pleural fluid are negative for tumor. In these cases, fluid is nonbloody and is not an exudate. When these elements and clinical judgment dictate that the effusion is not related to the tumor, the effusion should be excluded as a staging element and the patient should be staged T1, T2, or T3.*
		Regional Lymph Nodes (N)
[ ]	[ ]	NX Regional lymph nodes cannot be assessed
[ ]	[ ]	N0 No regional lymph node metastasis
[ ]	[ ]	N1 Metastasis to ipsilateral peribronchial and/or ipsilateral hilar lymph nodes and intrapulmonary nodes involved by direct extension of the primary tumor
[ ]	[ ]	N2 Metastasis to ipsilateral mediastinal and/or subcarinal lymph node(s)
[ ]	[ ]	N3 Metastasis in contralateral mediastinal, contralateral hilar, ipsilateral or contralateral scalene or supraclavicular lymph node(s)
		Distant Metastasis (M)
[ ]	[ ]	MX Distant metastasis cannot be assessed
[ ]	[ ]	M0 No distant metastasis
[ ]	[ ]	M1 Distant metastasis present (includes synchronous separate nodule[s] in a different lobe)

(continued on next page)

Clin	Path	Stage Grouping			
[ ]	[ ]	Occult	TX	N0	M0
[ ]	[ ]	0	Tis	N0	M0
[ ]	[ ]	IA	T1	N0	M0
[ ]	[ ]	IB	T2	N0	M0
[ ]	[ ]	IIA	T1	N1	M0
[ ]	[ ]	IIB	T2	N1	M0
			T3	N0	M0
[ ]	[ ]	IIIA	T1	N2	M0
			T2	N2	M0
			T3	N1	M0
			T3	N2	M0
[ ]	[ ]	IIIB	Any T	N3	M0
			T4	Any N	M0
[ ]	[ ]	IV	Any T	Any N	M1

Staged by ______________________ M.D.

______________________ Registrar

Date ______________________

Illustrations

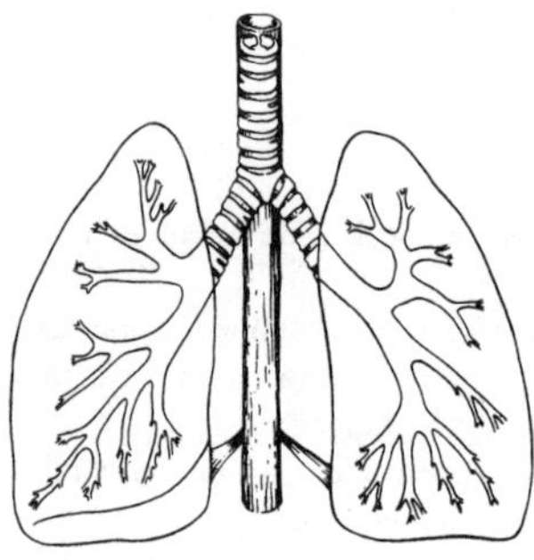

Show primary tumor, indicating size in cm (greatest diameter) and measurability:

EV = evaluable
ME = measurable
NE = nonevaluable

Show lymph node metastases.

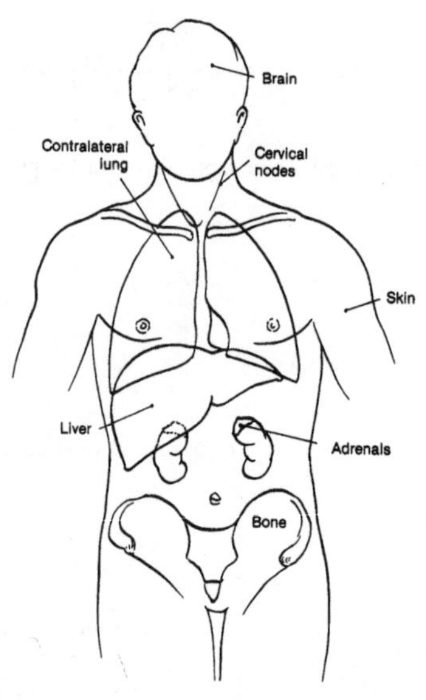

Distant metastases beyond hemiothorax. Indicate all known metastases.

Histopathologic Grade (G)

[ ] GX Grade cannot be assessed
[ ] G1 Well differentiated
[ ] G2 Moderately differentiated
[ ] G3 Poorly differentiated
[ ] G4 Undifferentiated

Lymph Nodes

Mediastinal:
- Peritracheal (including those that may be designated tracheobronchial, e.g., lower peritracheal, including azygos)
- Pretracheal and retrotracheal (including precarinal)
- Aortic (including subaortic, aorticopulmonary window, and periaortic, including ascending aorta or phrenic)
- Subcarinal
- Periesophageal
- Pulmonary ligament

Intrapulmonary:
- Hilar (proximal lobar)
- Peribronchial
- Intrapulmonary (including interlobar, lobar, segmental)

Histopathologic Type

There are four common types of lung cancer

Squamous cell carcinoma (epidermoid carcinoma)
- Variant: Spindle cell

Small cell carcinoma
- Oat cell carcinoma
- Intermediate cell type
- Combined oat cell carcinoma

Adenocarcinoma
- Acinar adenocarcinoma
- Papillary adenocarcinoma
- Bronchiolo-alveolar carcinoma
- Solid carcinoma with mucus formation

Large cell carcinoma
- Variants: Giant cell carcinoma
  Clear cell carcinoma

This classification applies only to carcinomas, including small cell carcinoma. The classification may be applied to those tumors classified as "undifferentiated carcinomas" with no special cell types identified. Sarcomas and other rare tumors are excluded because the relationship between disease extent and prognosis has not been established or does not pertain.

(continued on next page)

REGIONAL NODAL STATIONS FOR LUNG CANCER STAGING

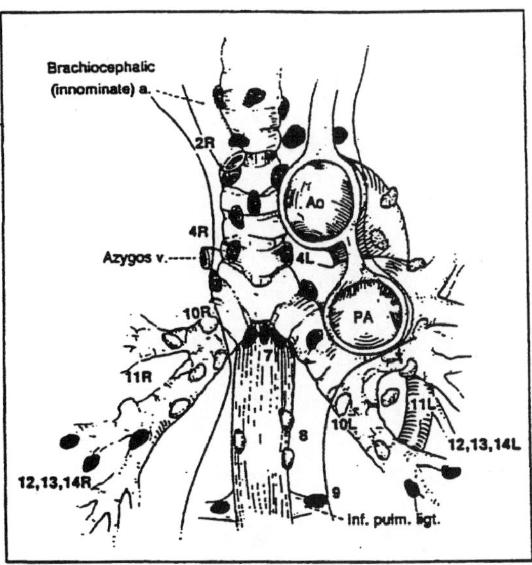

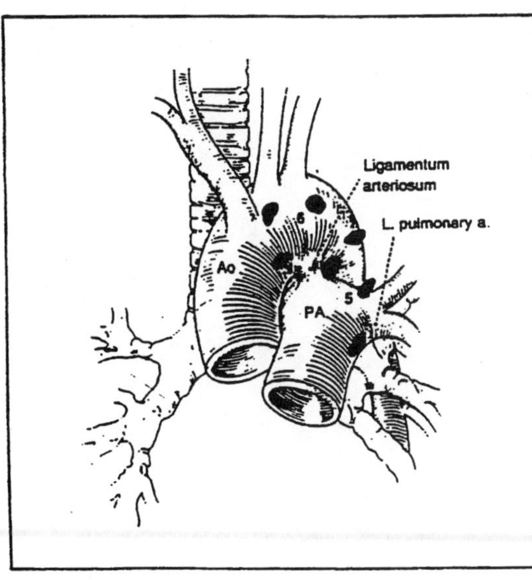

N_2 NODES
SUPERIOR MEDIASTINAL NODES

1 Highest Mediastinal

2 Upper Paratracheal

3 Pre- and Retrotracheal

4 Lower Paratracheal (including Azygos Nodes)

AORTIC NODES

5 Subaortic (A-P window)

6 Para-aortic (ascending aorta or phrenic)

INFERIOR MEDIASTINAL NODES

7 Subcarinal

8 Paraesophageal (below carina)

9 Pulmonary Ligament

N_1 NODES

10 Hilar

11 Interlobar

12 Lobar

13 Segmental

14 Subsegmental

Indicate on diagrams primary tumor and regional nodes involved.

20

Pleural Mesothelioma

(Tumors metastatic to the pleura and lung tumors that have extended to the pleural surfaces are not included.)

C38.4 Pleura

Mesotheliomas are relatively rare tumors that arise from the mesothelium that lines the pleural cavities. They represent less than 2% of all malignant tumors. Highly virulent, mesotheliomas are usually associated with long-term exposure to asbestos. While similar tumors can arise along the mesothelial surfaces in the abdomen or pericardial cavity, this staging system applies only to tumors that arise in the pleural cavities. Because these tumors are not common, a staging system was not published previously by the International Union Against Cancer or by the American Joint Committee on Cancer. For staging, the disease should be histologically confirmed. The initial symptoms may be nonspecific.

ANATOMY

Primary Site. The mesothelium covers the external surface of the lungs and the inside of the chest wall. It is usually composed of flat tightly connected cells no more than one layer thick.

Regional Lymph Nodes. The regional lymph nodes include:

Intrathoracic
Scalene
Supraclavicular

See Chapter 19 for a detailed list of intrathoracic lymph nodes. For pN, histologic examination of a mediastinal lymphadenectomy specimen will ordinarily include 6 or more regional lymph nodes.

RULES FOR CLASSIFICATION

This staging system serves both clinical and pathologic staging. Clinical staging depends on imaging, especially computed tomography scanning. Pathologic staging is based on surgical resection. The extent of disease before and after resection should be carefully documented. In some cases, complete N staging may not be possible, especially if tumor has encompassed the hilar and mediastinal structures.

DEFINITION OF TNM

Primary Tumor (T)

TX Primary tumor cannot be assessed
T0 No evidence of primary tumor
T1 Tumor limited to ipsilateral parietal and/or visceral pleura
T2 Tumor invades any of the following: ipsilateral lung, endothoracic fascia, diaphragm, pericardium
T3 Tumor invades any of the following: ipsilateral chest wall muscle, ribs, mediastinal organs or tissues

T4 Tumor directly extends to any of the following: contralateral pleura, lung, peritoneum, intra-abdominal organs, or cervical tissues

Regional Lymph Nodes (N)

NX Regional lymph nodes cannot be assessed
N0 No regional lymph node metastasis
N1 Metastasis in ipsilateral peribronchial and/or ipsilateral hilar lymph nodes, including direct extension
N2 Metastasis in ipsilateral mediastinal and/or subcarinal lymph node(s)
N3 Metastasis in contralateral mediastinal, contralateral hilar, ipsilateral or contralateral scalene, or supraclavicular lymph node(s)

Distant Metastasis (M)

MX Distant metastasis cannot be assessed
M0 No evidence of distant metastasis
M1 Distant metastasis

STAGE GROUPING

Stage I	T1	N0	M0
	T2	N0	M0
Stage II	T1	N1	M0
	T2	N1	M0
Stage III	T1	N2	M0
	T2	N2	M0
	T3	N0	M0
	T3	N1	M0
	T3	N2	M0
Stage IV	Any T	N3	M0
	T4	Any N	M0
	Any T	Any N	M1

HISTOPATHOLOGIC TYPE

This staging classification applies only to primary pleural mesothelioma. It does not apply to metastatic tumors or to lung tumors that have extended to the pleural surfaces.

BIBLIOGRAPHY

Bignon J, Brochard P, de Cremous H, et al: Contribution of epidemiology and biology to the comprehension of causes and mechanisms of mesothelioma. Int Trends in Gen Thoracic Surg 327–335, 1990

Borden EC: Mesothelioma: natural history and current therapeutic approaches. Curr Conc Oncol 5:3–8, 1983

Boutin C, Rey F, Gouvernet J, et al: Thoracoscopy in pleural malignant mesothelioma: a prospective study of 188 consecutive patients. Part 2: Prognosis and staging. Cancer 72:394–404, 1993.

Brunner J, Sordillo PP, Magill GB, et al: Malignant mesothelioma of the pleura. Review of 123 patients. Cancer 49:2431–2435, 1982

Dimitrov NV, McMahon SM, Carr DT: Multidisciplinary approach to management of patients with mesothelioma. Cancer Res 43:3974, 1983

Rusch VW: Clinical features and current treatment of diffuse malignant pleural mesothelioma (Review). Lung Cancer 12(Suppl 2):S127–146, 1995

Rusch V, Ginsberg RJ: New concepts in the staging of mesotheliomas. Int Trends in Gen Thoracic Surg 336–343, 1990

Sugarbaker DJ, Strauss GM, Lynch TJ, et al: Node status has prognostic significance in the multimodality therapy of diffuse malignant mesothelioma. J Clin Oncol 11:1172–1178, 1993

Tammilehto L, Kivisaari L, Salminen US, et al: Evaluation of the clinical TNM staging system for malignant pleural mesothelioma: an assessment in 88 patients. Lung Cancer 12:25–34, 1995

Data Form for Cancer Staging

Patient identification
Name ______
Address ______
Hospital or clinic number ______
Age ____ Sex ____ Race ______

Institution identification
Hospital or clinic ______
Address ______

Oncology Record

Anatomic site of cancer ______
Histologic type ______
Grade (G) ______
Date of classification ______

DEFINITIONS

Primary Tumor (T)

Clin	Path		
[ ]	[ ]	TX	Primary tumor cannot be assessed
[ ]	[ ]	T0	No evidence of primary tumor
[ ]	[ ]	T1	Tumor limited to ipsilateral parietal and/or visceral pleura
[ ]	[ ]	T2	Tumor invades any of the following: ipsilateral lung, endothoracic fascia, diaphragm, or pericardium
[ ]	[ ]	T3	Tumor invades any of the following: ipsilateral chest wall muscle, ribs, or mediastinal organs or tissues
[ ]	[ ]	T4	Tumor directly extends to any of the following: contralateral pleura, lung, peritoneum, intra-abdominal organs, or cervical tissues

Regional Lymph Nodes (N)

Clin	Path		
[ ]	[ ]	NX	Regional lymph nodes cannot be assessed
[ ]	[ ]	N0	No regional lymph node metastasis
[ ]	[ ]	N1	Metastasis in ipsilateral peribronchial and/or ipsilateral hilar lymph nodes, including direct extension
[ ]	[ ]	N2	Metastasis in ipsilateral mediastinal and/or subcarinal lymph node(s)
[ ]	[ ]	N3	Metastasis in contralateral mediastinal, contralateral hilar, ipsilateral or contralateral scalene, or supraclavicular lymph node(s)

Distant Metastasis (M)

Clin	Path		
[ ]	[ ]	MX	Distant metastasis cannot be assessed
[ ]	[ ]	M0	No evidence of distant metastasis
[ ]	[ ]	M1	Distant metastasis

Stage Grouping

Clin	Path	Stage	T	N	M
[ ]	[ ]	Stage I	T1	N0	M0
			T2	N0	M0
[ ]	[ ]	Stage II	T1	N1	M0
			T2	N1	M0
[ ]	[ ]	Stage III	T1	N2	M0
			T2	N2	M0
			T3	N0	M0
			T3	N1	M0
			T3	N2	M0
[ ]	[ ]	Stage IV	Any T	N3	M0
			T4	Any N	M0
			Any T	Any N	M1

Histopathologic Type

This staging classification applies only to primary pleural mesotheliomas. It does not apply to metastatic tumors or to lung tumors that have extended to the pleural surfaces.

Staged by ______ M.D.
______ Registrar

Date ______

MUSCULOSKELETAL SITES

21

Bone

(Primary malignant lymphoma, multiple myeloma, juxtacortical osteosarcoma, and juxtacortical chondrosarcoma are not included.)

C40.0 Long bones of upper limb, scapula, and associated joints
C40.1 Short bones of upper limb and associated joints
C40.2 Long bones of lower limb and associated joints
C40.3 Short bones of lower limb and associated joints
C40.8 Overlapping lesion of bones, joints, and articular cartilage of limbs
C40.9 Bone of limb, NOS
C41.0 Bones of skull and face and associated joints
C41.1 Mandible
C41.2 Vertebral column
C41.3 Rib, sternum, clavicle, and associated joints
C41.4 Pelvic bones, sacrum, coccyx, and associated joints
C41.8 Overlapping lesion of bones, joints, and articular cartilage
C41.9 Bone, NOS

This classification is used for all primary malignant tumors of bone except primary malignant lymphoma, multiple myeloma, juxtacortical osteosarcoma, and juxtacortical chondrosarcoma. Cases are categorized by histologic type (e.g., osteosarcoma, chondrosarcoma) and by histologic grade of differentiation.

ANATOMY

Primary Site. All bones of the skeleton.

Regional Lymph Nodes. The regional lymph nodes are those appropriate to the site of the primary tumor. For pN, histologic examination of a regional lymphadenectomy specimen will ordinarily include six or more regional lymph nodes.

Metastatic Sites. A metastatic site includes any site beyond the regional lymph nodes of the primary site. Spread to the lungs is frequent.

RULES FOR CLASSIFICATION

Clinical Staging. Clinical staging includes all relevant data prior to primary definitive therapy including physical examination, imaging, and biopsy. Clinical evaluation of the local extent of the tumor is currently best accomplished with imaging by computerized axial tomography (CAT) scan or magnetic resonance imaging (MRI). Although both of these techniques are very useful to evaluate cortical fracture and extraosseous extension, MRI is particularly valuable in determining the extent of marrow involvement of the tumor within the bone of origin. Furthermore, CAT scans of the chest are extremely useful for the detection of pulmonary metastasis.

The pathologic diagnosis is made on the basis of microscopic examination correlated with plain radiographs, CAT scan, and/or MRI. A specific diagnostic technique for small round cell tumors, or Ewing's tumor, is the presence of a specific chromosomal translocation between chromosomes 11 and 22: t(11;22) (q24;q12) or 21 and 22: t(21;22)(q21;q12).

Pathologic Staging. Pathologic staging includes all clinical staging data as well as pathologic data obtained from examination of a resected specimen sufficient to evaluate the highest T category, histopathologic type and grade, regional lymph nodes as appropriate, or distant metastasis. Since regional lymph node involvement from bone tumors is rare, the pathologic stage grouping includes any of the following combinations: pT pG pN pM, or pT pG cN cM, or cT cN pM.

DEFINITION OF TNM

Primary Tumor (T)

TX Primary tumor cannot be assessed
T0 No evidence of primary tumor
T1 Tumor confined within the cortex
T2 Tumor invades beyond the cortex

Regional Lymph Nodes (N)

NX Regional lymph nodes cannot be assessed
N0 No regional lymph node metastasis
N1 Regional lymph node metastasis

Note: Because of the rarity of lymph node involvement in sarcomas, the designation NX may not be appropriate and could be considered N0 if no clinical involvement is evident.

Distant Metastasis (M)

MX Distant metastasis cannot be assessed
M0 No distant metastasis
M1 Distant metastasis

HISTOPATHOLOGIC GRADE (G)

GX Grade cannot be assessed
G1 Well differentiated—Low Grade
G2 Moderately differentiated—Low Grade
G3 Poorly differentiated—High Grade
G4 Undifferentiated—High Grade

Note: Ewing's sarcoma is classified as G4.

STAGE GROUPING

Stage	G	T	N	M
Stage IA	G1,2	T1	N0	M0
Stage IB	G1,2	T2	N0	M0
Stage IIA	G3,4	T1	N0	M0
Stage IIB	G3,4	T2	N0	M0
Stage III	Not defined			
Stage IVA	Any G	Any T	N1	M0
Stage IVB	Any G	Any T	Any N	M1

HISTOPATHOLOGIC TYPE

A. Bone-forming
   1. Osteosarcoma (osteogenic sarcoma)
B. Cartilage-forming
   1. Chondrosarcoma
   2. Mesenchymal chondrosarcoma
C. Giant cell tumor, malignant
D. Ewing's sarcoma
E. Vascular tumors
   1. Hemangioendothelioma
   2. Hemangiopericytoma
   3. Angiosarcoma
F. Connective tissue tumors
   1. Fibrosarcoma
   2. Liposarcoma
   3. Malignant mesenchymoma
   4. Undifferentiated sarcoma
G. Other tumors
   1. Chordoma
   2. Adamantinoma of long bones

Primary malignant lymphoma, multiple myeloma, juxtacortical osteosarcoma, and juxtacortical chondrosarcoma are not included.

PROGNOSTIC FACTORS

Known prognostic factors for malignant bone tumors include: (1) the T-classification: T1 tumors have a better prognosis than T2 tumors; (2) histopathologic low grade (G1, G2) has a better prognosis than high grade (G3, G4); (3) location of the primary tumor: patients who have an anatomically resectable primary tumor

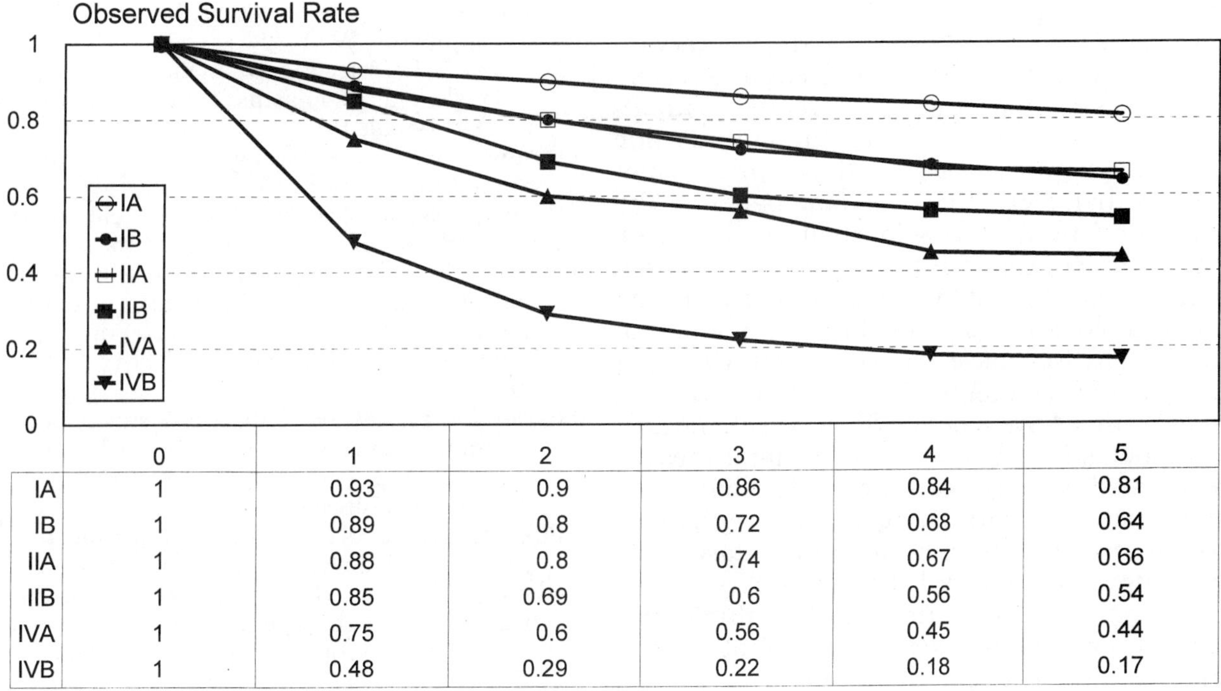

	0	1	2	3	4	5
IA	1	0.93	0.9	0.86	0.84	0.81
IB	1	0.89	0.8	0.72	0.68	0.64
IIA	1	0.88	0.8	0.74	0.67	0.66
IIB	1	0.85	0.69	0.6	0.56	0.54
IVA	1	0.75	0.6	0.56	0.45	0.44
IVB	1	0.48	0.29	0.22	0.18	0.17

A

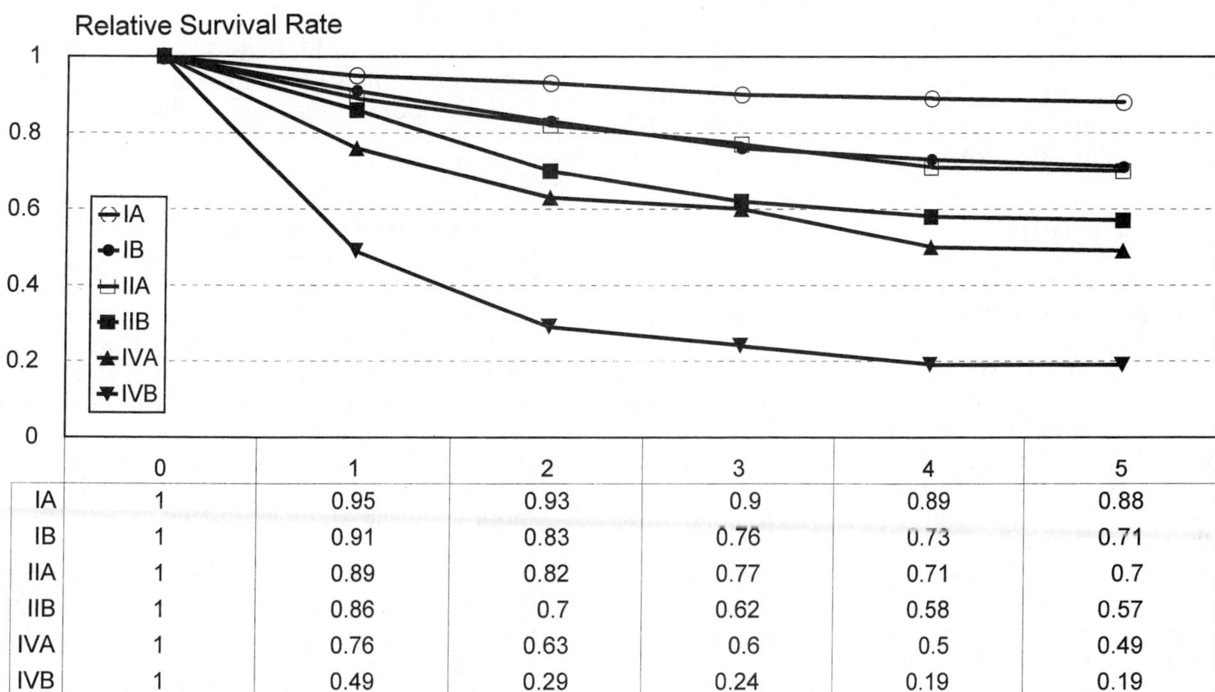

	0	1	2	3	4	5
IA	1	0.95	0.93	0.9	0.89	0.88
IB	1	0.91	0.83	0.76	0.73	0.71
IIA	1	0.89	0.82	0.77	0.71	0.7
IIB	1	0.86	0.7	0.62	0.58	0.57
IVA	1	0.76	0.63	0.6	0.5	0.49
IVB	1	0.49	0.29	0.24	0.19	0.19

B

FIG. 21-1. Observed **(A)** and relative **(B)** survival rates for 1,317 patients with bone cancer classified by the current AJCC staging classification. Data taken from the National Cancer Data Base (Commission on Cancer of the American College of Surgeons and the American Cancer Society) for the years 1985–1989. Stage IA includes 280 patients; Stage IB, 276; Stage IIA, 104; Stage IIB, 231; Stage IVA, 87; Stage IVB, 339.

have a better prognosis than those with a nonresectable tumor; (4) the size of the primary tumor is a prognostic factor for osteosarcoma and Ewing's sarcoma. Ewing's sarcoma patients with a tumor 8 cm or less in greatest dimension have a better prognosis than those with a tumor greater than 8 cm. Osteosarcoma patients with a tumor 15 cm or less in greatest dimension have a better prognosis than those with a tumor greater than 15 cm; (5) osteosarcomas with increased blood levels of alkaline phosphatase or lactic dehydrogenase are associated with poor prognosis; (6) patients who have a localized primary tumor have a better prognosis than those with metastases; (7) certain metastatic sites are associated with a poorer prognosis than other sites: bony or hepatic metastases convey a much worse prognosis than do lung metastases, and patients with solitary lung metastases have a better prognosis than those with multiple lung lesions; and (8) histologic response of the primary tumor to chemotherapy is a prognostic factor for osteosarcoma and Ewing's sarcoma. Those patients with a "good" response, > 90% tumor necrosis, have a better prognosis than those with less necrosis.

Figure 21-1 shows observed and relative survival rates for 1,317 patients with bone cancer for the years 1985–1989 classified by the AJCC staging classification.

BIBLIOGRAPHY

Aboulafia AJ, Mlawer MM: Surgical management of pelvic and extremity osteosarcoma. Cancer 71(10 Suppl):3358–3366, 1993

Bacci G, Avella M, McDonald D, et al: Serum lasctate dehydrogenase (LDH) as a tumor marker in Ewing's sarcoma. Tumori 74(6):649–655, 1988

Bacci G, Dallari D, Battistini A, et al: The prognostic value of serum alkaline phosphatase in osteosarcoma of the limbs. Chirurgia Degli Organi di Movimento 77(2):171–180, 1992

Bacci G, Ferrari S, Sangiorgi L, et al: Prognostic significance of serum lactate dehydrogenase in patients with osteosarcoma of the extremities. J Chemo 6(3):204–210, 1994

Bacci G, Picci P, Ferrari S, et al: Prognostic significance of serum alkaline phosphatase measurements in patients with osteosarcoma treated with adjuvant or neoadjuvant chemotherapy. Cancer 71(4):1224–1230, 1993

Beahrs OH, Henson DE, Hutter RVP, Kennedy BJ (Eds.): American Joint Committee on Cancer: Manual for staging of cancer, 4th ed. Philadelphia: JB Lippincott, 1992

Berquist TH: Magnetic resonance imaging of primary skeletal neoplasms. Radiol Clin North Am 31(2):411–424, 1993

Denny, CT: Gene rearrangements in Ewing's sarcoma. Cancer Invest 14(1):83–88, 1996

Evans R, Nesbit M, Askin F, et al: Local recurrence, rate and sites of metastases, and time to relapse as a function of treatment regimen, size of primary and surgical history in 62 patients presenting with nonmetastatic Ewing's sarcoma of the pelvic bones. Int J Radiat Oncol Biol Phys 11:129–136, 1985

Farley FA, Healey JH, Caparros-Sison B, et al: Lactase dehydrogenase as a tumor marker for recurrent disease in Ewing's sarcoma. Cancer 59(7):1245–1248, 1987

Fukuma H: Report to UICC TNM/Project Marker Committee. Geneva, Switzerland, May 3-4, 1994

Glasser DB, Lane JM, Huvos, AG, et al: Survival, prognosis and therapeutic response in osteosarcoma: The Memorial Hospital Experience. Cancer 67:698–708, 1992

Hayes FA, Thompson EI, Meyer WH, et al: Therapy for localized Ewing's sarcoma of bone. J Clin Oncol 7(2):208–213, 1989

Link MP, Goorin AM, Horowitz M, et al: Adjuvant chemotherapy of high-grade osteosarcoma of the extremity. Updated results of the Multi-Institutional Osteosarcoma Study. Clin Orthop 270:8–14, 1991

Liu PP, Leung KS, Kumta SM, et al: Bone-specific alkaline phosphatase in plasma as tumour marker for osteosarcoma. Oncology 53(4):275–280, 1996

Picci P, Rougraff B, Bucci G, et al: Prognostic significance of histopathologic response to chemotherapy in nonmetastatic Ewing's sarcoma of the extremity. J Clin Oncol 11:1763–1769, 1983

Raymond AK, Chawla SP, Cariasco CH, et al: Osteosarcoma chemotherapy effect: a prognostic factor. Sem Diag Pathol 4:212–236, 1987

Schajowicz F: Histological typing of bone tumours, 2nd ed. WHO histological classification of tumours. Berlin-Heidelberg-New York: Springer-Verlag, 1993

Schima W, Amann G, Stiglbauer R, et al: Preoperative staging of osteosarcoma: efficacy of MR imaging in detecting joint involvement. Amer J Roentgenology 163(5):1171–1175, 1994

Scully SP, Temple HT, O Keefe RJ, et al: Role of surgical resection in pelvic Ewing's sarcoma. J Clin Oncol 13(9):2336–2341, 1995

Ward WG, Mikaelian K, Dorey F, et al: Pulmonary metastases of stage IIB extremity osteosarcoma and subsequent pulmonary metastases. J Clin Oncol 12(9):1849–1858, 1994

Data Form for Cancer Staging

Patient identification
Name ____________________
Address ____________________
Hospital or clinic number ____________________
Age ____ Sex ____ Race ____________________

Institution identification
Hospital or clinic ____________________
Address ____________________

Oncology Record

Anatomic site of cancer ____________________
Histologic type ____________________
Grade (G) ____________________
Date of classification ____________________

Clin	Path	DEFINITIONS	
		Primary Tumor (T)	
[ ]	[ ]	TX	Primary tumor cannot be assessed
[ ]	[ ]	T0	No evidence of primary tumor
[ ]	[ ]	T1	Tumor confined within the cortex
[ ]	[ ]	T2	Tumor invades beyond the cortex
[ ]	[ ]	T2a	Tumor 8 cm or less in greatest dimension
[ ]	[ ]	T2b	Tumor more than 8 cm in greatest dimension
		Regional Lymph Nodes (N)	
[ ]	[ ]	NX	Regional lymph nodes cannot be assessed
[ ]	[ ]	N0	No regional lymph node metastasis
[ ]	[ ]	N1	Regional lymph node metastasis
		Because of the rarity of lymph node involvement in sarcomas the designation NX may not be appropriate and could be considered N0.	
		Distant Metastasis (M)	
[ ]	[ ]	MX	Distant metastasis cannot be assessed
[ ]	[ ]	M0	No distant metastasis
[ ]	[ ]	M1	Distant metastasis
		Histopathologic Grade (G)	
[ ]	[ ]	GX	Grade cannot be assessed
[ ]	[ ]	G1	Well differentiated—Low Grade
[ ]	[ ]	G2	Moderately differentiated—Low Grade
[ ]	[ ]	G3	Poorly differentiated—High Grade
[ ]	[ ]	G4	Undifferentiated—High Grade
		Ewing' sarcoma is classified as G4.	

Clin	Path	Stage Grouping				
[ ]	[ ]	IA	G1, 2	T1	N0	M0
[ ]	[ ]	IB	G1, 2	T2	N0	M0
[ ]	[ ]	IIA	G3, 4	T1	N0	M0
[ ]	[ ]	IIB	G3, 4	T2	N0	M0
[ ]	[ ]	III	Not defined			
[ ]	[ ]	IVA	Any G	Any T	N1	M0
[ ]	[ ]	IVB	Any G	Any T	Any N	M1

Histopathologic Type

A. Bone-forming
   1. Osteosarcoma (osteogenic sarcoma)
B. Cartilage-forming
   1. Chondrosarcoma
   2. Mesenchymal chondrosarcoma
C. Giant cell tumor, malignant
D. Ewing' sarcoma
E. Vascular tumors
   1. Hemangioendothelioma
   2. Hemangiopericytoma
   3. Angiosarcoma
F. Connective tissue tumors
   1. Fibrosarcoma
   2. Liposarcoma
   3. Malignant mesenchymoma
   4. Undifferentiated sarcoma
G. Other tumors
   1. Chordoma
   2. Adamantinoma of long bones

Staged by ____________________ **M.D.**
____________________ **Registrar**

Date ____________________

22

Soft Tissue Sarcoma

(Kaposi's sarcoma, dermatofibrosarcoma [protuberans], fibrosarcoma grade I [desmoid tumor], and sarcoma arising from the dura mater, brain, parenchymatous organs or hollow viscera are not included.)

C38.0 Heart
C38.1 Anterior mediastinum
C38.2 Posterior mediastinum
C38.3 Mediastinum, NOS
C38.8 Overlapping lesion of heart, mediastinum, and pleura

C47.0 Peripheral nerves and autonomic nervous system of head, face, and neck
C47.1 Peripheral nerves and autonomic nervous system of upper limb and shoulder
C47.2 Peripheral nerves and autonomic nervous system of lower limb and hip
C47.3 Peripheral nerves and autonomic nervous system of thorax
C47.4 Peripheral nerves and autonomic nervous system of abdomen
C47.5 Peripheral nerves and autonomic nervous system of pelvis
C47.6 Peripheral nerves and autonomic nervous system of trunk, NOS
C47.8 Overlapping lesion of peripheral nerves and autonomic nervous system
C47.9 Autonomic nervous system, NOS

C48.0 Retroperitoneum
C48.1 Specified parts of peritoneum
C48.2 Peritoneum, NOS
C48.8 Overlapping lesion of retroperitoneum and peritoneum

C49.0 Connective, subcutaneous, and other soft tissues of head, face, and neck
C49.1 Connective, subcutaneous, and other soft tissues of upper limb and shoulder
C49.2 Connective, subcutaneous, and other soft tissues of lower limb and hip
C49.3 Connective, subcutaneous, and other soft tissues of thorax
C49.4 Connective, subcutaneous, and other soft tissues of abdomen
C49.5 Connective, subcutaneous and other soft tissues of pelvis
C49.6 Connective, subcutaneous, and other soft tissues of trunk, NOS
C49.8 Overlapping lesion of connective, subcutaneous, and other soft tissues
C49.9 Connective, subcutaneous, and other soft tissues, NOS

The staging system applies to all soft tissue sarcomas except Kaposi's sarcoma, dermatofibrosarcoma, and desmoid type of fibrosarcoma grade 1. Excluded from the staging system are those sarcomas arising within the confines of the dura mater, including the brain, and sarcomas arising in parenchymatous organs and from hollow viscera. For the purposes of classification, we would adhere to the NIH recommendation of age 16 and above to be considered adult, but with the strong emphasis that the treatment decision be made by those with expertise. For example: rhabdomyosarcoma may well be treated with a pediatric regimen up to the age of 25, whereas low grade fibrosarcoma in a 14 year old might be treated with an adult surgical-only approach. Data to support this system are based on current available analysis from multiple institutions and these are the recommendations based on an AJCC task force on soft tissue sarcoma.

In the analysis, it was determined that, in addition to clinical information, the histologic type, grade, and tumor size and depth are essential for a meaningful staging system. The histologic diagnosis identifying the type of tumor and the pathologist's assessment of the inherent extent of malignancy (differentiation of the tumor) are fundamentals on which the staging is based.

Determination of the histologic grade and type of tumor is also required for staging soft tissue sarcomas and must be established by a qualified pathologist working with an adequate sample of the tumor.

Present data suggest that site itself should not be a component of the staging system, but all data should be reported specifically as to site. Generic grouping of site is accepted with extremity and superficial trunk being combined, and viscera, including all the intra-abdominal viscera, but reported where enough numbers exist, by divisions into various components of the gastrointestinal trace. Lung and genitourinary sarcomas should be grouped separately, as should any specific sites wherever possible, e.g., uterus.

Site Groups for Soft Tissue Sarcoma

Head and neck
Extremity and superficial trunk
Visceral
Retroperitoneal and lung, pleural, mediastinal
Breast
Other

STAGING OF SOFT TISSUE SARCOMA

Inclusions. The present staging system applies to soft tissue sarcomas. Primary sarcomas can arise from a variety of soft tissues. These tissues include fibrous connective tissue, fat, smooth or striated muscle, vascular tissue, and peripheral neural tissue as well as undifferentiated mesenchyme.

Regional Lymph Nodes. Involvement of regional lymph nodes by soft tissue is uncommon in adults. While nodal disease should be recorded in the staging system, it will have limited impact because of infrequency. When a regional lymph node dissection is done, for pN, histologic examination of a regional lymphadenectomy specimen will ordinarily include 6 or more regional lymph nodes.

Metastatic Sites. Metastatic sites for soft tissue sarcoma are highly dependent on the original site of the primary lesion. For example, the vast majority of patients with extremity lesions will have a primary site of metastasis to the lung. Patients with visceral lesions are more likely to have a primary site of metastasis in the liver. Conversely, a patient presenting with a metastasis of a sarcoma in the liver is most likely to have a primary visceral leiomyosarcoma (Fig. 22-1).

RULES FOR CLASSIFICATION

Clinical Staging. Clinical staging is dependent on characteristics of T, N, and M. For the majority of patients, N will not be an issue. T is divided into patients with lesions either 5 cm or less, or more than 5 cm in greatest dimension, but wherever possible, three-dimensional measurements should be provided. These can be readily calculated, described clinically, or subsequently measured radiologically. In the ex-

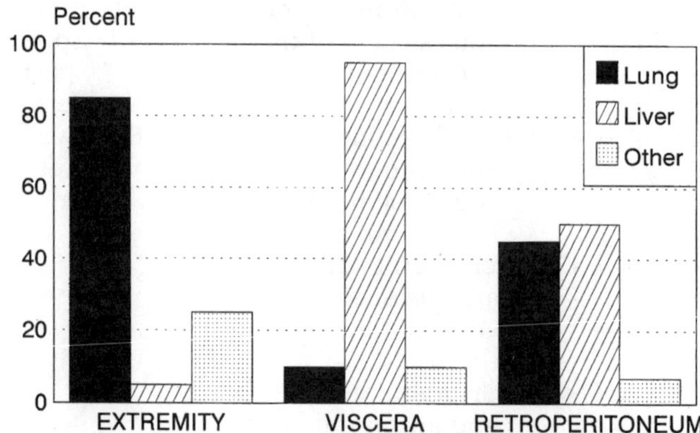

Fig. 22-1. Lung, liver, and all other metastases by primary site of soft tissue sarcoma: retroperitoneum, viscera, and extremity. From Memorial Sloan Kettering Cancer Center (MSKCC), 1982–1987.

tremity this will best be done by MRI; in other sites by either CT or MRI. Metastatic disease should be described according to the most likely sites of metastasis, as described above.

Pathologic Staging. Pathologic staging requires delineation of histopathologic type and subtype, along with the use of immunohistochemistry for accurate definition. Pathologic (pTNM) staging consists of the removal and pathologic evaluation of the primary tumor, histopathologic grade, and regional lymph nodes or distant metastases as indicated. Since regional lymph node involvement is rare in adult soft tissue sarcomas, pathologic stage grouping consists of pT pN pM, pT cN cM, or cT cN pM.

Definition of T. While size is currently designated as ≤ 5 cm or > 5 cm, particular emphasis should be placed, in sites other than the extremity or superficial trunk, on providing size measurements, preferably volume determinants. Size should be seen as a continuous variable, with 5 cm merely an arbitrary division that allows better characterization.

Historically, size has been considered a subcategory of grade, i.e., in previous systems a small (< 5 cm) high grade lesion would be considered as Stage III. The present system proposes to define size better according to its association with superficial or deep, and does not include small lesions as advanced stage.

Depth. Superficial is defined as lack of any involvement of the superficial investing muscular fascia in extremity lesions. For practical purposes, all retroperitoneal and visceral lesions will be deep lesions.

Depth (superficial or deep) is an independent variable, should be included in the system, and will include the following definitions:

1. Superficial
   a. Lesion does not involve superficial fascia.
2. Deep
   a. Lesion is deep to or invades the superficial (investing) fascia.
   b. All intraperitoneal visceral lesions or lesions with major vessel invasion, intrathoracic lesions, and the majority of head and neck tumors are considered deep.
3. Depth should be a subcategory of tumor size (T):
   a. Tumor ≤ 5 cm: T1a = superficial, T1b = deep
   b. Tumor > 5 cm: T2a = superficial, T2b = deep

Nodal Disease. Nodal involvement is rare in adult soft tissue sarcomas but has a very poor prognosis when evident. These patients do have a poor prognosis and the outcome of patients with N1 disease is the same as those with M1 disease. In assigning stage group, patients whose nodal status is not determined to be positive for tumor, either clinically or pathologically, should be designated as N0.

Grade. Grade should be assigned. Various grading systems exist. The present system of grading 1 through 4 would seem preferable. In those institutions where grading is high versus low, grades 1 and 2 would be considered low grade, and grades 3 and 4 high grade. For the clinician it is clear that division into two categories of high and low grade is simpler in recording all data. However, grade is a continuous biological variable and so it is difficult to assign arbitrary divisions. The following grading system is preferred:

GX Grade cannot be assessed
G1 Well differentiated
G2 Moderately differentiated
G3 Poorly differentiated
G4 Undifferentiated

Restaging of Recurrent Tumors. When a patient enters a clinical trial and requires restaging for recurrence, the same staging should be used. However, any report should include data on whether patients have primary lesions, or lesions that have undergone previous treatment and had subsequent recurrence. Identification and reporting of etiologic factors such as radiation exposure and familial syndromes is to be encouraged. These may be part of prognostication and therapeutic decision-making in the future.

Summary of Changes from Previous Staging System

The stage grouping is now simplified:

a. Subdivisions of the tumor (T) category would be used to designate superficial and deep lesions.
b. Pathologic stage grouping includes pT and cN0.
c. Presence of positive nodes (N1) is considered Stage IV.

Validation. Validation of this staging system is illustrated by the fact that the local recurrence rate is similar for all three stages. (Table 22-1) For this reason any of these patients can be incorporated into studies that examine the consequences of adjuvant therapy for local recurrence. Figure 22-2, however, emphasizes the value of staging in discriminating in terms of overall survival: p = 0.0001. Stage I lesions have a very small chance of going on to disease-dependent death, while stages II and III show a progressive difference. (Table 22-1) These figures are based on large numbers (194 patients in Stage I, 484 patients in Stage II, and 341 patients in Stage III), all obtained from a primary data base, presenting as primary lesions and managed in one institution. There is a poor prognosis for patients with nodal or disseminated metastases.

DEFINITION OF TNM

Primary Tumor (T)

TX Primary tumor cannot be assessed
T0 No evidence of primary tumor
T1 Tumor 5 cm or less in greatest dimension
  T1a superficial tumor
  T1b deep tumor
T2 Tumor more than 5 cm in greatest dimension
  T2a superficial tumor
  T2b deep tumor

Note: Superficial tumor is located exclusively above the superficial fascia without invasion of the fascia; deep tumor is located either exclusively beneath the superficial fascia, or superficial to the fascia with invasion of or through the fascia, or superficial and beneath the fascia. Retroperitoneal, mediastinal, and pelvic sarcomas are classified as deep tumors.

Regional Lymph Nodes (N)

NX Regional lymph nodes cannot be assessed
N0 No regional lymph node metastasis
N1 Regional lymph node metastasis

Table 22-1. Five Year Rate

STAGE	FREEDOM FROM LOCAL RECURRENCE	DISEASE-FREE SURV.	OVERALL SURVIVAL
I	79.09%	77.91%	98.79%
II	75.16%	63.63%	81.80%
III	74.46%	36.27%	51.65%

[1] Low grade <5 cm/deep/low grade >5 cm superficial.
[2] Low grade >5 cm/deep/high grade <5 cm/high grade >5 cm superficial.
[3] High grade >5 cm/deep.
Local recurrence, disease-free, and overall survival by Stage. Source: Memorial Sloan Kettering Cancer Center (MSKCC), 1992.

Distant Metastasis (M)

MX Distant metastasis cannot be assessed
M0 No distant metastasis
M1 Distant metastasis

HISTOPATHOLOGIC GRADE

GX Grade cannot be assessed
G1 Well differentiated
G2 Moderately differentiated
G3 Poorly differentiated
G4 Undifferentiated

STAGE GROUPING

Stage I				
A (Low grade, small, superficial and deep)	G1-2,	T1a-1b,	N0,	M0
B (Low grade, large, superficial)	G1-2,	T2a,	N0,	M0
Stage II				
A (Low grade, large, deep)	G1-2,	T2b,	N0,	M0
B (High grade, small, superficial, deep)	G3-4,	T1a-1b,	N0,	M0
C (High grade, large, superficial)	G3-4,	T2a,	N0,	M0
Stage III (High grade, large, deep)	G3-4,	T2b,	N0,	M0
Stage IV (any metastasis)	any G,	any T,	N1,	M0
	any G,	any T,	N0,	M1

HISTOPATHOLOGIC TYPE

Tumors included in the soft tissue category are listed below with the appropriate ICD-O morphology rubrics:

Alveolar soft-part sarcoma (9581/3)
Angiosarcoma (9120/3)
Epithelioid sarcoma (8804/3)
Extraskeletal chondrosarcoma (9220/3)
Extraskeletal osteosarcoma (9180/3)
Fibrosarcoma (8810/3)
Leiomyosarcoma (8890/3)
Liposarcoma (8850/3)
Malignant fibrous histiocytoma (8830/3)

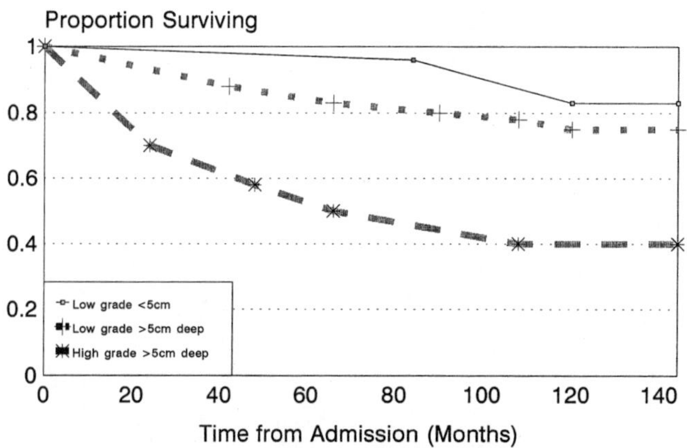

Fig. 22-2. Kaplan-Meier survival curves. Probability of overall survival by stage. From Memorial Sloan Kettering Cancer Center (MSKCC), 1982–1987.

Malignant hemangiopericytoma (9150/3)
Malignant mesenchymoma (8890/3)
Malignant schwannoma (9560/3)
Rhabdomyosarcoma (8900/3)
Synovial sarcoma (9040/3)
Sarcoma, NOS (8800/3)

The following histological types of tumors are not included: Kaposi's sarcoma, dermatofibrosarcoma (protuberans), fibrosarcoma grade I (desmoid tumor), and sarcoma arising from the dura mater, brain, parenchymatous organs or hollow viscera.

PROGNOSTIC FACTORS

Neurovascular and Bone Invasion

In earlier staging systems, neurovascular and bone invasion by soft tissue sarcomas had been included as a determinant of stage. It is not included in the current staging system and no plans are proposed to change it at the present time. Nevertheless, neurovascular and bone invasion should always be reported where possible, and studies are needed to determine whether or not such invasion is an independent prognostic factor.

Molecular Markers

Molecular markers are progressively being evaluated as determinants of outcome. At the present time, however, insufficient data exist to include specific molecular markers in the staging system. Nevertheless, studies are required to allow continued validation of such molecular markers.

Similar commentary should be made about the current identification of genetic abnormalities identified by chromosomal analysis. For the present time, molecular and genetic markers should be considered as definitions of specific histopathologic subtypes rather than determinants of stage.

BIBLIOGRAPHY

Brennan MR: Management of extremity soft tissue sarcoma. Eur J Surgical Oncology 16:520–531, 1990

Castro EB, Hajdr, SI, Fortner JG: Surgical therapy of fibrosarcoma of extremities. Arch Surg 107: 284–286, 1973

Enzinger FM, Lattes R, Torloni H: Histological typing of soft tissue tumors. International histological classification of tumors, No. 3. Geneva: World Health Organization, 1969

Enzinger FM, Shiraki M: Alveolar rhabdomyosarcoma: an analysis of 110 cases. Cancer 24:18–31, 1969

Fong Y, Coit DG, Woodruff JM, et al: Lymph note metastasis from soft tissue sarcoma: analysis of data from a prospective data base of 1772 sarcoma patients. Ann Surg 217:72, 1993

Greer RJ, Woodruff J, Casper ES, et al: Management of small soft tissue sarcoma of the extremity in adults. Arch Surg 127:1285–1289, 1992

Hajdu SI: Pathology of soft tissue tumours. Philadelphia: Lea & Febiger, 1979

Heise HW, Myers MH, Russell WO, et al: Recurrence-free survival time for surgically-treated soft tissue sarcoma patients. Cancer 57:172–177, 1986

Mazeron JJ, Suit HM: Lymph nodes as a site of metastasis from sarcomas of the soft tissue. Cancer 60:1800, 1987

Pritchard DJ, Soule EH, Taylor WF, et al: Fibrosarcoma: a clinicopathologic and statistical study of 199 tumors of the soft tissues of the extremities and trunk. Cancer 33(3): 888–897, 1974

Russell WO, Cohen J, Enzinger F, et al: a clinical and pathological staging system for soft tissue sarcomas. Cancer 40:1562–1570, 1977

Weingrad DN, Rosenberg SA: Early lymphatic spread of osteogenic and soft tissue sarcoma. Surgery 84:231, 1978

Weiss SW: Histological typing of soft tissue tumours. WHO international histological classification of tumours, 2nd ed. Berlin-Heidelberg-New York: Springer-Verlag, 1994

Data Form for Cancer Staging

Patient identification
Name ______
Address ______
Hospital or clinic number ______
Age ____ Sex ____ Race ______

Institution identification
Hospital or clinic ______
Address ______

Oncology Record

Anatomic site of cancer ______
Histologic type ______
Grade (G) ______
Date of classification ______

DEFINITIONS

Primary Tumor (T)

Clin	Path		
[ ]	[ ]	TX	Primary tumor cannot be assessed
[ ]	[ ]	T0	No evidence of primary tumor
[ ]	[ ]	T1	Tumor 5 cm or less in greatest dimension
[ ]	[ ]	T1a	superficial tumor
[ ]	[ ]	T1b	deep tumor
[ ]	[ ]	T2	Tumor more than 5 cm in greatest dimension
[ ]	[ ]	T2a	superficial tumor
[ ]	[ ]	T2b	deep tumor

Superficial tumor is located exclusively above the superficial fascia without invasion of the fascia; deep tumor is located either exclusively beneath the superficial fascia, or superficial to the fascia with invasion of or through the fascia, or superficial and beneath the fascia. Retroperitoneal, mediastinal, and pelvic sarcomas are classified as deep tumors.

Regional Lymph Nodes (N)

Clin	Path		
[ ]	[ ]	NX	Regional lymph nodes cannot be assessed*
[ ]	[ ]	N0	No regional lymph node metastasis
[ ]	[ ]	N1	Regional lymph node metastasis

** Because of the rarity of lymph node involvement in sarcomas, the designation NX may not be appropriate and could be considered N0 if no clinical involvement is evident.*

Distant Metastasis (M)

Clin	Path		
[ ]	[ ]	MX	Distant metastasis cannot be assessed
[ ]	[ ]	M0	No distant metastasis
[ ]	[ ]	M1	Distant metastasis

Histopathologic Grade (G)

Clin	Path		
[ ]	[ ]	GX	Grade cannot be assessed
[ ]	[ ]	G1	Well differentiated
[ ]	[ ]	G2	Moderately differentiated
[ ]	[ ]	G3	Poorly differentiated
[ ]	[ ]	G4	Undifferentiated

Stage Grouping

Clin	Path	Stage		
[ ]	[ ]	Stage I		
		A	(Low grade, small, superficial and deep)	G1-2, T1a-1b, N0, M0
		B	(Low grade, large, superficial)	G1-2, T2a, N0, M0
[ ]	[ ]	Stage II		
		A	(Low grade, large, deep)	G1-2, T2b, N0, M0
		B	(High grade, small, superficial, deep)	G3-4, T1a-1b, N0, M0
		C	(High grade, large, superficial)	G3-4, T2a, N0, M0
[ ]	[ ]	Stage III		
			(High grade, large, deep)	G3-4, T2b, N0, M0
[ ]	[ ]	Stage IV		any G, any T, N1, M0
			(any metastasis)	any G, any T, N0, M1

Staged by ______ M.D.
______ Registrar
Date ______

(continued on next page)

Histopathologic Type

Tumors included in the soft tissue category are listed below with the appropriate ICD-O morphology rubrics:

Alveolar soft-part sarcoma (9581/3)
Angiosarcoma (9120/3)
Epithelioid sarcoma (8804/3)
Extraskeletal chondrosarcoma (9220/3)
Extraskeletal osteosarcoma (9180/3)
Fibrosarcoma (8810/3)
Leiomyosarcoma (8890/3)
Liposarcoma (8850/3)
Malignant fibrous histiocytoma (8830/3)
Malignant hemangiopericytoma (9150/3)
Malignant mesenchymoma (8890/3)
Malignant schwannoma (9560/3)
Rhabdomyosarcoma (8900/3)
Synovial sarcoma (9040/3)
Sarcoma, NOS (8800/3)

The following histologic types of tumors are not included: Kaposi's sarcoma, dermatofibrosarcoma (protuberans), fibrosarcoma grade I (desmoid tumor), and sarcoma arising from the dura mater, brain, parenchymatous organs or hollow viscera.

SKIN

23

Carcinoma of the Skin (Excluding Eyelid, Vulva, and Penis)

C44.0 Skin of lip, NOS
C44.2 External ear
C44.3 Skin of other and unspecified parts of the face
C44.4 Skin of scalp and neck
C44.5 Skin of trunk
C44.6 Skin of upper limb and shoulder
C44.7 Skin of lower limb and hip
C44.8 Overlapping lesion
C44.9 Skin, NOS

C63.2 Scrotum

This chapter applies to nonmelanomatous cancers of the skin, which are predominantly squamous cell carcinomas and basal cell carcinomas. Skin cancers are related to solar exposure and are relatively common, although their frequency varies with geographic longitude. For example, they occur in 143 individuals per 100,000 population in the Southern United States versus only 25 per 100,000 in the Northern United States. Higher rates are found in Australia and New Zealand and the incidence generally is rising rapidly. Basal cell carcinomas are the most common cancer in humans, and are two to three times more common than squamous cell carcinomas of the skin. For the most part nonmelanomatous skin cancers have a good prognosis. Refer to Chapter 40 for staging of carcinoma of the eyelid and Chapter 24 for malignant melanoma of the skin.

ANATOMY

Primary Site. The skin is made up of three layers, an outermost epidermis, a middle dermis, and an inner subcutis. The epidermis consists predominately of stratified squamous epithelium, the outermost layer of which is keratinized. The innermost layer consists primarily of germinative cells and scattered melanocytes. The dermis is made up of connective tissue and elastic fibers immersed in an amorphous matrix of mucoproteins and mucopolysaccharides. The subcutis is predominantly adipose tissue.

The sebaceous and other glands of the skin, collectively called adnexal structures, are found in the dermis and adjacent subcutaneous tissue. All of the components of the skin (epidermis, dermis, and adnexal structures), can give rise to malignant neoplasms. The most common skin cancers, basal cell and squamous cell, are derived respectively from the germinative (inner epidermal) and keratinizing (outer epidermal) layers of the epidermis.

Cancers of the skin most commonly arise on those surfaces exposed to sunlight (including the face, ears, hands, and scalp) and the role of sunlight in the induction of cutaneous cancer has been well described. Approximately four-fifths of all cutaneous squamous cell cancers and approximately two-thirds of all basal cell cancers occur in sun-exposed skin. The relatively few squamous cell cancers that arise on skin not exposed to the sun, such as the truncal regions and on the extremities, usually arise within previously traumatized and ulcerated skin, i.e., at sites of burns and chronic ulcers. This is especially true of tumors arising in the skin of most darkly pigmented races.

Skin cancers rarely cause symptoms. Signs vary depending upon the local site of origin and the type of precursor lesion, i.e., cutaneous ulcer, vaccination site, actinic keratosis, or chronically irritated skin. Squamous cell tumors developing at the site of actinic keratoses begin as flat, red, scaling slightly elevated plaques. Induration, which is absent in actinic keratoses develops early in squamous cell cancer. Further aging is associated with thickening of the plaque, ulceration, and bleeding. Lip lesions are often quite innocuous in appearance, tending to occur without thickness or elevation. Ulceration occurs late, often after metastases have occurred. High risk tumors are also found on the scalp, ears, eyelids, and nose.

Basal cell cancers appear early as firm translucent papules coursed by firm telangiectatic blood vessels. Central areas of crusting and depression, associated with ulceration, appear late. Bleeding may be described in early as well as late lesions. Pigmentation occurs in dark skinned individuals. Morphea type tumors may look and feel like localized patches of scleroderma, and are without telangiectasia or measurable elevation.

Primary Growth. Local extension is the predominant mode of growth of nonmelanomatous skin cancers. Basal cell carcinomas that remain untreated for long periods will eventually erode adjacent structures, such as bone, and into local vasculature. Spread to adjacent and/or distant sites such as brain and lung may follow. Perineural invasion by both squamous cell and basal cell cancers is sometimes observed in chronic lesions of the head and neck.

Regional Lymph Nodes. Although skin cancers characteristically spread by local extension, involvement of regional lymph nodes infrequently occurs. The specific lymph node chains involved by disease depends on the location of the primary lesion, as tumors are passively borne along with the "draining" lymphatic fluid, usually to the geographically closest node(s). In this context, the inguinal nodes are considered the regional basin; the iliac nodes are considered sites of distant metastasis and should be coded as M1. For pN, histologic examination of a regional lymphadenectomy specimen will ordinarily include 6 or more regional lymph nodes.

Hematogenously Borne Metastases. Basal cell and squamous cell cancers that arise in actinically damaged skin are relatively slow growing and rarely metastasize. Metastases are more likely to arise from those lesions that originate in chronically injured skin sites. However, in addition to a increasing incidence of squamous cell cancer, there now appears to be a comparable increase in aggressive (metastasizing) lesions arising in sun-exposed skin. Tumors that metastasize are usually present for decades before metastases are observed. The most common metastatic site is the lung, especially for squamous cell carcinomas. Other sites of distant spread are unusual.

RULES FOR CLASSIFICATION

The clinical and pathologic classifications are identical. However, pathologic staging uses the symbol p as a prefix.

Clinical Staging. The assessment of skin cancer is based upon inspection and palpation of the involved area and the regional lymph nodes. Imaging studies of the underlying bony structures is important, especially for lesions of the scalp if the lesion is fixed to underlying structures.

Pathologic Staging. Complete resection of the entire site is required. Confirmation of lymph node involvement is also necessary. The degree of malignancy of squamous cell cancer of the skin generally is related to the degree of anaplasia viewed histopathologically within the tumor. Benign or low grade tumors show considerable cell differentiation, uniform cell size, infrequent cellular mitoses and nuclear irregularity, and intact intercellular bridges. Highly malignant tumors show opposite histopathologic signs. Depth of invasion also correlates with degree of tumor malignancy. Diversity of structure as revealed histopathologically does not appear to relate to the degree of malignancy of basal cell carcinoma.

DEFINITION OF TNM

Definitions for clinical (cTNM) and pathologic (pTNM) classifications are the same.

Primary Tumor (T)

TX Primary tumor cannot be assessed
T0 No evidence of primary tumor
Tis Carcinoma *in situ*
T1 Tumor 2 cm or less in greatest dimension
T2 Tumor more than 2 cm but not more than 5 cm in greatest dimension
T3 Tumor more than 5 cm in greatest dimension
T4 Tumor invades deep extradermal structures (i.e., cartilage, skeletal muscle, or bone)

Note: In the case of multiple simultaneous tumors, the tumor with the highest T category will be classified and the number of separate tumors will be indicated in parentheses, e.g., T2 (5).

Regional Lymph Nodes (N)

NX Regional lymph nodes cannot be assessed
N0 No regional lymph node metastasis
N1 Regional lymph node metastasis

Distant Metastasis (M)

MX Distant metastasis cannot be assessed
M0 No distant metastasis
M1 Distant metastasis

STAGE GROUPING

Stage 0	Tis	N0	M0
Stage I	T1	N0	M0
Stage II	T2	N0	M0
	T3	N0	M0
Stage III	T4	N0	M0
	Any T	N1	M0
Stage IV	Any T	Any N	M1

HISTOPATHOLOGIC TYPE

The classification applies only to carcinomas of the skin, primarily squamous cell and basal cell varieties. It also applies to the adenocarcinomas that develop from sweat or sebaceous glands and a spindle cell variant of squamous cell carcinoma. There should be microscopic verification of the disease to permit division of cases by histologic type. A form of *in situ* carcinoma or intraepidermal carcinoma is often referred to as Bowen's disease. This lesion should be coded as Tis. Squamous cell tumors may also be described as verrucous.

HISTOPATHOLOGIC GRADE (G)

GX Grade cannot be assessed
G1 Well differentiated
G2 Moderately differentiated
G3 Poorly differentiated
G4 Undifferentiated

PROGNOSTIC FACTORS

In squamous cell carcinoma, tumor aggressiveness correlates well with tumor size, duration, location, origin, and degree of anaplasia. Large tumors are usually present for long periods or are rapidly growing. Long-standing tumors tend to grow extensively and invade other structures, such as local vasculature, or nervous tissue. Tumors of the scalp, ears, lips, nose and eyelids readily invade subcutaneous tissue and have a greater risk of subclinical tumor extension.

Anaplastic tumors readily tend to invade locally and to metastasize earlier than well-differentiated tumors regardless of location. Tumors that arise in non-sun-exposed skin usually develop in areas of precursor lesions other than actinic keratoses or in chronic cutaneous ulcerations, or simply chronically irritated skin.

Metastases from basal cell carcinomas are rare. However, basal cell cancers are often locally destructive. Destructiveness is related to a number of factors that include: (a) tumor-stroma interdependence; (b) contact inhibition; (c) host/cell mediated immunity; (d) host/humoral immunity; (e) host immune system reactivity to sunlight; (f) locally induced biochemical reactions; (g) degree of attachment between cancer cells and surrounding stroma; and (h) status of tumor cell locomotor reactivity.

BIBLIOGRAPHY

Chuang T-Y, Heinrich LA, Schultz MD, et al: PUVA and skin cancer: a historical cohort study on 492 patients. J Am Acad Dermatol 26:173–177, 1992

Czarnecki D, Collins M, Meehan C, et al: Basal cell carcinoma in temperate and tropical Australia. Int J Cancer 50:874–875, 1992

Czarnecki D, Obrien T, Meehan CJ: Nonmelanoma skin cancer: number of cancers and their distribution in outpatients. Int J Dermatol 33:416–417, 1994

Czarnecki D, Staples M, Mar A, et al: Metastases from squamous cell carcinomas of the skin in southern Australia. Dermatology 189:52–54, 1994

Haenzel W: Variations in skin cancer incidence within the United States. Nat Cancer Inst Monograph 10:225, 1963

Kwa RE, Campana K, Moy RL: Biology of cutaneous squamous cell carcinoma. J Am Acad Dermatol 26:1–26, 1992

Lund HZ: How often does squamous cell carcinoma of the skin metastasize? Arch Dermatol 92:635–637, 1965

McDonald CJ: Malignant neoplasms of the skin. In Calabresi P, Schein PS (Eds.), Medical oncology. New York: McGraw-Hill; 517–543, 1993

Moan J, Dalback A: The relationship between skin cancers, solar radiation and ozone depletion. Br J Cancer 65:916–921, 1992

Scotto J, Fearst R, Fraumeni JF: Incidence of nonmelanoma skin cancer in the United States. NIH Publication No. 83-2433. Washington, D.C.: US Department of Health and Human Services, 1983

CARCINOMA OF THE SKIN (EXCLUDING EYELID, VULVA, AND PENIS)

Data Form for Cancer Staging

Patient identification
Name ______
Address ______
Hospital or clinic number ______
Age ____ Sex ____ Race ______

Institution identification
Hospital or clinic ______
Address ______

Oncology Record

Anatomic site of cancer ______
Histologic type ______
Grade (G) ______
Date of classification ______

DEFINITIONS

Primary Tumor (T)

Clin	Path		
[ ]	[ ]	TX	Primary tumor cannot be assessed
[ ]	[ ]	T0	No evidence of primary tumor
[ ]	[ ]	Tis	Carcinoma *in situ*
[ ]	[ ]	T1	Tumor 2 cm or less in greatest dimension
[ ]	[ ]	T2	Tumor more than 2 cm but not more than 5 cm in greatest dimension
[ ]	[ ]	T3	Tumor more than 5 cm in greatest dimension
[ ]	[ ]	T4	Tumor invades deep extradermal structures, i.e., cartilage, skeletal muscle or bone

In the case of multiple simultaneous tumors, the tumor with the highest T category will be classified and the number of separate tumors will be indicated in parentheses, e.g., T2 (5).

Regional Lymph Nodes (N)

Clin	Path		
[ ]	[ ]	NX	Regional lymph nodes cannot be assessed
[ ]	[ ]	N0	No regional lymph node metastasis
[ ]	[ ]	N1	Regional lymph node metastasis

Distant Metastasis (M)

Clin	Path		
[ ]	[ ]	MX	Distant metastasis cannot be assessed
[ ]	[ ]	M0	No distant metastasis
[ ]	[ ]	M1	Distant metastasis

Stage Grouping

Clin	Path	Stage	T	N	M
[ ]	[ ]	0	Tis	N0	M0
[ ]	[ ]	I	T1	N0	M0
[ ]	[ ]	II	T2	N0	M0
			T3	N0	M0
[ ]	[ ]	III	T4	N0	M0
			Any T	N1	M0
[ ]	[ ]	IV	Any T	Any N	M1

Histopathologic Grade (G)

[ ] GX Grade cannot be assessed
[ ] G1 Well differentiated
[ ] G2 Moderately differentiated
[ ] G3 Poorly differentiated
[ ] G4 Undifferentiated

Illustrations

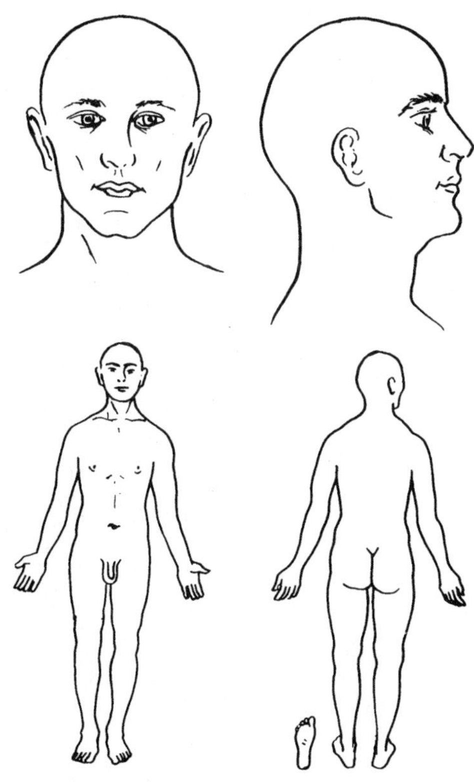

Indicate on diagram primary tumor and regional nodes involved.

Histopathologic Type

The classification applies only to carcinomas of the skin, primarily squamous cell and basal cell varieties. It also applies to the adenocarcinomas that develop from sweat or sebaceous glands and a spindle cell variant of squamous cell carcinoma. There should be microscopic verification of the disease to permit division of cases by histologic type. A form of *in situ* carcinoma or intraepidermal carcinoma is often referred to as Bowen's disease. This lesion should be coded as Tis. Squamous cell tumors may also be described as verrucous.

Staged by ______ **M.D.**
______ **Registrar**
Date ______

24

Malignant Melanoma of the Skin

C44.0 Skin of lip, NOS
C44.1 Eyelid
C44.2 External ear
C44.3 Skin of other and unspecified parts of face
C44.4 Skin of scalp and neck
C44.5 Skin of trunk
C44.6 Skin of upper limb and shoulder
C44.7 Skin of lower limb and hip
C44.8 Overlapping lesion of skin
C44.9 Skin, NOS

C51.0 Vulva

C60.9 Penis

C63.2 Scrotum

Malignant melanomas occur most commonly in fair-skinned persons, often those who have a history of sun exposure. Individuals who have genetically-determined hypersensitivity to ultraviolet irradiation (e.g., as in xeroderma pigmentosum) have a substantial risk of developing these neoplasms. Melanomas may take origin in any skin site, including the palms, soles, and nail beds. Most commonly they arise *de novo,* but approximately 15% are derived from pre-existing melanocytic nevi, such as "giant hairy" congenital nevi. Rarely, melanomas originate in the mucous membranes of the oral cavity, nasopharynx, vagina, urethra, anal canal, esophagus, bronchi, and biliary tree. In approximately one-third of patients who present with disseminated metastatic disease, the primary site of disease may not be found despite extensive clinical evaluation, and may be presumed to have regressed spontaneously. Improved detection and management of "early" melanomas has significantly lessened the mortality from such lesions over the past 20 years.

The staging classification for malignant melanoma presented herein applies only to primary cutaneous melanocytic malignancies.

ANATOMY

Primary Sites. As mentioned above, cutaneous malignant melanoma can originate in virtually any skin site, although it does so by far most commonly in sun-exposed areas (i.e., head and neck, arms, back, and legs). Multiple primary tumors may occur synchronously or metachronously, and these may be difficult to distinguish from epidermotropic metastases.

Regional Lymph Nodes. Spread of disease to regional nodes occurs not infrequently. The specific lymph node chains involved by disease depends on the location of the primary lesion, as tumors are passively borne along with the "draining" lymphatic fluid, usually to the geographically closest node(s). Melanomas also commonly metastasize through the lymphatics in a "satellitotic" fashion to the adjacent skin and subcutaneous tissues. In this context, it should be recognized that occasional melanomas yield *intraepidermal* ("pagetoid") metastases that cannot be distinguished from multiple new primary tumors by the pathologist. For pN, histologic examination of a regional lymphadenectomy specimen will ordinarily include 6 or more regional lymph nodes.

Distant Metastases. Malignant melanomas have the potential for widespread metastasis. Often a multiplicity of organs and tissues (particularly the liver, bones, lungs, and brain) are affected. In fact, no anatomic site is immune to involvement by these neoplasms. "Thick" tumors (> 1.5 mm) and/or involved regional lymph nodes frequently predict distant metastases. But, some so-called "thin" (< 0.76 mm) melanomas, by virtue of being in their vertical growth phase (*vide infra*), may skip regional lymph nodes and metastasize first to the viscera. Sometimes, metastases may not become clinically apparent for many years (up to 30) after initial diagnosis.

For staging purposes, two "M" substage categories—identified as "a" and "b"—are included. Metastases to the skin, subcutaneous tissues, or lymph nodes outside the scope of regional lymph node drainage are considered M1a disease. Secondary involvement of other distant sites—often labeled "visceral metastases"—is coded as M1b disease. This distinction is justified by the more favorable therapeutic response of patients who have only dermal, subcutaneous, or nodal metastases of their primary tumors.

RULES FOR CLASSIFICATION

Clinical Staging. The "length by width" classification of tumor size that correlates with prognosis for most tumor types is not useful for malignant melanomas. Instead, it is the thickness (i.e., the third primary tumor dimension) that predicts outcome. Consequently, clinical "T" classification is usually not possible. Excisional biopsy and histopathologic interpretation of primary lesions are necessary for proper staging. Ulceration of the primary lesion typically is associated with a worse prognosis, and should be recorded for that reason, but its presence does not alter the staging procedure.

Pathologic Staging. Histopathologic staging of primary cutaneous melanomas is based on the microscopic measurement of both (a) the absolute thickness of the tumor—the "Breslow" system—and (b) the relative depth of invasion (as compared to the position of normal tissue structures: the tips of the rete ridges (i.e., the papillary dermis), the superior and inferior reticular dermis and the subcutis)—the "Clark" system. Both the "Breslow" thickness (in mm) and the "Clark" level of invasion have been shown to have prognostic import. In case of discrepancy between the T category that would be assigned by the "Breslow" and "Clark" methods, the numerically greater value is used for the pT category. [Specifically, the maximal thickness of the tumor is measured with an ocular micrometer *at a right angle to the surface of the skin over the tumor mass.* The upper reference point is the superficial aspect of the granular cell layer of the epidermis, or the *base* of the lesion if the tumor is ulcerated. The lower reference point is the deepest point of tumor invasion. This may be represented by the leading edge of the lesion "in continuity," or "detached" cell groups deep to the epicenter of the mass.] Because evaluation of the entire primary tumor and adjacent normal skin is mandatory to find the thickest/deepest part, "shave" and punch biopsies should be avoided. Regional nodes should be carefully evaluated, if they are available, and the number of involved nodes should be identified and compared to the total number of lymph nodes removed. If the extent of the primary lesion is not evident because of previous intervention, distortion introduced by the surgical procedure or histopathologic processing, the tumor is coded "TX." If no primary site can be found despite an appropriate search (i.e., the primary regressed spontaneously), the tumor is coded "T0."

"Satellite" lesions and subcutaneous nodules within 2 cm of the primary tumor are considered extensions of the primary mass and coded pT4b. Satellite lesions and cutaneous and subcutaneous metastases more than 2 cm away from the primary tumor (but within the pathway to the regional lymph nodes which serve the primary site) are coded as "in-transit metastases" (N2b).

DEFINITION OF TNM

Both the level of invasion and the maximum thickness determine the T classification and should be recorded. In case of discrepancy between tumor thickness and level, the pT category is based on the less favorable finding.

Satellite lesions or cutaneous and subcutaneous metastases more than 2 cm from the primary tumor but not beyond the site of the pri-

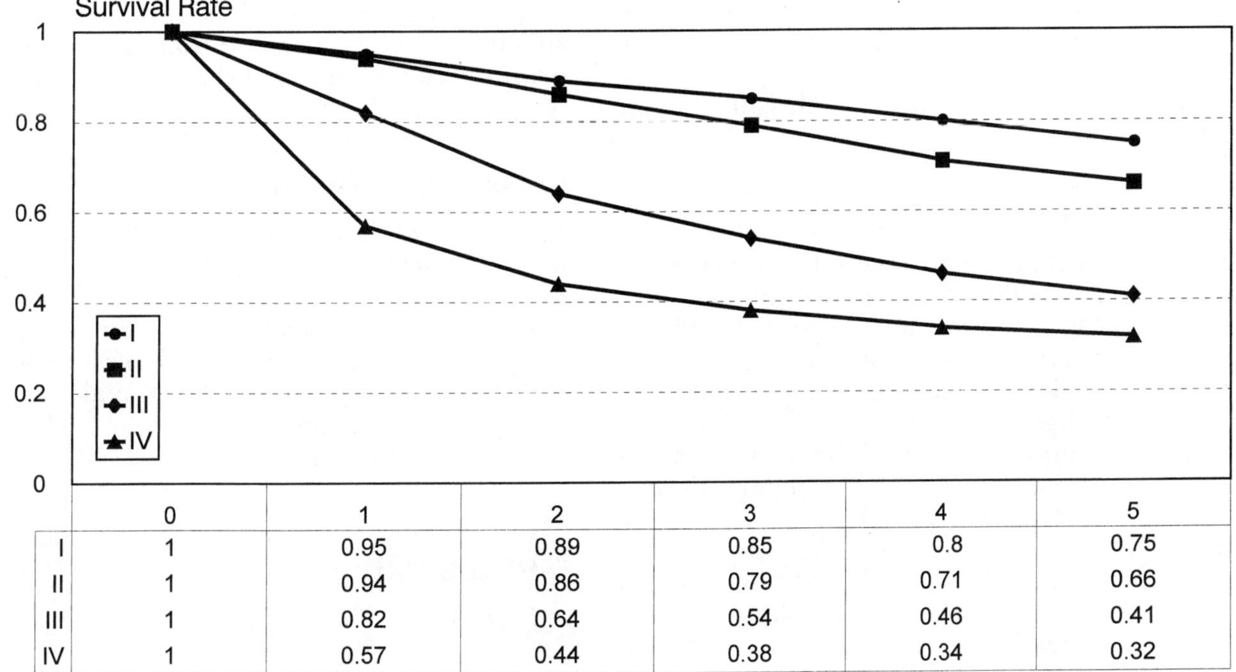

	0	1	2	3	4	5
I	1	0.95	0.89	0.85	0.8	0.75
II	1	0.94	0.86	0.79	0.71	0.66
III	1	0.82	0.64	0.54	0.46	0.41
IV	1	0.57	0.44	0.38	0.34	0.32

A

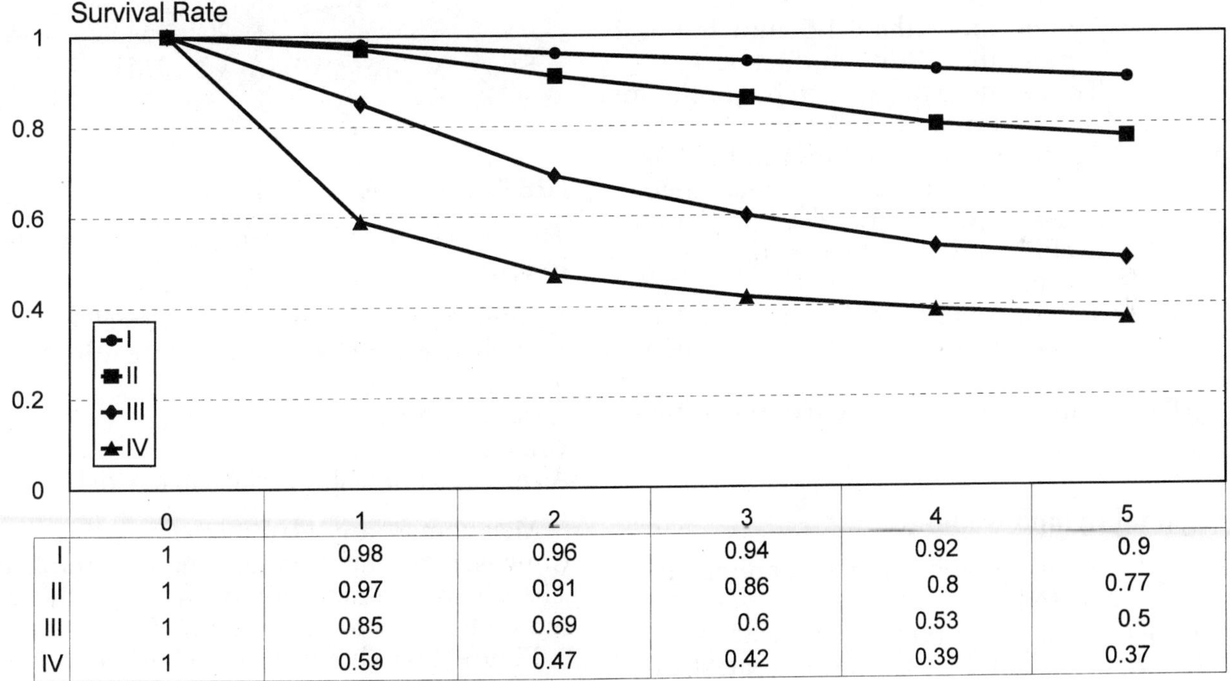

	0	1	2	3	4	5
I	1	0.98	0.96	0.94	0.92	0.9
II	1	0.97	0.91	0.86	0.8	0.77
III	1	0.85	0.69	0.6	0.53	0.5
IV	1	0.59	0.47	0.42	0.39	0.37

B

FIG. 24-1. Observed **(A)** and relative **(B)** survival rates for 31,879 patients with malignant melanoma classified by the current AJCC staging classification. Data taken from the National Cancer Data Base (Commission on Cancer of the American College of Surgeons and the American Cancer Society) for the years 1985–1989. Stage I includes 21,979 patients; Stage II, 4,570; Stage III, 3,341; Stage IV, 1,592.

mary lymph node drainage are considered "in-transit metastases" and are listed under the N categories.

The extent of tumor is classified after excision.

Primary Tumor (pT)

pTX Primary tumor cannot be assessed
pT0 No evidence of primary tumor
pTis Melanoma *in situ* (atypical melanocytic hyperplasia, severe melanocytic dysplasia), not an invasive malignant lesion (Clark's Level I)
pT1 Tumor 0.75 mm or less in thickness and invades the papillary dermis (Clark's Level II)
pT2 Tumor more than 0.75 mm but not more than 1.5 mm in thickness and/or invades to papillary-reticular dermal interface (Clark's Level III)
pT3 Tumor more than 1.5 mm but not more than 4 mm in thickness and/or invades the reticular dermis (Clark's Level IV)
 pT3a Tumor more than 1.5 mm but not more than 3 mm in thickness
 pT3b Tumor more than 3 mm but not more than 4 mm in thickness
pT4 Tumor more than 4 mm in thickness and/or invades the subcutaneous tissue (Clark's Level V) and/or satellite(s) within 2 cm of the primary tumor
 pT4a Tumor more than 4 mm in thickness and/or invades the subcutaneous tissue
 pT4b Satellite(s) within 2 cm of the primary tumor

Regional Lymph Nodes (N)

NX Regional lymph nodes cannot be assessed
N0 No regional lymph node metastasis
N1 Metastasis 3 cm or less in greatest dimension in any regional lymph node(s)
N2 Metastasis more than 3 cm in greatest dimension in any regional lymph node(s) and/or in-transit metastasis
 N2a Metastasis more than 3 cm in greatest dimension in any regional lymph node(s)
 N2b In-transit metastasis
 N2c Both (N2a and N2b)

Note: In-transit metastasis involves skin or subcutaneous tissue more than 2 cm from the primary tumor but not beyond the regional lymph nodes.

Distant Metastasis (M)

MX Distant metastasis cannot be assessed
M0 No distant metastasis
M1 Distant metastasis
 M1a Metastasis in skin or subcutaneous tissue or lymph node(s) beyond the regional lymph nodes
 M1b Visceral metastasis

STAGE GROUPING

Stage 0	pTis	N0	M0
Stage I	pT1	N0	M0
	pT2	N0	M0
Stage II	pT3	N0	M0
Stage III	pT4	N0	M0
	Any pT	N1	M0
	Any pT	N2	M0
Stage IV	Any pT	Any N	M1

HISTOPATHOLOGIC TYPE

The types of malignant melanoma are as follows:

Lentigo maligna (Hutchinson's freckle)
Radial spreading (superficial spreading)
Nodular
Acral lentiginous
Unclassified
A rare desmoplastic variant also exists.

Melanomas are identified according to site (mucosal, ocular, vaginal, anal, urethral, etc.). The staging classification described in this chapter applies only to those arising in the skin.

Figure 24-1 shows observed and relative survival rates for 31,879 patients with malignant melanoma for the years 1985–1989 classified by the AJCC staging classification.

BIBLIOGRAPHY

Aitchison TC, Sirel JM, Watt DC, et al: Prognostic trees to aid prognosis in patients with cutaneous malignant melanoma. Scottish Melanoma Group. Br Med J 311(7019):1536–1541, 1995

Balch C, Soong SJ, Shaw H, et al: An analysis of prognostic factors in 8500 patients with cutaneous melanoma. In Balch C, Houghton A, Milton G (Eds.), Cutaneous melanoma, 2nd ed. Philadelphia: JB Lippincott; 165–187, 1992

Breslow A: Thickness, cross-sectional areas, and depth of invasion in the prognosis of cutaneous melanoma. Ann Surg 172:902–908, 1970

Clark WH Jr, From L, Bernardino E, et al: The histogenesis and biologic behavior of primary human malignant melanomas of the skin. Cancer Res 29:705–726, 1969

Gamel JW, George SL, Stanley WE, et al: Skin melanoma: cured fraction and survival time as functions of thickness, site, histologic type, age, and sex. Cancer 72:1219–1223, 1993

Hermanek P, Blinov NN: Malignant melanoma of the skin. In Hermanek P, Gospodarowicz MK, Henson DE, et al (Eds.): Prognostic factors in cancer. Berlin, Springer-Verlag; 152–164, 1995

Sugihara T, Yoshida T, Kokubu I, et al: Prognostic evaluation of cutaneous malignant melanoma based on the pTNM classification. J Dermatol 21:953–959, 1994

MALIGNANT MELANOMA OF THE SKIN

Data Form for Cancer Staging

Patient identification
Name ______
Address ______
Hospital or clinic number ______
Age ____ Sex ____ Race ______

Institution identification
Hospital or clinic ______
Address ______

Oncology Record

Anatomic site of cancer ______
Histologic type ______
Grade (G) ______
Date of classification ______

Clin	Path	DEFINITIONS	
		Primary Tumor (pT)	
[ ]	[ ]	pTX	Primary tumor cannot be assessed
[ ]	[ ]	pT0	No evidence of primary tumor
[ ]	[ ]	pTis	Melanoma *in situ* (atypical melanocytic hyperplasia, severe melanocytic dysplasia, not an invasive lesion) (Clark's Level I)
[ ]	[ ]	pT1	Tumor 0.75 mm or less in thickness and invades the papillary dermis (Clark's Level II)
[ ]	[ ]	pT2	Tumor more than 0.75 mm but not more than 1.5 mm in thickness and/or invades to papillary-reticular dermal interface (Clark's Level III)
[ ]	[ ]	pT3	Tumor more than 1.5 mm but not more than 4 mm in thickness and/or invades the reticular dermis (Clark's Level IV)
[ ]	[ ]	pT3a	Tumor more than 1.5 mm but not more than 3 mm in thickness
[ ]	[ ]	pT3b	Tumor more than 3 mm but not more than 4 mm in thickness
[ ]	[ ]	pT4	Tumor more than 4 mm in thickness and/or invades the subcutaneous tissue (Clark's Level V) and/or satellite(s) within 2 cm of the primary tumor
[ ]	[ ]	pT4a	Tumor more than 4 mm in thickness and/or invades the subcutaneous tissue
[ ]	[ ]	pT4b	Satellite(s) within 2 cm of primary tumor
		Regional Lymph Nodes (N)	
[ ]	[ ]	NX	Regional lymph nodes cannot be assessed
[ ]	[ ]	N0	No regional lymph node metastasis
[ ]	[ ]	N1	Metastasis 3 cm or less in greatest dimension in any regional lymph node(s)
[ ]	[ ]	N2	Metastasis more than 3 cm in greatest dimension in any regional lymph node(s) and/or in-transit metastasis
[ ]	[ ]	N2a	Metastasis more than 3 cm in greatest dimension in any regional lymph node(s)
[ ]	[ ]	N2b	In-transit metastasis
[ ]	[ ]	N2c	Both (N2a and N2b)
		Distant Metastasis (M)	
[ ]	[ ]	MX	Distant metastasis cannot be assessed
[ ]	[ ]	M0	No distant metastasis
[ ]	[ ]	M1	Distant metastasis
[ ]	[ ]	M1a	Metastasis in skin or subcutaneous tissue or lymph node(s) beyond the regional lymph nodes
[ ]	[ ]	M1b	Visceral metastasis

Stage Grouping

Clin	Path	Stage	T	N	M
[ ]	[ ]	0	pTis	N0	M0
[ ]	[ ]	I	pT1	N0	M0
			pT2	N0	M0
[ ]	[ ]	II	pT3	N0	M0
[ ]	[ ]	III	pT4	N0	M0
			Any pT	N1	M0
			Any pT	N2	M0
[ ]	[ ]	IV	Any pT	Any N	M1

Staged by ______ **M.D.**
______ **Registrar**
Date ______

(continued on next page)

Histopathologic Type

The types of malignant melanoma are as follows:

Lentigo maligna (Hutchinson's freckle)
Radial spreading (superficial spreading)
Nodular
Acral lentiginous
Unclassified

A rare desmoplastic variant also exists.
Melanomas are identified according to site (mucosal, ocular, vaginal, anal, urethral, and so forth). The staging classification described in this chapter applies only to those arising in the skin.

Sites of Distant Metastasis

[ ] Pulmonary PUL
[ ] Osseous OSS
[ ] Hepatic HEP
[ ] Brain BRA
[ ] Lymph nodes LYM
[ ] Bone marrow MAR
[ ] Pleura PLE
[ ] Peritoneum PER
[ ] Skin SKI
[ ] Other OTH

Depth of Invasion

[ ] Level I (not a melanoma and further characterization is not necessary)
[ ] Level II
[ ] Level III
[ ] Level IV
[ ] Level V

Other description ____________________
Maximal thickness (mm) ____________________
Size of primary lesion (check diagram) ____________________

Extent of primary lesion (include all pigmentation) ____________________

Size in greatest diameter _____ cm

Illustrations

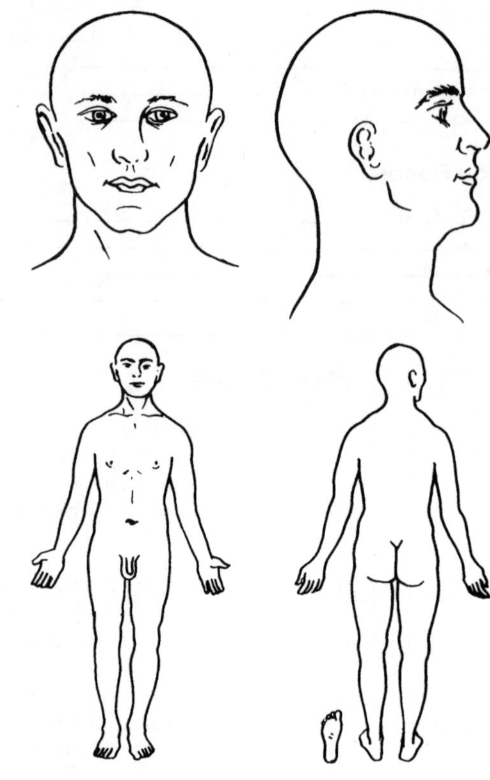

Indicate on diagram primary tumor and regional nodes involved.

25

Breast

C50.0 Nipple
C50.1 Central portion breast
C50.2 Upper-inner quadrant breast
C50.3 Lower-inner quadrant breast
C50.4 Upper-outer quadrant breast
C50.5 Lower-outer quadrant breast
C50.6 Axillary tail breast
C50.8 Overlapping lesion breast
C50.9 Breast, NOS

The following TNM definitions and stage groupings for carcinoma of the breast are the same for the American Joint Committee on Cancer (AJCC) and the Union Internationale Contre le Cancer (UICC)/TNM projects. This staging system for carcinoma of the breast applies to infiltrating (including microinvasive) and *in situ* carcinomas. Microscopic confirmation of the diagnosis is mandatory and the histologic type and grade of carcinoma should be recorded.

ANATOMY

Primary Site. The mammary gland, situated on the anterior chest wall, is composed of glandular tissue within a dense fibroareolar stroma. The glandular tissue consists of approximately 20 lobes, each of which terminates in a separate excretory duct in the nipple.

Regional Lymph Nodes. The breast lymphatics drain by way of three major routes: axillary, transpectoral, and internal mammary. Intramammary lymph nodes are considered with, and coded as, axillary lymph nodes for staging purposes. Metastasis to any other lymph node is considered distant (M1), including supraclavicular, cervical, or contralateral internal mammary. (Please refer to diagram.) The regional lymph nodes are:

1. Axillary (ipsilateral): interpectoral (Rotter's) nodes and lymph nodes along the axillary vein and its tributaries which may be (but are not required to be) divided into the following levels:
   (i) Level I (low-axilla): lymph nodes lateral to the lateral border of pectoralis minor muscle.
   (ii) Level II (mid-axilla): lymph nodes between the medial and lateral borders of the pectoralis minor muscle and the interpectoral (Rotter's) lymph nodes.
   (iii) Level III (apical axilla): lymph nodes medial to the medial margin of the pectoralis minor muscle including those designated as subclavicular, infraclavicular, or apical.

Note: Intramammary lymph nodes are coded as axillary lymph nodes.

2. Internal mammary (ipsilateral): lymph nodes in the intercostal spaces along the edge of the sternum in the endothoracic fascia.

REGIONAL LYMPH NODES

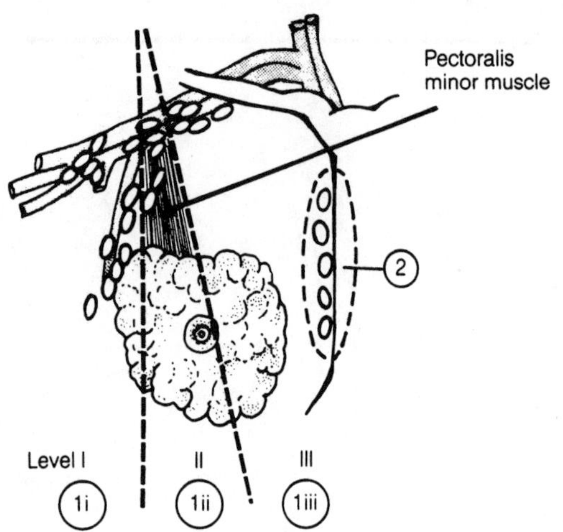

Any other lymph node metastasis is coded as a distant metastasis (M1), including supraclavicular, cervical, or contralateral internal mammary lymph nodes.

Metastatic Sites. All distant visceral sites are potential sites of metastasis. The four major sites of involvement are bone, lung, brain, and liver, but this widely metastasizing disease has been found in many other sites.

RULES FOR CLASSIFICATION

Clinical Staging. Clinical staging includes physical examination, with careful inspection and palpation of the skin, mammary gland, and lymph nodes (axillary, supraclavicular, and cervical), imaging, and pathologic examination of the breast *or* other tissues to establish the diagnosis of breast carcinoma. The extent of tissue examined pathologically for clinical staging is less than that required for pathologic staging (see Pathologic Staging). Appropriate operative findings are elements of clinical staging, including the size of the primary tumor and chest wall invasion, and the presence or absence of regional or distant metastasis.

Pathologic Staging. Pathologic staging includes all data used for clinical staging, surgical exploration and resection as well as pathologic examination of the primary carcinoma, including not less than excision of the primary carcinoma with no macroscopic tumor in any margin of resection by pathologic examination. A case can be classified pT for pathologic stage grouping if there is only microscopic, but not macroscopic, involvement at the margin. If there is tumor in the margin of resection by macroscopic examination, it is coded TX because the extent of the primary tumor cannot be assessed. If there is no clinical evidence of axillary metastasis, resection of at least the low axillary lymph nodes (Level I), that is, those lymph nodes located lateral to the lateral border of the pectoralis minor muscle should be performed for pathologic (pN) classification. Such a resection will ordinarily include 6 or more lymph nodes. Metastatic nodules in the fat adjacent to the mammary carcinoma within the breast, without evidence of residual lymph node tissue, are classified as regional lymph node metastases (N). Pathologic stage grouping includes any of the following combinations: pT pN pM, or pT pN cM, or cT cN pM.

TNM CLASSIFICATION

Primary Tumor

The clinical measurement used for classifying the primary tumor (T) is the one judged to be most accurate for that particular case (e.g., physical examination or imaging such as a mammogram). The pathologic tumor size for classification (T) is a measurement of *only the invasive component.* For example, if there is a 4.0 cm intraductal component and a 0.3 cm invasive component, the tumor is classified T1a. The size of the primary tumor is measured for T-classification before any tissue is removed for special studies, such as for estrogen receptors.

Microinvasion of Breast Carcinoma

Microinvasion is the extension of cancer cells beyond the basement membrane into the adjacent tissues with no focus more than 0.1 cm in greatest dimension. When there are multiple foci of microinvasion, the size of only the largest focus is used to classify the microinvasion. (Do not use the sum of all the individual foci.) The presence of multiple foci of microinvasion should be noted, as it is with multiple larger invasive carcinomas.

Multiple Simultaneous Ipsilateral Primary Carcinomas

The following guidelines are used when classifying multiple simultaneous ipsilateral primary (infiltrating, macroscopically measurable) carcinomas. These criteria do not apply to one macroscopic carcinoma associated with multiple separate microscopic foci.

1. Use the largest primary carcinoma to classify T.
2. Enter into the record that this is a case of multiple simultaneous ipsilateral primary carcinomas. Such cases should be analyzed separately.

Simultaneous Bilateral Breast Carcinomas

Each carcinoma is staged as a separate primary carcinoma in a separate organ.

Inflammatory Carcinoma

Inflammatory carcinoma is a clinicopathologic entity characterized by diffuse brawny induration of the skin of the breast with an erysipeloid edge, usually without an underlying palpable mass. Radiologically there may be a detectable mass and characteristic thickening of the skin over the breast. This clinical presentation is due to tumor embolization of dermal lymphatics. The tumor of inflammatory carcinoma is classified T4d.

Paget's Disease of the Nipple

Paget's disease of the nipple without an associated tumor mass (clinical) or invasive carcinoma (pathologic) is classified Tis. Paget's disease with a demonstrable mass (clinical) or an invasive component (pathologic) is classified according to the size of the tumor mass or invasive component.

Skin of Breast

Dimpling of the skin, nipple retraction, or any other skin change except those described under T4b and T4d may occur in T1, T2, or T3 without changing the classification.

Chest Wall

Chest wall includes ribs, intercostal muscles, and serratus anterior muscle but not pectoral muscle.

DEFINITION OF TNM

Definitions for classifying the primary tumor (T) are the same for clinical and for pathologic classification. The telescoping method of classification can be applied. If the measurement is made by physical examination, the examiner will use the major headings (T1, T2, or T3). If other measurements, such as mammographic or pathologic, are used, the telescoped subsets of T1 can be used.

Primary Tumor (T)

TX Primary tumor cannot be assessed
T0 No evidence of primary tumor
Tis Carcinoma *in situ:* Intraductal carcinoma, lobular carcinoma *in situ,* or Paget's disease of the nipple with no tumor.
T1 Tumor 2 cm or less in greatest dimension
  T1mic Microinvasion 0.1 cm or less in greatest dimension
  T1a Tumor more than 0.1 but not more than 0.5 cm in greatest dimension
  T1b Tumor more than 0.5 cm but not more than 1 cm in greatest dimension
  T1c Tumor more than 1 cm but not more than 2 cm in greatest dimension
T2 Tumor more than 2 cm but not more than 5 cm in greatest dimension
T3 Tumor more than 5 cm in greatest dimension
T4 Tumor of any size with direct extension to (a) chest wall or (b) skin, only as described below.
  T4a Extension to chest wall
  T4b Edema (including peau d'orange) or ulceration of the skin of the breast or satellite skin nodules confined to the same breast
  T4c Both (T4a and T4b)
  T4d Inflammatory carcinoma (see definition of inflammatory carcinoma in the introduction)

Note: Paget's disease associated with a tumor is classified according to the size of the tumor.

Regional Lymph Nodes (N)

NX Regional lymph nodes cannot be assessed (e.g., previously removed)
N0 No regional lymph node metastasis
N1 Metastasis to movable ipsilateral axillary lymph node(s)
N2 Metastasis to ipsilateral axillary lymph node(s) fixed to one another or to other structures

N3 Metastasis to ipsilateral internal mammary lymph node(s)

Pathologic Classification (pN)

- pNX Regional lymph nodes cannot be assessed (e.g., previously removed, or not removed for pathologic study)
- pN0 No regional lymph node metastasis
- pN1 Metastasis to movable ipsilateral axillary lymph node(s)
  - pN1a Only micrometastasis (none larger than 0.2 cm)
  - pN1b Metastasis to lymph node(s), any larger than 0.2 cm
    - pN1bi Metastasis in 1 to 3 lymph nodes, any more than 0.2 cm and all less than 2 cm in greatest dimension
    - pN1bii Metastasis to 4 or more lymph nodes, any more than 0.2 cm and all less than 2 cm in greatest dimension
    - pN1biii Extension of tumor beyond the capsule of a lymph node metastasis less than 2 cm in greatest dimension
    - pN1biv Metastasis to a lymph node 2 cm or more in greatest dimension
- pN2 Metastasis to ipsilateral axillary lymph nodes that are fixed to one another or to other structures
- pN3 Metastasis to ipsilateral internal mammary lymph node(s)

Distant Metastasis (M)

- MX Distant metastasis cannot be assessed
- M0 No distant metastasis
- M1 Distant metastasis (includes metastasis to ipsilateral supraclavicular lymph node[s])

STAGE GROUPING

Stage 0	Tis	N0	M0
Stage I	T1*	N0	M0
Stage IIA	T0	N1	M0
	T1*	N1**	M0
	T2	N0	M0
Stage IIB	T2	N1	M0
	T3	N0	M0
Stage IIIA	T0	N2	M0
	T1*	N2	M0
	T2	N2	M0
	T3	N1	M0
	T3	N2	M0
Stage IIIB	T4	Any N	M0
	Any T	N3	M0
Stage IV	Any T	Any N	M1

**Note:* T1 includes T1mic

***Note:* The prognosis of patients with N1a is similar to that of patients with pN0.

HISTOPATHOLOGIC TYPE

The histologic types are the following:

Carcinoma, NOS (not otherwise specified)
Ductal
- Intraductal (*in situ*)
- Invasive with predominant intraductal component
- Invasive, NOS (not otherwise specified)
- Comedo
- Inflammatory
- Medullary with lymphocytic infiltrate
- Mucinous (colloid)
- Papillary
- Scirrhous
- Tubular
- Other

Lobular
- *In situ*
- Invasive with predominant *in situ* component
- Invasive

Nipple
- Paget's disease, NOS (not otherwise specified)
- Paget's disease with intraductal carcinoma
- Paget's disease with invasive ductal carcinoma

Other
- Undifferentiated carcinoma

HISTOPATHOLOGIC GRADE (G)

- GX Grade cannot be assessed
- G1 Well differentiated
- G2 Moderately differentiated

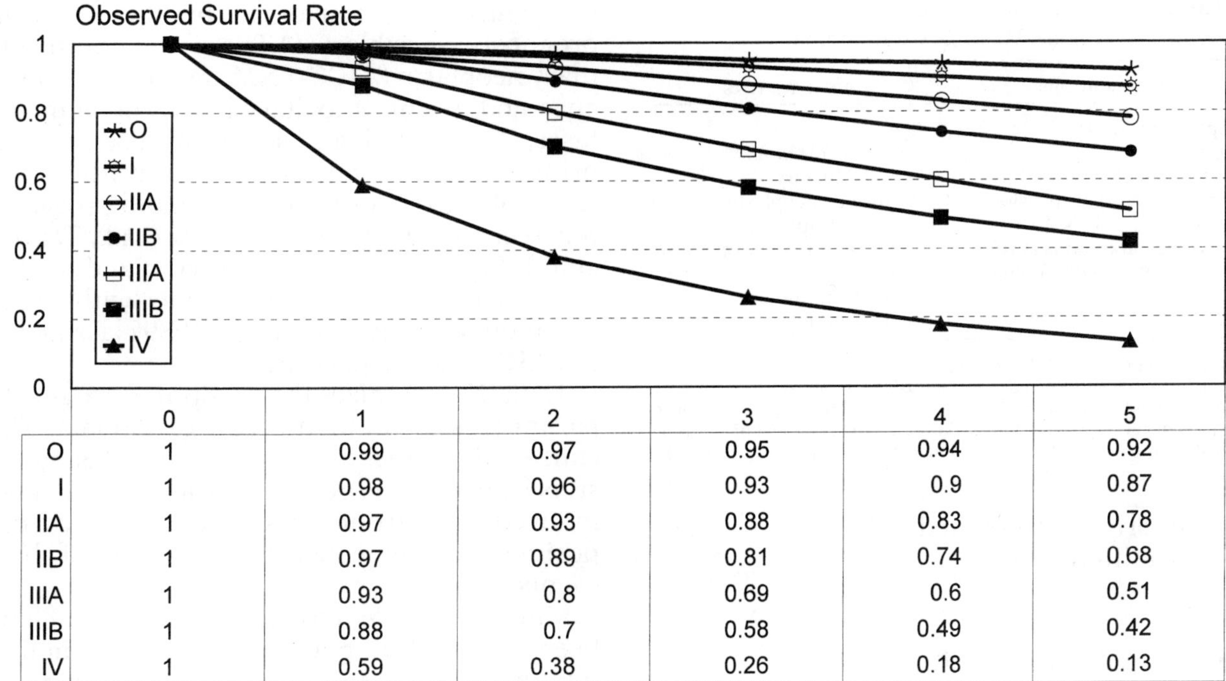

	0	1	2	3	4	5
O	1	0.99	0.97	0.95	0.94	0.92
I	1	0.98	0.96	0.93	0.9	0.87
IIA	1	0.97	0.93	0.88	0.83	0.78
IIB	1	0.97	0.89	0.81	0.74	0.68
IIIA	1	0.93	0.8	0.69	0.6	0.51
IIIB	1	0.88	0.7	0.58	0.49	0.42
IV	1	0.59	0.38	0.26	0.18	0.13

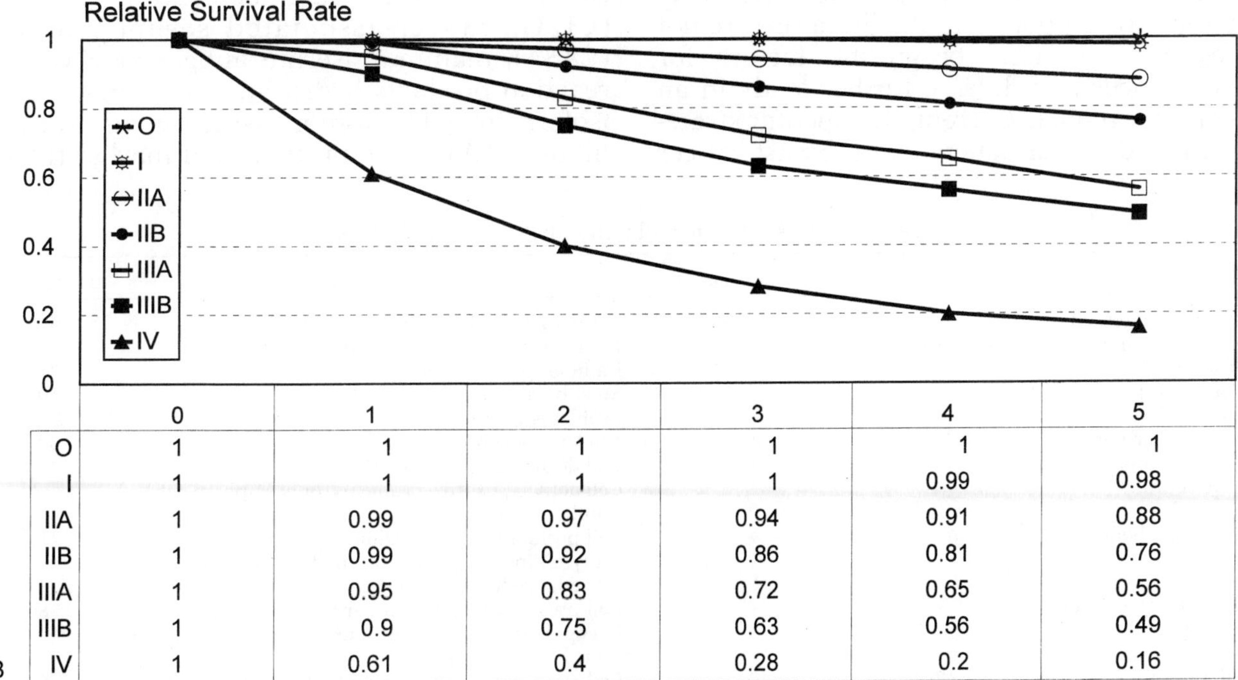

	0	1	2	3	4	5
O	1	1	1	1	1	1
I	1	1	1	1	0.99	0.98
IIA	1	0.99	0.97	0.94	0.91	0.88
IIB	1	0.99	0.92	0.86	0.81	0.76
IIIA	1	0.95	0.83	0.72	0.65	0.56
IIIB	1	0.9	0.75	0.63	0.56	0.49
IV	1	0.61	0.4	0.28	0.2	0.16

FIG. 25-1. Observed **(A)** and relative **(B)** survival rates for 50,383 patients with breast carcinoma classified by the current AJCC staging classification. Data taken from the National Cancer Data Base (Commission on Cancer of the American College of Surgeons and the American Cancer Society) for the year 1989. Stage 0 includes 5,686 patients; Stage I, 21,604; Stage IIA, 10,412; Stage IIB, 5,673; Stage IIIA, 1,864; Stage IIB, 2,035; Stage IV, 3,109.

Table 25-1. Traditional Prognostic Parameters for Human Mammary Carcinoma

TUMOR FACTORS	HOST FACTORS
Lymph node status	Age
Tumor size	Menopausal status
Histologic/nuclear grade	Familial history
Lymphatic/vascular invasion	Previous neoplastic disease
Pathologic stage (TNM)	Immunosuppression
Steroid receptor status (ER/PR)	Host inflammatory response
DNA content (ploidy, S-phase)	Nutrition
EIC (*in situ*)	Prior chemotherapy
	Prior radiation

ER = estrogen receptor; PR = progesterone receptor; EIC = extensive intraductal component (associated with invasive carcinoma).
(From Bland KI, Konstadoulakis MM, Vezeridis MP, Wanebo HJ: Oncogene protein coexpression: value of Ha-ras, c-myc, c-fos, and p53 as prognostic discriminants for breast carcinoma. Ann Surg 1995;221:706-720)

G3 Poorly differentiated
G4 Undifferentiated

PROGNOSTIC FACTORS

A proliferation of prognostic factors for breast cancer is evident in that currently approximately 80 putative prognostic variables have been reported for humans with this tumor. Factors that are supported in the literature are not necessarily the final prognostic factors for breast cancer and deserve further study in an integrative model. Current therapeutic strategies for individual patients with breast cancer frequently are determined by the following prognostic variables: (1) The size (T) of the primary neoplasm (AJCC-TNM stage); (2) the presence and extent of axillary lymph node metastases; (3) Pathologic stage of disease after primary therapy; and (4) The presence or absence of estrogen receptor (ER) and progesterone receptor (PR) activity (Clark et al., Tandon et al.). Figure 25-1 shows observed and relative survival rates for 50,383 patients with breast carcinoma for the years 1985–1989 classified by the AJCC staging classification.

Table 25-1 itemizes the traditional prognostic parameters for human breast carcinoma. This cancer, like other mammalian neoplasms, results from a series of genetic alterations ("hits") induced by environment stimuli, genetic predisposition, or by concurrent activity of both events.

Multiple serum biochemical markers have been included as potential prognostic indicators and have been reviewed by Stenman and Heikkinen and by Werner et al. These serum proteins include the breast mucin markers CA15-3, CA549, CAM26, CAM29, the adenocarcinoma marker carcinoembryonic antigen (CEA), cancer-associated serum antigen (CASA), mammary serum antigen (MSA), the reaction products hydroxyproline, ferritin and isoferritin (p43), tumor-associated trypsin inhibitor (TATI), the proliferation marker tissue

Table 25-2. Anatomic and Cellular Prognostic Factors

NAME	LITERATURE SUPPORT	PROPERTIES	REFERENCES[b]
Tumor size, extent (T)	+	Pathologic more reliable than clinical	47
Regional lymph node involvement (N)	+	Pathologic more reliable than clinical	9
Metastasis (M)	+	Radiographic tests acceptable	31
Histology: Type	+	Most breast cancer is ductal	19
Grade	+	Problems with uniformity of criteria	7, 21, 27
Chromatin	+	Nuclear morphology	33
Tumor necrosis	+	Cell degeneration and death	20
Mitotic counts	+	Cell activity, fixative problems, only M-phase cells	13, 30
DNA ploidy	0	Conflicting results	36
Thymidine labeling index	+	Cell proliferation, thymidine a DNA precursor, thymidine analogue 5-bromodeoxyuridine also used, predicts recurrence	39, 41, 56
S-phase; flow cytometry	+	Cell proliferation, no standardized cut-off point	36
Ki-67 antibody	+	Recognizes nuclear antigen expressed only in proliferating cells	64, 67
Proliferating cell nuclear antigen (PCNA)	0	Cell cycle-dependent protein that accumulates in the nucleus of replicating cells during S-phase, conflicting results	6
Angiogenesis[a]	+	Related to tumor angiogenesis factors	66
Peritumoral lymphatic vessel invasion	+	Significant for relapse-free survival but not overall survival	19

+ Well supported; 0 equivocal support.
[a] Factor VIII-related antigen and CD31 are vascular detection techniques for quantifying tumor angiogenesis. Basic fibroblast growth factor is an angiogenic peptide and can be measured in the urine [40]. The degree to correlation between vascular antigens and angiogenic peptide in tumor angiogenesis is not known.
[b] (From Burke HB, Hutter RVP, Henson DE. Breast carcinoma. In: Prognostic Factors in Cancer, Hermanek P, Gospodarowicz MK, Henson DE, Hutter RVP, Sobin LH (editors). Union Internationale Contre le Cancer. New York: Springer-Verlag, 1995:165-176.)

polypeptide antigen (TPA), C-reactive protein (CRP), orosomucoid, and erythrocyte sedimentation rate (ESR) (Burke et al., 1995). The majority of these serum proteins represent a nonspecific host response to tissue damage initiated by the neoplasm. Although approved for application in clinical practice, the predominant utilization of these markers has been in investigatory studies. The indiscriminate use of these tumor-derived proteins is ill-advised, as the available research suggests that the majority of these markers lack adequate sensitivity and specificity for prediction of outcome. However, identification of elevation specific to the cancerous growth is of value when sequential testing is utilized for the purposes of quantification of tumor burden, monitoring of disease, and determination of therapeutic outcome (Burke et al.).

Table 25-2 identifies anatomic and cellular prognostic factors that have been identified and that support their application in the search for new prognostic factors. Additionally, the identification of genetic mutations and gene deletions/substitutions are an integral part of active research models that are being clinically applied internationally. Integration of oncogene protein discriminants into prognostic models that have previously shown value to predict outcome include Ha-ras, c-myc, c-fos, c-erbB-2 (HER-2/neu), NME-1, and int-2. Moreover, mutation of the tumor suppressor gene TP53 (p53) on chromosome 17p has been extensively studied and represents a common genetic mutation for multiple human neoplasms, including breast carcinogenesis. In 1993, the AJCC adopted criteriafor definition of a prognostic factor thatinclude:

I. Statistically significant, i.e., its prognostic value only rarely occurs by chance;
II. Independent, i.e., retains its prognostic value when combined with other factors; and
III. Clinically relevant, i.e., has a major impact on prognostic accuracy.

Subsequent to this adoption of definition, the College of American Pathologists (CAP) convened a multidisciplinary conference in 1994 and placed further emphasis on the sensitivity of these prognostic factors and their subsets to predict outcome when judged as relevant prognostic factors by managing physicians. Group I includes prognostic variables well-supported biologically and clinically in the scientific literature. Such examples include TNM variables, histologic type, grade (histologic/nuclear), and steroid receptor activity (estrogen, progesterone). Group II was divided into two subsets of prognostic factors extensively studied both clinically and biologically. Group IIA utilized factors commonly applied in clinical trials, e.g., proliferative markers such as percent S-phase fraction and Ki-67 (M1B1), and mitotic index (thymidine-labeling indices). When expanded to the biological subset, Group IIB includes prognostic factors for which biologic and clinically correlative studies had been completed; however, this subset had few outcome studies (e.g., c-erbB-2 (HER-2/neu), p53, angiogenesis and vascular invasion [lymphatic/venous]). Finally, Group III represents factors that are clinically relevant and, therefore, have major implications for accuracy relative to prognosis. Group III includes some of the anatomic and cellular prognostic factors and the molecular-genetic prognostic factors that do not conform to Group I and II. With the enlarging literature relative to molecular and genetic translational research, it is highly probable that these factors will give increasing application to build prognostic models that are highly accurate for evaluation of tumor phenotype and accurately predict disease-free and overall survival outcomes when integrated with anatomic and cellular prognostic factors (Bland et al.).

BIBLIOGRAPHY

Beahrs OH, Henson DE, Hutter RVP, Myers M (Eds.): American Joint Committee on Cancer: manual for staging of cancer, 3rd ed. Philadelphia: JB Lippincott, 1988

Beahrs OH, Myers M (Eds.): American Joint Committee on Cancer: manual for staging of cancer, 2nd ed. Philadephia: JB Lippincott, 1983

Bland KI, Konstadoulakis MM, Vezeridis MP, et al: Oncogene protein co-expression: value of Ha-ras, c-myc, c-fos, and p53 as prognostic discriminants for breast carcinoma. Ann Surg 221:706–720, 1995

Burke HB, Hutter RVP, Henson DE: Breast carcinoma. In Hermanek P, Gospodarowicz MK, Henson DE, Hutter RVP, Sobin LH (Eds.), Prognostic factors in cancer, Union Internationale Contre le Cancer. New York: Springer-Verlag; 165–176, 1995

Clark GM, McGuire WL, Hubay CA, et al: Progesterone receptor as a prognostic factor in stage II breast cancer. N Engl J Med 309:1343–1347, 1983

Harmer MH: UICC TNM classification of malignant tumors, 3rd ed. Berlin: Springer-Verlag, 1982

Henson DE: Future directions for the AMCC. Cancer 69(6 Suppl):1639–1644, 1992

Henson DE et al: Relationship among outcome, stage of disease, and histologic grade for 22,616 cases of breast cancer: the basis for a prognostic index. Cancer 68:2142–2149, 1991

Histologic Typing of Breast Tumours, 2nd ed. WHO International histological classification of tumours. Geneva: World Health Organization, 1981

Hutter RVP: At last—worldwide agreement on staging of cancer. Arch Surg 122:1235–1239, 1987

Kiricuta IC: Correspondence. Eur J Surg Onc 19:393–395, 1993

Nachlas MM: Irrationality in the management of breast cancer. I. The staging system. Cancer 68:681–690, 1991

Russo J et al: The pathology of breast cancer: staging and prognostic indicators. JAMWA 47:181–187, 1992

Silverstein MJ et al: Prognostic classification of breast ductal carcinoma *in situ*. The Lancet 345:1154–1157, 1995

Sobin LH, Wittekind C: UICC/TNM classification of malignant tumors, 5th ed. New York: Wiley, 1997

Sorensen ME: Managing care in breast cancer staging: routine bone scan is not indicated. Proceedings ASCO 13:70(Abstr), 1994

Spiessl B, Beahrs OH, Hermanek P, et al: UICC/TNM Atlas: illustrated guide to the TNM/pTNM classification of malignant tumors, 3rd ed, 2nd revision. Berlin: Springer-Verlag, 1992

Stelling CB: Breast cancer staging with contrast material-enhanced MR imaging: should it change patient treatment? Radiology 196:16–19, 1995

Stenman U, Heikkinen R: Serum markers for breast cancer. Scand J Clin Lab Invest 206:52–59, 1991

Tandon AK, Clark GM, Chamness GC, et al: HER-2/neu oncogene protein and prognosis in breast cancer. J Clin Oncol 7:1120–1128, 1989

Werner M, Faser C, Silverberg M: Clinical utility and validation of emerging biochemical markers for mammary adenocarcinoma. Clin Chem 39:2386–2396, 1993

World Health Organization: International histological classification of tumours, 2nd ed. Berlin-Heidelberg-New York: Springer-Verlag, 1988 to 1997

World Health Organization: ICD-O International classification of diseases for oncology, 2nd ed. Geneva: World Health Organization, 1990

Data Form for Cancer Staging

Patient identification
Name ____________________
Address ____________________
Hospital or clinic number ____________________
Age ____ Sex ____ Race ____________________

Institution identification
Hospital or clinic ____________________
Address ____________________

Oncology Record

Anatomic site of cancer ____________________
Histologic type ____________________
Grade (G) ____________________
Date of classification ____________________

Clin	Path	DEFINITIONS	
		Primary Tumor (T)	
[ ]	[ ]	TX	Primary tumor cannot be assessed
[ ]	[ ]	T0	No evidence of primary tumor
[ ]	[ ]	Tis	Carcinoma *in situ:* Intraductal carcinoma, lobular carcinoma *in situ,* or Paget's disease of the nipple with no tumor
[ ]	[ ]	T1	Tumor 2 cm or less in greatest dimension
[ ]	[ ]	pT1mic	Microinvasion 0.1 cm or less in greatest dimension
[ ]	[ ]	T1a	Tumor more than 0.1 cm but not more than 0.5 cm in greatest dimension
[ ]	[ ]	T1b	More than 0.5 cm but not more than 1 cm in greatest dimension
[ ]	[ ]	T1c	More than 1 cm but not more than 2 cm in greatest dimension
[ ]	[ ]	T2	Tumor more than 2 cm but not more than 5 cm in greatest dimension
[ ]	[ ]	T3	Tumor more than 5 cm in greatest dimension
[ ]	[ ]	T4	Tumor of any size with direct extension to (a) chest wall or (b) skin, only as described below
[ ]	[ ]	T4a	Extension to chest wall
[ ]	[ ]	T4b	Edema (including peau d'orange) or ulceration of the skin of breast or satellite skin nodules confined to same breast
[ ]	[ ]	T4c	Both (T4a and T4b)
[ ]	[ ]	T4d	Inflammatory carcinoma
		Paget's disease associated with a tumor is classified according to the size of the tumor.	
		Regional Lymph Nodes (N)	
[ ]	[ ]	NX	Regional lymph nodes cannot be assessed (e.g., previously removed)
[ ]	[ ]	N0	No regional lymph node metastasis
[ ]	[ ]	N1	Spread to movable ipsilateral axillary lymph node(s)
[ ]	[ ]	N2	Spread to ipsilateral axillary lymph node(s) fixed to one another or to other structures
[ ]	[ ]	N3	Spread to ipsilateral internal mammary lymph node(s)
		Pathologic Classification (pN)	
	[ ]	pNX	Regional lymph nodes cannot be assessed (e.g., previously removed, or not removed for pathologic study)
	[ ]	pN0	No regional lymph node metastasis
	[ ]	pN1	Metastasis to movable ipsilateral axillary lymph node(s)
	[ ]	pN1a	Only micrometastasis (none larger than 0.2 cm)
	[ ]	pN1b	Metastasis to lymph nodes, any larger than 0.2 cm
	[ ]	pN1bi	Metastasis in 1 to 3 lymph nodes, any more than 0.2 cm and all less than 2 cm in greatest dimension
	[ ]	pN1bii	Metastasis to 4 or more lymph nodes, any more than 0.2 cm and all less than 2 cm in greatest dimension
	[ ]	pN1biii	Extension of tumor beyond the capsule of a lymph node metastasis less than 2 cm in greatest dimension
	[ ]	pN1biv	Metastasis to a lymph node 2 cm or more in greatest dimension
	[ ]	pN2	Metastasis to ipsilateral axillary lymph nodes that are fixed to one another or to other structures
	[ ]	pN3	Metastasis to ipsilateral internal mammary lymph node(s)
		Distant Metastasis (M)	
[ ]	[ ]	MX	Distant metastasis cannot be assessed
[ ]	[ ]	M0	No distant metastasis
[ ]	[ ]	M1	Distant metastasis (includes metastasis to ipsilateral superclavicular lymph node(s))

(continued on next page)

Stage Grouping

Clin	Path	Stage	T	N	M
[ ]	[ ]	0	Tis	N0	M0
[ ]	[ ]	I	T1*	N0	M0
[ ]	[ ]	IIA	T0	N1	M0
			T1*	N1**	M0
			T2	N0	M0
[ ]	[ ]	IIB	T2	N1	M0
			T3	N0	M0
[ ]	[ ]	IIIA	T0	N2	M0
			T1*	N2	M0
			T2	N2	M0
			T3	N1	M0
			T3	N2	M0
[ ]	[ ]	IIIB	T4	Any N	M0
			Any T	N3	M0
[ ]	[ ]	IV	Any T	Any N	M1

**T1 includes pT1mic.*
***The prognosis of patients with N1a is similar to that of patients with pN0.*

Staged by ______________________________ M.D.

______________________________ Registrar

Date ______________________________

Illustrations

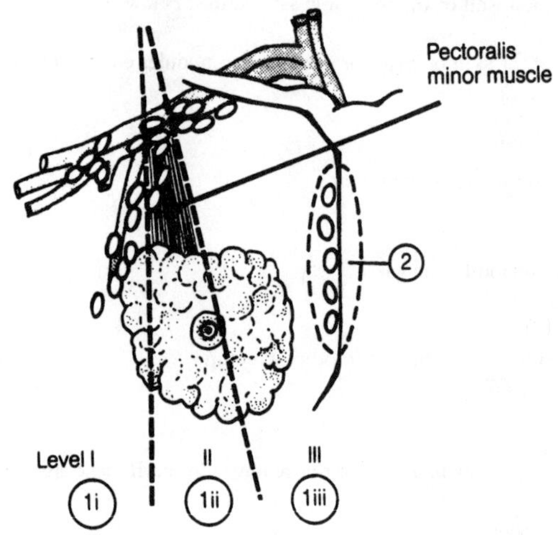

Histopathologic Grade (G)

[ ] GX Grade cannot be assessed
[ ] G1 Well differentiated
[ ] G2 Moderately differentiated
[ ] G3 Poorly differentiated
[ ] G4 Undifferentiated

Histopathologic Type

The histologic types are the following:
Carcinoma, NOS (not otherwise specified)
Ductal
- Intraductal (*in situ*)
- Invasive with predominant intraductal component
- Invasive, NOS (not otherwise specified)
- Comedo
- Inflammatory
- Medullary with lymphocytic infiltrate
- Mucinous (colloid)
- Papillary
- Scirrhous
- Tubular
- Other

Lobular
- *In situ*
- Invasive with predominant *in situ* component
- Invasive

Nipple
- Paget's disease, NOS (not otherwise specified)
- Paget's disease with intraductal carcinoma
- Paget's disease with invasive ductal carcinoma

Other
- Undifferentiated carcinoma

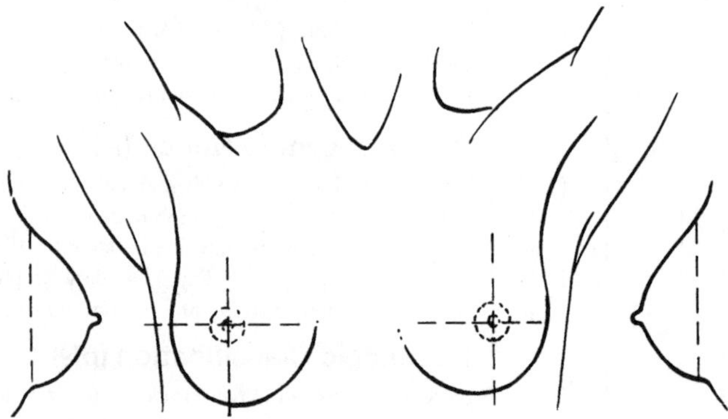

Indicate on diagram primary tumor and regional nodes involved.

GYNECOLOGIC SITES

Cervix uteri, corpus uteri, ovary, vagina, vulva, fallopian tube, and gestational trophoblastic disease are the sites included in this section. Cervix uteri and corpus uteri were among the first sites to be classified by the TNM system. The League of Nations stages for carcinoma of the cervix have been used with minor modifications for nearly 50 years, and, because these are accepted by the Federation Internationale de Gynecologie et d'Obstetrique (FIGO), the TNM categories have been defined to correspond to the FIGO stages. Some amendments have been made in collaboration with FIGO, and the classifications now published have the approval of FIGO, the American Joint Committee on Cancer (AJCC), and all other national TNM committees of the Union Internationale Contre le Cancer (UICC).

The AJCC has worked closely with the FIGO in classification of cancer at gynecologic sites. Staging of malignant tumors is essentially the same and stages are comparable with the two systems.

26

Vulva

(Mucosal malignant melanoma is not included.)

C51.0 Labium majus
C51.1 Labium minus
C51.2 Clitoris
C51.8 Overlapping lesion
C51.9 Vulva, NOS

Cases should be classified as carcinoma of the vulva when the primary site of the growth is in the vulva. Tumors present in the vulva as secondary growths from either a genital or extra-genital site should be excluded. This classification does not apply to mucosal malignant melanoma. There should be histologic confirmation of the tumor.

ANATOMY

Primary Site. The vulva is the anatomic area immediately external to the vagina.

Regional Lymph Nodes. The femoral and inguinal nodes are the sites of regional spread. For pN, histologic examination of an inguinal lymphadenectomy specimen will ordinarily include 6 or more lymph nodes.

Metastatic Sites. This includes any site beyond the area of the regional lymph nodes. Internal iliac, external iliac, and common iliac lymph nodes are now considered as distant metastasis.

DEFINITION OF TNM

Vulvar cancer is surgically staged and final diagnosis is dependent upon thorough histopathologic evaluation of the operative specimen (vulva and lymph nodes).

Primary Tumor (T)

TX Primary tumor cannot be assessed
T0 No evidence of primary tumor
Tis Carcinoma *in situ* (preinvasive carcinoma)
T1 Tumor confined to the vulva or vulva and perineum, 2 cm or less in greatest dimension.
  T1a Tumor confined to the vulva or vulva and perineum, 2 cm or less in greatest dimension, and with stromal invasion no greater than 1 mm.*
  T1b Tumor confined to the vulva or vulva and perineum, 2 cm or less in greatest dimension, and with stromal invasion greater than 1 mm.*
T2 Tumor confined to the vulva or vulva and perineum, more than 2 cm in greatest dimension
T3 Tumor of any size with adjacent spread to the lower urethra and/or vagina or anus
T4 Tumor invades any of the following: upper urethral mucosa, bladder mucosa, rectal mucosa, or is fixed to the pubic bone

**Note:* The depth of invasion is defined as the measurement of the tumor from the epithelial-stromal junction of the adjacent most superficial dermal papilla to the deepest point of invasion.

Regional Lymph Nodes (N)

NX Regional lymph nodes cannot be assessed
N0 No regional lymph node metastasis
N1 Unilateral regional lymph node metastasis
N2 Bilateral regional lymph node metastasis

Distant Metastasis (M)

MX Distant metastasis cannot be assessed
M0 No distant metastasis
M1 Distant metastasis (including pelvic lymph node metastasis)

STAGE GROUPING

Stage 0	Tis	N0	M0
Stage IA	T1a	N0	M0
Stage IB	T1b	N0	M0
Stage II	T2	N0	M0
Stage III	T1	N1	M0
	T2	N1	M0
	T3	N0	M0
	T3	N1	M0
Stage IVA	T1	N2	M0
	T2	N2	M0
	T3	N2	M0
	T4	Any N	M0
Stage IVB	Any T	Any N	M1

HISTOPATHOLOGIC TYPE

Squamous cell carcinoma is the most frequent form of cancer of the vulva. This classification does not apply to mucosal malignant melanoma.

The histopathologic types are:

Vulvar intraepithelial neoplasia, grade III
Squamous cell carcinoma *in situ*
Squamous cell carcinoma
Verrucous carcinoma
Paget's disease of vulva
Adenocarcinoma, NOS
Basal cell carcinoma, NOS
Bartholin's gland carcinoma

HISTOPATHOLOGIC GRADE (G)

GX Grade cannot be assessed
G1 Well differentiated
G2 Moderately differentiated
G3 Poorly differentiated
G4 Undifferentiated

PROGNOSTIC FACTORS

Vulvar cancer is a surgically-staged entity. This allows staging to identify very specifically tumor volume in regards to the primary disease, as well as status of the lymph nodes. Therefore, surgical staging is the most important prognostic factor in vulvar cancer. Other commonly evaluated items such as histological type, differentiation, DNA ploidy, and S-phase fraction analysis, as well as age, are not uniformly identified as important prognostic factors in vulvar cancer.

Data Form for Cancer Staging

Patient identification
Name ____________
Address ____________
Hospital or clinic number ____________
Age ____ Sex ____ Race ____________

Institution identification
Hospital or clinic ____________
Address ____________

Oncology Record

Anatomic site of cancer ____________
Histologic type ____________
Grade (G) ____________
Date of classification ____________

DEFINITIONS

Primary Tumor (T)

Clin	Path		
[ ]	[ ]	TX	Primary tumor cannot be assessed
[ ]	[ ]	T0	No evidence of primary tumor
[ ]	[ ]	Tis	Carcinoma *in situ* (preinvasive carcinoma)
[ ]	[ ]	T1	Tumor confined to the vulva or vulva and perineum, 2 cm or less in greatest dimension
[ ]	[ ]	T1a	Tumor confined to the vulva or vulva and perineum, 2 cm or less in greatest dimension, and with stromal invasion no greater than 1 mm*
[ ]	[ ]	T1b	Tumor confined to the vulva or vulva and perineum, 2 cm or less in greatest dimension, and with stromal invasion greater than 1 mm*
[ ]	[ ]	T2	Tumor confined to the vulva or vulva and perineum, more than 2 cm in greatest dimension
[ ]	[ ]	T3	Tumor of any size with adjacent spread to the lower urethra and/or vagina or anus
[ ]	[ ]	T4	Tumor invades any of the following: upper urethral mucosa, bladder mucosa, rectal mucosa; or is fixed to the pubic bone

** The depth of invasion is defined as the measurement of the tumor from the epithelial-stromal junction of the adjacent most superficial dermal papilla to the deepest point of invasion.*

Regional Lymph Nodes (N)

Clin	Path		
[ ]	[ ]	NX	Regional lymph nodes cannot be assessed
[ ]	[ ]	N0	No regional lymph node metastasis
[ ]	[ ]	N1	Unilateral regional lymph node metastasis
[ ]	[ ]	N2	Bilateral regional lymph node metastasis

Distant Metastasis (M)

Clin	Path		
[ ]	[ ]	MX	Distant metastasis cannot be assessed
[ ]	[ ]	M0	No distant metastasis
[ ]	[ ]	M1	Distant metastasis (including pelvic lymph node metastasis)

Stage Grouping

AJCC/UICC/FIGO

Clin	Path	Stage	T	N	M
[ ]	[ ]	0	Tis	N0	M0
[ ]	[ ]	IA	T1a	N0	M0
[ ]	[ ]	IB	T1b	N0	M0
[ ]	[ ]	II	T2	N0	M0
[ ]	[ ]	III	T1	N1	M0
			T2	N1	M0
			T3	N0	M0
			T3	N1	M0
[ ]	[ ]	IVA	T1	N2	M0
			T2	N2	M0
			T3	N2	M0
			T4	Any N	M0
[ ]	[ ]	IVB	Any T	Any N	M1

Staged by ____________ M.D.
____________ Registrar
Date ____________

(continued on next page)

Histopathologic Grade (G)

[ ] GX Grade cannot be assessed
[ ] G1 Well differentiated
[ ] G2 Moderately differentiated
[ ] G3 Poorly differentiated
[ ] G4 Undifferentiated

Histopathologic Type

Squamous cell carcinoma is the most frequent form of cancer of the vulva. This classification does not apply to mucosal malignant melanoma.

The histopathologic types are:

Vulvar intraepithelial neoplasia, grade III
Squamous cell carcinoma *in situ*
Squamous cell carcinoma
Verrucous carcinoma
Paget's disease of the vulva
Adenocarcinoma, NOS
Basal cell carcinoma, NOS
Bartholin's gland carcinoma

Illustrations

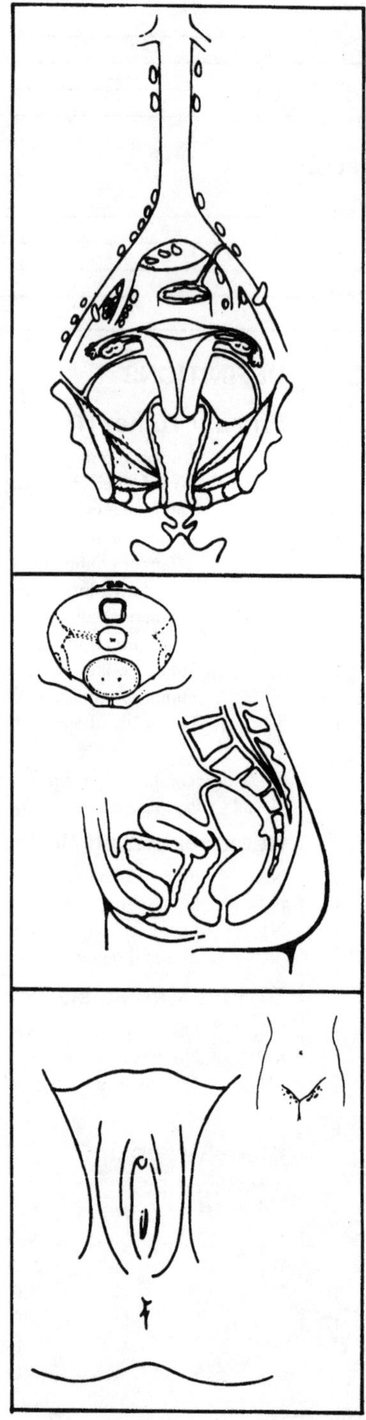

Indicate on diagrams primary tumor and regional nodes involved.

27

Vagina

C52.9 Vagina

ANATOMY

Primary Site. The vagina extends from the vulva upward to the uterine cervix. Cases should be classified as carcinoma of the vagina when the primary site of the growth is in the vagina. Tumors present in the vagina as secondary growths from either genital or extragenital sites should be excluded. A growth that has extended to the portio and reached the area of the external os should always be allotted to carcinoma of the cervix. A growth limited to the urethra should be classified as carcinoma of the urethra. Tumor involving the vulva should be classified as carcinoma of the vulva. There should be histologic verification of the disease. The vagina is drained by lymphatics, toward the pelvic nodes in its upper two-thirds and toward the inguinal nodes in the lower third. The most common sites of distant spread include the lungs and skeleton. The rules for staging are similar to those for carcinoma of the cervix.

Regional Lymph Nodes. The regional lymph nodes are as follows:

Femoral (lower third only)
Inguinal (lower third only)
Common iliac
Internal iliac
External iliac
Hypogastric (obturator)
Pelvic, NOS (upper two-thirds only)
For pN, histologic examination of a pelvic lymphadenectomy specimen will ordinarily include 10 or more lymph nodes.

Metastatic Sites. The most common sites of distant spread include the lungs and skeleton.

RULES FOR CLASSIFICATION

The classification applies to primary carcinoma only.

A tumor that has extended to the portio and reached the external os should be classified as carcinoma of the cervix.

A tumor involving the vulva should be classified as carcinoma of the vulva.

There should be histologic confirmation of the disease. Any unconfirmed cases must be reported separately.

Clinical Staging. All data available prior to first definitive treatment should be used.

Pathologic Staging. In addition to data used for clinical staging, additional information available from examination of the resected specimen is to be used.

DEFINITION OF TNM

The definitions of the T categories correspond to the several stages accepted by The Federation Internationale de Gynecologie et d'Obstetrique (FIGO). Both systems are included for comparison.

Primary Tumor (T)

TNM categories	FIGO stages	
TX		Primary tumor cannot be assessed
T0		No evidence of primary tumor
Tis	0	Carcinoma *in situ*
T1	I	Tumor confined to vagina
T2	II	Tumor invades paravaginal tissues but not to pelvic wall

T3	III	Tumor extends to pelvic wall
T4*	IVA	Tumor invades mucosa of the bladder or rectum and/or extends beyond the true pelvis (Bullous edema is not sufficient evidence to classify a tumor as T4.)
M1	IVB	Distant metastasis

**Note:* If the bladder mucosa is not involved, the tumor is Stage III.

Regional Lymph Nodes (N)

NX Regional lymph nodes cannot be assessed
N0 No regional lymph node metastasis
N1 Pelvic or inguinal lymph node metastasis

Distant Metastasis (M)

MX Distant metastasis cannot be assessed
M0 No distant metastasis
M1 Distant metastasis

pTNM Pathologic Classification

The pT, pN, and pM categories correspond to the T, N, and M categories.

STAGE GROUPING

Stage 0	Tis	N0	M0
Stage I	T1	N0	M0
Stage II	T2	N0	M0
Stage III	T1	N1	M0
	T2	N1	M0
	T3	N0	M0
	T3	N1	M0
Stage IVA	T4	Any N	M0
Stage IVB	Any T	Any N	M1

HISTOPATHOLOGIC TYPE

Squamous cell carcinoma is the most common type of cancer occurring in the vagina but infrequently an adenocarcinoma may occur.

HISTOPATHOLOGIC GRADE (G)

GX Grade cannot be assessed
G1 Well differentiated
G2 Moderately differentiated
G3 Poorly differentiated
G4 Undifferentiated

PROGNOSTIC FACTORS

Because of the rarity of this cancer, there are no known prognostic factors other than anatomic staging.

Data Form for Cancer Staging

Patient identification
Name ______
Address ______
Hospital or clinic number ______
Age ____ Sex ____ Race ______

Institution identification
Hospital or clinic ______
Address ______

Oncology Record

Anatomic site of cancer ______
Histologic type ______
Grade (G) ______
Date of classification ______

Clin	Path	TNM categories	FIGO stage	DEFINITIONS
				Primary Tumor (T)
[ ]	[ ]	TX		Primary tumor cannot be assessed
[ ]	[ ]	T0		No evidence of primary tumor
[ ]	[ ]	Tis	0	Carcinoma *in situ*
[ ]	[ ]	T1	I	Tumor confined to vagina
[ ]	[ ]	T2	II	Tumor invades paravaginal tissues but not to pelvic wall
[ ]	[ ]	T3	III	Tumor extends to pelvic wall
[ ]	[ ]	T4*	IVA	Tumor invades mucosa of the bladder or rectum and/or extends beyond the true pelvis (Bullous edema is not sufficient evidence to classify a tumor as T4.)
[ ]	[ ]	M1	IVB	Distant metastasis
		** If the bladder mucosa is not involved the tumor is stage III.*		
				Regional Lymph Nodes (N)
[ ]	[ ]	NX		Regional lymph nodes cannot be assessed
[ ]	[ ]	N0		No regional lymph node metastasis
[ ]	[ ]	N1		Pelvic or inguinal lymph node metastasis
		** If the bladder mucosa is not involved the tumor is stage III.*		
				Distant Metastasis (M)
[ ]	[ ]	MX		Distant metastasis cannot be assessed
[ ]	[ ]	M0		No distant metastasis
[ ]	[ ]	M1		Distant metastasis

Stage Grouping

AJCC/UICC/FIGO

Clin	Path	Stage	T	N	M
[ ]	[ ]	0	Tis	N0	M0
[ ]	[ ]	I	T1	N0	M0
[ ]	[ ]	II	T2	N0	M0
[ ]	[ ]	III	T1	N1	M0
			T2	N1	M0
			T3	N0	M0
			T3	N1	M0
[ ]	[ ]	IVA	T4	Any N	M0
[ ]	[ ]	IVB	Any T	Any N	M1

Staged by ______ M.D.
______ Registrar
Date ______

(continued on next page)

Histopathologic Type

Squamous cell carcinoma is the most common type of cancer occurring in the vagina but infrequently an adenocarcinoma may occur.

Histopathologic Grade (G)

[ ] GX Grade cannot be assessed
[ ] G1 Well differentiated
[ ] G2 Moderately differentiated
[ ] G3 Poorly differentiated
[ ] G4 Undifferentiated

Illustrations

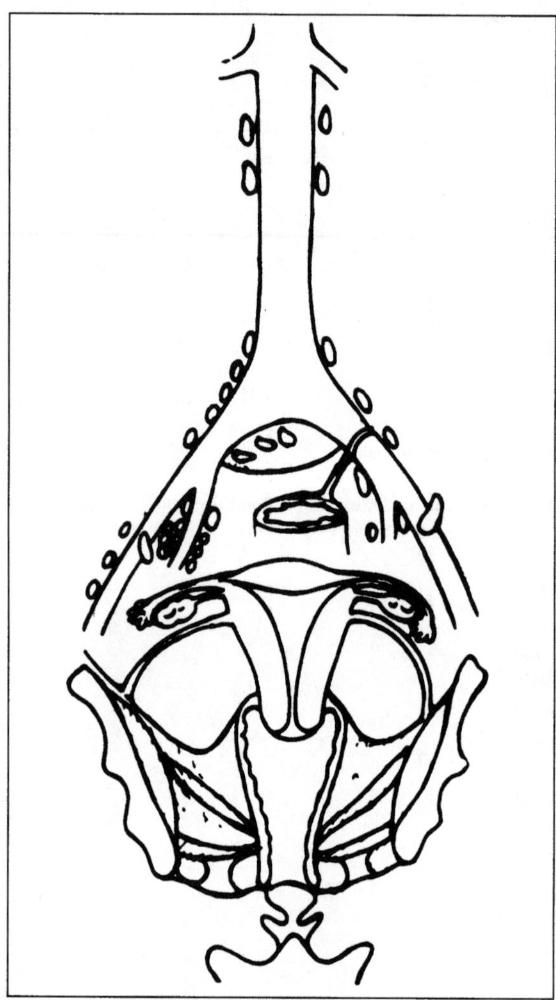

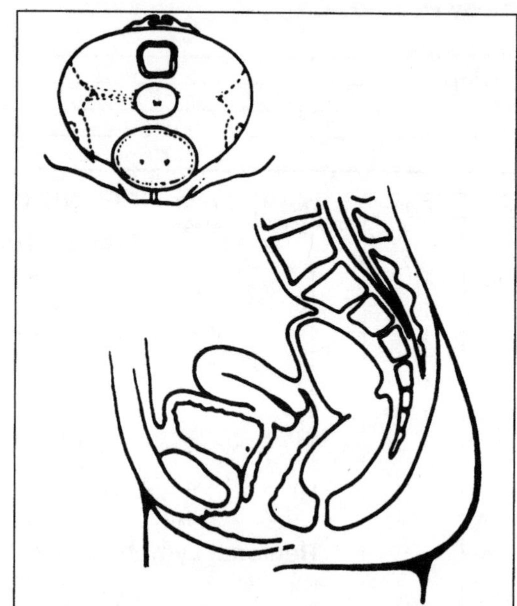

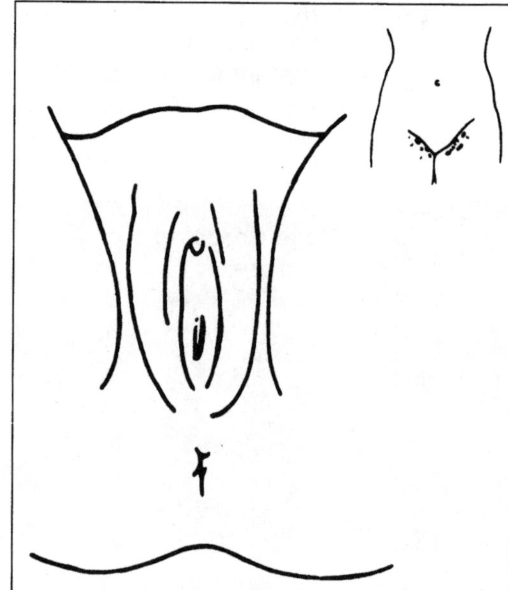

Indicate on diagrams primary tumor and regional nodes involved.

28

Cervix Uteri

C53.0 Endocervix
C53.1 Exocervix
C53.8 Overlapping lesion
C53.9 Cervix uteri

ANATOMY

Primary Site. The cervix is the lower third of the uterus. It is roughly cylindrical in shape, projects through the upper anterior vaginal wall, and communicates with the vagina through an orifice called the external os. Cancer of the cervix may originate on the vaginal surface or in the canal.

Regional Lymph Nodes. The cervix is drained by preureteral, postureteral, and uterosacral routes into the following regional lymph nodes:

Parametrial
Paracervical
Hypogastric (obturator)
Common iliac
External iliac
Internal iliac
Sacral
Presacral

For pN, histologic examination of a pelvic lymphadenectomy specimen will ordinarily include 10 or more lymph nodes. Para-aortic node involvement is considered distant metastasis and is coded M1.

Metastatic Sites. The most common sites of distant spread include the aortic and mediastinal nodes, lungs, and skeleton.

RULES FOR CLASSIFICATION

The classification applies only to carcinoma. There should be histologic confirmation of the disease.

Clinical Staging. Careful clinical examination should be performed in all cases, preferably by an experienced examiner and with anesthesia. The clinical staging must not be changed because of subsequent findings. When there is doubt as to which stage a particular cancer should be allocated, the earlier stage is mandatory. The following examinations are permitted: palpation, inspection, colposcopy, endocervical curettage, hysteroscopy, cystoscopy, proctoscopy, intravenous urography, and x-ray examination of the lungs and skeleton. Suspected bladder or rectal involvement must be confirmed by biopsy and histology. Optional examinations include lymphangiography, arteriography, venography, laparoscopy, and other imaging methods. Because these are not yet generally available and because the interpretation of results is variable, the findings of optional studies should not be the basis for changing the clinical staging.

Pathologic Staging. In cases treated by surgical procedures, the pathologist's findings in the removed tissues can be the basis for extremely accurate statements on the extent of disease. These findings should not be allowed to change the clinical staging but should be recorded in the manner described for the pathologic staging of disease. The pTNM nomenclature is appropriate for this purpose. Infrequently, hysterectomy is carried out in the presence of unsuspected extensive invasive cervical carcinoma. Such cases cannot be clinically staged or included in therapeutic statistics, but it is desirable that they be reported separately. Only if the rules for clinical staging are strictly observed will it be possible to compare results among clinics and by differing modes of therapy.

Anatomic Subsites

Endocervix
Exocervix

DEFINITION OF TNM

The definitions of the T categories correspond to the several stages accepted by The Federation Internationale de Gynecologie et d'Obstetrique (FIGO). Both systems are included for comparison.

Primary Tumor (T)

TNM categories	FIGO stages	
TX	-	Primary tumor cannot be assessed
T0	-	No evidence of primary tumor
Tis	-	Carcinoma *in situ*
T1	I	Cervical carcinoma confined to uterus (extension to corpus should be disregarded)
T1a	IA	Invasive carcinoma diagnosed only by microscopy. All macroscopically visible lesions—even with superficial invasion—are T1b/IB. Stromal invasion with a maximal depth of 5.0 mm measured from the base of the epithelium and a horizontal spread of 7.0 mm or less. Vascular space involvement, venous or lymphatic, does not affect classification
T1a1	IA1	Measured stromal invasion 3.0 mm or less in depth and 7.0 mm or less in horizontal spread
T1a2	IA2	Measured stromal invasion more than 3.0 mm and not more than 5.0 mm with a horizontal spread 7.0 mm or less
T1b	IB	Clinically visible lesion confined to the cervix or microscopic lesion greater than T1a2/IA2
T1b1	IB1	Clinically visible lesion 4.0 cm or less in greatest dimension
T1b2	IB2	Clinically visible lesion more than 4.0 cm in greatest dimension
T2	II	Cervical carcinoma invades beyond uterus but not to pelvic wall or to the lower third of vagina
T2a	IIA	Tumor without parametrial invasion
T2b	IIB	Tumor with parametrial invasion
T3	III	Tumor extends to the pelvic wall, and/or involves the lower third of the vagina, and/or causes hydronephrosis or nonfunctioning kidney
T3a	IIIA	Tumor involves lower third of the vagina, no extension to pelvic wall
T3b	IIIB	Tumor extends to pelvic wall and/or causes hydronephrosis or nonfunctioning kidney
T4	IVA	Tumor invades mucosa of the bladder or rectum, and/or extends beyond true pelvis (Bullous edema is not sufficient to classify a tumor as T4)
M1	IVB	Distant metastasis

Regional Lymph Nodes (N)

NX Regional lymph nodes cannot be assessed
N0 No regional lymph node metastasis
N1 Regional lymph node metastasis

Distant Metastasis (M)

MX Distant metastasis cannot be assessed
M0 No distant metastasis
M1 Distant metastasis

pTNM Pathologic Classification

The pT, pN, and pM categories correspond to the T, N, and M categories.

STAGE GROUPING

Stage 0	Tis	N0	M0
Stage IA1	T1a1	N0	M0
Stage IA2	T1a2	N0	M0
Stage IB1	T1b1	N0	M0
Stage IB2	T1b2	N0	M0
Stage IIA	T2a	N0	M0
Stage IIB	T2b	N0	M0
Stage IIIA	T3a	N0	M0
Stage IIIB	T1	N1	M0
	T2	N1	M0
	T3a	N1	M0
	T3b	Any N	M0
Stage IVA	T4	Any N	M0
Stage IVB	Any T	Any N	M1

HISTOPATHOLOGIC TYPE

Cases should be classified as carcinoma of the cervix if the primary growth is in the cervix. All histologic types must be included. Grading is encouraged but is not a basis for modifying the stage groupings. When surgery is the primary treatment, the histologic findings permit the case to have pathologic staging. In this, the pTNM nomenclature is to be used. All tumors are to be microscopically verified.

The histopathologic types are:

Cervical intraepithelial neoplasia, grade III
Squamous cell carcinoma *in situ*
Squamous cell carcinoma
  Invasive
  Keratinizing
  Nonkeratinizing
  Verrucous
Adenocarcinoma *in situ*
Adenocarcinoma *in situ,* endocervical type
Adenocarcinoma, invasive
Endometrioid adenocarcinoma
Clear cell adenocarcinoma
Adenosquamous carcinoma
Adenoid cystic carcinoma
Small cell carcinoma
Undifferentiated carcinoma

HISTOPATHOLOGIC GRADE (G)

GX Grade cannot be assessed
G1 Well differentiated
G2 Moderately differentiated
G3 Poorly differentiated
G4 Undifferentiated

PROGNOSTIC FACTORS

Multiple other factors have been evaluated including histologic features, DNA ploidy, S-phase fraction, oncogenes as well as HPV status. Of note is the fact that all of these appear to be controversial with no general agreement reached as regards to whether or not they may be significant. One exception may be the HPV status. Current data would suggest that up to 90% of squamous cervical cancer contains HPV, most frequently types 16 and 18. When prognosis is evaluated in regards to HPV status, it is interesting to note that those who are HPV negative tend to have a poorer prognosis than those who are HPV positive.

Data Form for Cancer Staging

Patient identification
Name ______
Address ______
Hospital or clinic number ______
Age ____ Sex ____ Race ______

Institution identification
Hospital or clinic ______
Address ______

Oncology Record

Anatomic site of cancer ______
Histologic type ______
Grade (G) ______
Date of classification ______

Clin	Path	TNM categories	FIGO* stage	DEFINITIONS
				Primary Tumor (T)
[ ]	[ ]	TX		Primary tumor cannot be assessed
[ ]	[ ]	T0		No evidence of primary tumor
[ ]	[ ]	Tis		Carcinoma *in situ*
[ ]	[ ]	T1	I	Cervical carcinoma confined to uterus (extension to corpus should be disregarded)
[ ]	[ ]	T1a	IA	Invasive carcinoma diagnosed only by microscopy. All macroscopically visible lesions—even with superficial invasion—are T1b/IB. Stromal invasion with a maximal depth of 5.0 mm measured from the base of the epithelium and a horizontal spread of 7.0 mm or less. Vascular space involvement, venous or lymphatic, does not affect classification.
[ ]	[ ]	T1a1	IA1	Measured stromal invasion 3.0 mm or less in depth and 7.0 mm or less in horizontal spread.
[ ]	[ ]	T1a2	IA2	Measured stromal invasion more than 3.0 mm and not more than 5.0 mm with a horizontal spread 7.0 mm or less.
[ ]	[ ]	T1b	IB	Clinically visible lesion confined to the cervix or microscopic lesion greater than T1a2/IA2.
[ ]	[ ]	T1b1	IB1	Clinically visible lesion 4.0 cm or less in greatest dimension.
[ ]	[ ]	T1b2	IB2	Clinically visible lesion more than 4.0 cm in greatest dimension.
[ ]	[ ]	T2	II	Cervical carcinoma invades beyond uterus but not to pelvic wall or to the lower third of vagina
[ ]	[ ]	T2a	IIA	Tumor without parametrial invasion
[ ]	[ ]	T2b	IIB	Tumor with parametrial invasion
[ ]	[ ]	T3	III	Tumor extends to pelvic wall and/or involves lower third of vagina and/or causes hydronephrosis or nonfunctioning kidney
[ ]	[ ]	T3a	IIIA	Tumor involves lower third of vagina, no extension to pelvic wall
[ ]	[ ]	T3b	IIIB	Tumor extends to pelvic wall and/or causes hydronephrosis or nonfunctioning kidney
[ ]	[ ]	T4	IVA	Tumor invades mucosa of the bladder or rectum, and/or extends beyond true pelvis. (Bullous edema is not sufficient to classify a tumor as T4.)
[ ]	[ ]	M1	IVB	Distant metastasis
		Regional Lymph Nodes (N)		
[ ]	[ ]	NX		Regional lymph nodes cannot be assessed
[ ]	[ ]	N0		No regional lymph node metastasis
[ ]	[ ]	N1		Regional lymph node metastasis
		Distant Metastasis (M)		
[ ]	[ ]	MX		Presence of distant metastasis cannot be assessed
[ ]	[ ]	M0		No distant metastasis
[ ]	[ ]	M1		Distant metastasis

(continued on next page)

Clin	Path	Stage Grouping			
		AJCC/UICC/FIGO			
[ ]	[ ]	0	Tis	N0	M0
[ ]	[ ]	IA1	T1a1	N0	M0
[ ]	[ ]	IA2	T1a2	N0	M0
[ ]	[ ]	IB1	T1b1	N0	M0
[ ]	[ ]	IB2	T1b2	N0	M0
[ ]	[ ]	IIA	T2a	N0	M0
[ ]	[ ]	IIB	T2b	N0	M0
[ ]	[ ]	IIIA	T3a	N0	M0
[ ]	[ ]	IIIB	T1	N1	M0
			T2	N1	M0
			T3a	N1	M0
			T3b	Any N	M0
[ ]	[ ]	IVA	T4	Any N	M0
[ ]	[ ]	IVB	Any T	Any N	M1

**FIGO: Federation International de Gynecologie et d'Obstetrique*

Staged by ______________________________ M.D.

______________________________ Registrar

Date ______________________________

Histopathologic Grade (G)

[ ] GX Grade cannot be assessed
[ ] G1 Well differentiated
[ ] G2 Moderately differentiated
[ ] G3 Poorly differentiated
[ ] G4 Undifferentiated

Histopathologic Type

Cases should be classified as carcinoma of the cervix if the primary growth is in the cervix. All histologic types must be included. Grading is encouraged but is not a basis for modifying the stage groupings. When surgery is the primary treatment, the histologic findings permit the case to have pathologic staging. In this, the pTNM nomenclature is to be used. All tumors are to be microscopically verified.

The histopathologic types are:

Cervical intraepithelial neoplasia, grade III
Squamous cell carcinoma *in situ*
Squamous cell carcinoma
  Keratinizing
  Nonkeratinizing
  Verrucous
Adenocarcinoma *in situ*
Adenocarcinoma *in situ*, endocervical type
Adenocarcinoma, invasive
Endometroid adenocarcinoma
Clear cell adenocarcinoma
Adenosquamous carcinoma
Adenoid cystic carcinoma
Small cell carcinoma
Undifferentiated carcinoma

Illustrations

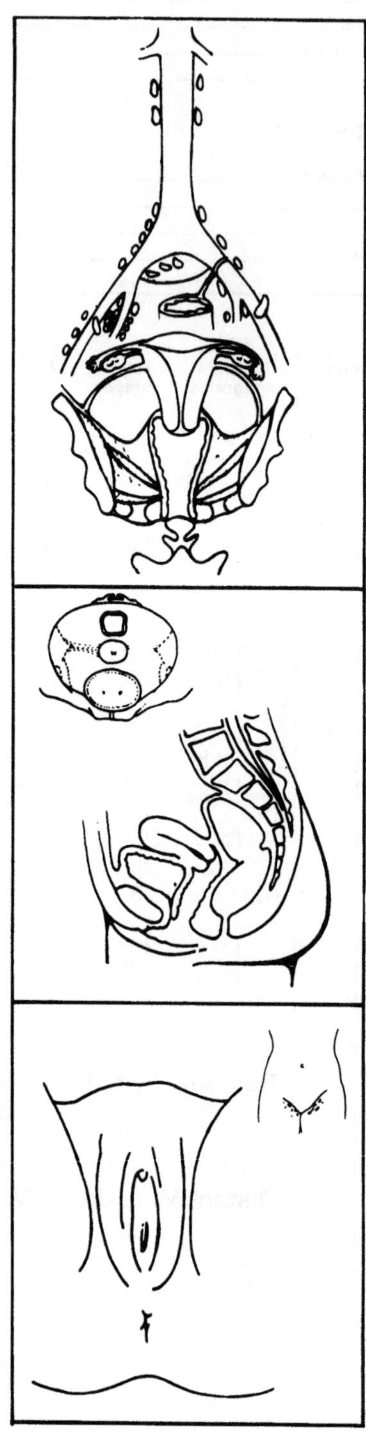

Indicate on diagrams primary tumor and regional nodes involved.

29

Corpus Uteri

C54.0 Isthmus uteri
C54.1 Endometrium
C54.2 Myometrium
C54.3 Fundus uteri
C54.8 Overlapping lesion
C54.9 Corpus uteri

C55.9 Uterus, NOS

ANATOMY

Primary Site. The upper two-thirds of the uterus above the level of the internal cervical os is called the corpus. The fallopian tubes enter at the upper lateral corners of a pear-shaped body. The portion of the muscular organ that is above a line joining the tubo-uterine orifices is often referred to as the fundus.

Regional Lymph Nodes. The regional lymph nodes are the:

Para-aortic
Hypogastric (obturator)
Common iliac
Internal iliac
External iliac
Parametrial
Sacral

For pN, histologic examination of a pelvic lymphadenectomy specimen will ordinarily include 10 or more lymph nodes.

Metastatic Sites. The vagina and lung are the common metastatic sites.

RULES FOR CLASSIFICATION

The classification applies only to carcinoma. There should be histologic verification and grading of the tumor.

Because corpus cancer is now surgically staged, procedures previously used for determination of stages are no longer applicable, such as the finding of fractional dilatation and curettage (D&C) to differentiate between stage I and stage II.

It is appreciated that there may be a small number of patients with corpus cancer who will be treated primarily with radiation therapy. If that is the case, the clinical staging adopted by The Federation Internationale de Gynecologie et d'Obstetrique (FIGO) in 1971 would still apply, but designation of that staging system would be noted.

Ideally, width of the myometrium should be measured along with the width of tumor invasion.

DEFINITION OF TNM

The definitions of the T categories correspond to the several stages accepted by FIGO. FIGO stages are further subdivided by histologic grade of tumor; i.e., Stage IC G2. Both systems are included for comparison.

Primary Tumor (T)

TNM categories	FIGO stages	
TX		Primary tumor cannot be assessed
T0		No evidence of primary tumor
Tis		Carcinoma *in situ*
T1	I	Tumor confined to corpus uteri
T1a	IA	Tumor limited to endometrium

T1b	IB	Tumor invades up to or less than one-half of the myometrium
T1c	IC	Tumor invades to more than one-half of the myometrium
T2	II	Tumor invades cervix but does not extend beyond uterus
T2a	IIA	Endocervical glandular involvement only
T2b	IIB	Cervical stromal invasion
T3	III	Local and/or regional spread as specified in T3a, b, and/or N1 and FIGO IIIA, B, and C below
T3a	IIIA	Tumor involves serosa and/or adnexa (direct extension or metastasis) and/or cancer cells in ascites or peritoneal washings
T3b	IIIB	Vaginal involvement (direct extension or metastasis)
N1	IIIC	Metastasis to the pelvic and/or para-aortic lymph nodes
T4	IVA	Tumor invades bladder mucosa and/or bowel mucosa (Bullous edema is not sufficient to classify a tumor as T4)
M1	IVB	Distant metastasis.(*Excluding* metastasis to vagina, pelvic serosa, or adnexa. *Including* metastasis to intra-abdominal lymph nodes other than para-aortic, and/or inguinal lymph nodes.)

Regional Lymph Nodes (N)

NX Regional lymph nodes cannot be assessed
N0 No regional lymph node metastasis
N1 Regional lymph node metastasis

Distant Metastasis (M)

MX Distant metastasis cannot be assessed
M0 No distant metastasis
M1 Distant metastasis

pTNM Pathologic Classification

The pT, pN, and pM categories correspond to the T, N, and M categories.

STAGE GROUPING

Stage 0	Tis	N0	M0
Stage IA	T1a	N0	M0
Stage IB	T1b	N0	M0
Stage IC	T1c	N0	M0
Stage IIA	T2a	N0	M0
Stage IIB	T2b	N0	M0
Stage IIIA	T3a	N0	M0
Stage IIIB	T3b	N0	M0
Stage IIIC	T1	N1	M0
	T2	N1	M0
	T3a	N1	M0
	T3b	N1	M0
Stage IVA	T4	Any N	M0
Stage IVB	Any T	Any N	M1

HISTOPATHOLOGIC TYPE

The histopathologic types are:

Endometrioid carcinoma
- Adenocarcinoma
- Adenoacanthoma (adenocarcinoma with squamous metaplasia)
- Adenosquamous carcinoma (mixed adenocarcinoma and squamous cell carcinoma)

Mucinous adenocarcinoma
Serous adenocarcinoma
Clear cell adenocarcinoma
Squamous cell carcinoma
Undifferentiated carcinoma

HISTOPATHOLOGIC GRADE (G)

GX Grade cannot be assessed
G1 Well differentiated
G2 Moderately differentiated
G3-4 Poorly differentiated or undifferentiated

Histopathology—Degree of Differentiation

Cases of carcinoma of the corpus should be grouped with regard to the degree of differentiation of the adenocarcinoma as follows:

G1 5% or less of a nonsquamous or nonmorular solid growth pattern
G2 6% to 50% of a nonsquamous or nonmorular solid growth pattern
G3 more than 50% of a nonsquamous or nonmorular solid growth pattern

Notes on Pathologic Grading:

1. Notable nuclear atypia, inappropriate for the architectural grade, raises the grade of a grade 1 or grade 2 tumor by 1.
2. In serous and clear cell adenocarcinomas, nuclear grading takes precedent.

3. Adenocarcinomas with squamous differentiation are graded according to the nuclear grade of the glandular component.

PROGNOSTIC FACTORS

Historically, factors such as grade of the tumor, and depth of myometrial invasion have long been recognized as important prognostic factors. In some studies using multivariate analysis, they lose their significance. Histopathology has also been considered to be important in that if a squamous component is present, particularly if malignant, it carries the worse prognosis. Current evaluation of data would suggest that having a squamous component (either benign or malignant) does not impact upon the prognosis as differentiation of the adeno component appears to be the important criteria. It is well-recognized that a papillary serous adenocarcinoma is a worse prognostic factor even when disease appears to be limited to the uterus. Other histologic features such as vascular space involvement does appear to be important, in that in multivariant analysis, these patients tend to have a higher incidence of extrauterine disease and, therefore, a worse prognosis. One patient-related factor appears to be important and that is the age of the patient. The older the patient, the worse the prognosis.

It is well-recognized in endometrial cancer that there are two phenotypic types. Classic (estrogen-related) appears in the nulliparous, obese white patient who may have a late menopause. These patients tend to have a well-differentiated superficially invasive cancer and excellent prognosis. The other phenotypic type appears not to be related to estrogen factors and is seen in the multiparous patient who is thin, many times African-American, and tends to have a poorly differentiated deeply invasive cancer with a high incidence of extrauterine disease and resultant poor prognosis. The reason for the discrepancy between these two types is unclear.

Tumor ploidy has been evaluated in this cancer and appears to be related to survival and recurrence. Hormone receptor status has also in some studies been noted to be prognostically significantly. In some studies, receptor status and multivariant analysis appears to be more important then grade of tumor or depth of invasion. Receptor status appears to correlate with extrauterine disease.

Data Form for Cancer Staging

Patient identification
Name ______
Address ______
Hospital or clinic number ______
Age ___ Sex ___ Race ______

Institution identification
Hospital or clinic ______
Address ______

Oncology Record

Anatomic site of cancer ______
Histologic type ______
Grade (G) ______
Date of classification ______

DEFINITIONS

Primary Tumor (T)

Clin	Path	TNM categories	FIGO* stage	
[ ]	[ ]	TX		Primary tumor cannot be assessed
[ ]	[ ]	T0		No evidence of primary tumor
[ ]	[ ]	Tis		Carcinoma *in situ*
[ ]	[ ]	T1	I	Tumor confined to corpus uteri
[ ]	[ ]	T1a	IA	Tumor limited to endometrium
[ ]	[ ]	T1b	IB	Tumor invades up to or less than one-half of the myometrium
[ ]	[ ]	T1c	IC	Tumor invades to more than one-half of the myometrium
[ ]	[ ]	T2	II	Tumor invades cervix but does not extend beyond uterus
[ ]	[ ]	T2a	IIA	Endocervical glandular involvement only
[ ]	[ ]	T2b	IIB	Cervical stromal invasion
[ ]	[ ]	T3	III	Local and/or regional spread as specified in T3a, b, and/or N1 and FIGO IIIA, B and C below
[ ]	[ ]	T3a	IIIA	Tumor involves serosa and/or adnexa (direct extension or metastasis) and/or cancer cells in ascites or peritoneal washings
[ ]	[ ]	T3b	IIIB	Vaginal involvement (direct extension or metastasis)
[ ]	[ ]	N1	IIIC	Metastasis to the pelvic and/or para-aortic lymph nodes
[ ]	[ ]	T4	IVA	Tumor invades bladder mucosa and/or bowel mucosa (Bullous edema is not sufficient to classify a tumor as T4.)
[ ]	[ ]	M1	IVB	Distant metastasis. (*Excluding* metastasis to vagina, pelvic serosa or adnexa. *Including* metastasis to intra-abdominal lymph nodes other than para-aortic, and/or inguinal lymph nodes.)

Regional Lymph Nodes (N)

Clin	Path		
[ ]	[ ]	NX	Regional lymph nodes cannot be assessed
[ ]	[ ]	N0	No regional lymph node metastasis
[ ]	[ ]	N1	Regional lymph node metastasis

Distant Metastasis (M)

Clin	Path		
[ ]	[ ]	MX	Distant metastasis cannot be assessed
[ ]	[ ]	M0	No distant metastasis
[ ]	[ ]	M1	Distant metastasis

Stage Grouping

AJCC/UICC/FIGO

Clin	Path	Stage	T	N	M
[ ]	[ ]	0	Tis	N0	M0
[ ]	[ ]	IA	T1a	N0	M0
[ ]	[ ]	IB	T1b	N0	M0
[ ]	[ ]	IC	T1c	N0	M0
[ ]	[ ]	IIA	T2a	N0	M0
		IIB	T2b	N0	M0
[ ]	[ ]	IIIA	T3a	N0	M0
[ ]	[ ]	IIIB	T3b	N0	M0
[ ]	[ ]	IIIC	T1	N1	M0
			T2	N1	M0
			T3a	N1	M0
			T3b	N1	M0
[ ]	[ ]	IVA	T4	Any N	M0
[ ]	[ ]	IVB	Any T	Any N	M1

*FIGO: *Federation Internationale de Gynecologie et d'Obstetrique*

Staged by ______ **M.D.**
______ **Registrar**
Date ______

(continued on next page)

Histopathologic Type

The histopathologic types are:

Endometrioid carcinoma
- Adenocarcinoma
- Adenoacanthoma (adenocarcinoma with squamous metaplasia)
- Adenosquamous carcinoma (mixed adenocarcinoma and squamous cell carcinoma)

Mucinous adenocarcinoma
Serous adenocarcinoma
Clear cell adenocarcinoma
Squamous cell carcinoma
Undifferentiated carcinoma

Histopathologic Grade (G)

[ ] GX Grade cannot be assessed
[ ] G1 Well differentiated
[ ] G2 Moderately differentiated
[ ] G3-G4 Poorly differentiated or undifferentiated

Illustrations

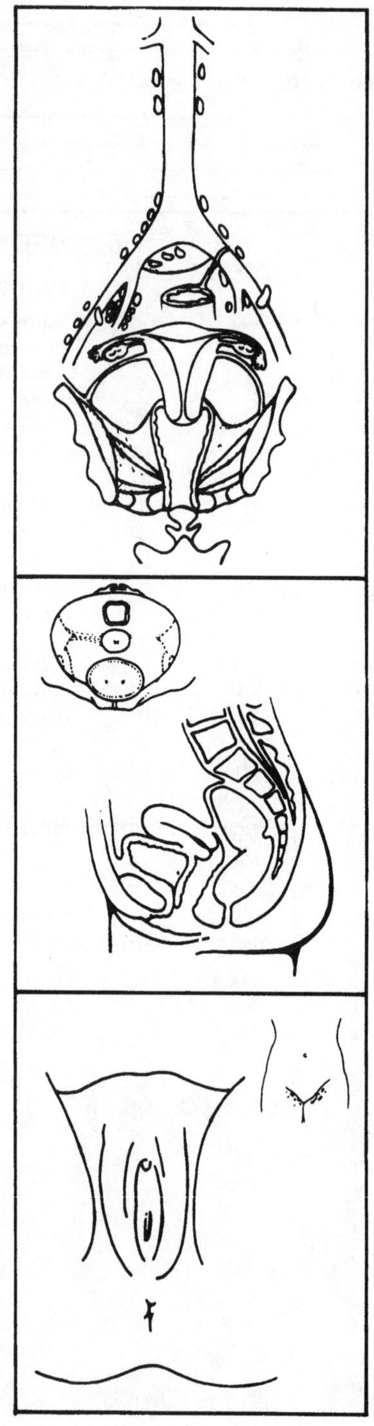

Indicate on diagrams primary tumor and regional nodes involved.

30

Ovary

C56.9 Ovary

ANATOMY

Primary Site. Ovaries are a pair of solid bodies, flattened ovoids 2 to 4 cm in diameter, that are connected by a peritoneal fold to the broad ligament and by the infundibulopelvic ligament to the lateral wall of the pelvis.

Regional Lymph Nodes. The lymphatic drainage occurs by the utero-ovarian and round ligament trunks and an external iliac accessory route into the following regional nodes:

External iliac
Common iliac
Hypogastric (obturator)
Lateral sacral
Para-aortic
Inguinal
Pelvic, NOS
Retroperitoneal, NOS

For pN, histologic examination of a pelvic lymphadenectomy specimen will ordinarily include 10 or more lymph nodes.

Metastatic Sites. The peritoneum, including the omentum and pelvic and abdominal viscera are common sites for seeding. Diaphragmatic and liver surface involvement are common. Pulmonary and pleural involvement are frequently seen. Liver capsule and peritoneal metastases are T3/Stage III.

RULES FOR CLASSIFICATION

Ovarian cancer is surgically staged. There should be histologic confirmation of the disease. Operative findings prior to tumor debulking determine stage which may be modified by histopathologic, as well as clinical or radiologic evaluation. Laparotomy and resection of the ovarian mass, as well as hysterectomy, form the basis for staging. Biopsies of all suspicious sites such as omentum, mesentery, liver, diaphragm, pelvic, and para-aortic nodes are required. The final histologic findings after surgery (and cytologic ones when available) are to be considered in the staging. Clinical studies include routine radiology of the chest. Computed tomography (CT) may be helpful in both initial staging and follow-up of tumors.

Clinical-Diagnostic Staging. Although clinical studies similar to those for other sites may be used, the establishment of a diagnosis requires surgical evaluation. A laparotomy is the most widely accepted procedure in surgical-pathologic staging. Clinical studies may include routine radiography of chest and abdomen, liver studies, and hemograms.

Surgical-Evaluative Staging. Laparotomy and biopsy of all suspected sites of involvement provide the basis for staging. Histologic and cytologic data are required.

Postsurgical Treatment—Pathologic Staging. This should include laparotomy and resection of ovarian masses, as well as hysterectomy. Biopsies of all suspicious sites, such as the omentum, mesentery, liver, diaphragm, and pelvic and para-aortic nodes are required. Pleural effusions should be documented by cytology.

Retreatment Staging. Second-look laparotomies and laparoscopy are being evaluated because of the limitation of routine pelvic and abdominal examinations in detecting early recurrence. Other optional and investigative procedures include ultrasound and CT. All suspected recurrences need biopsy confirmation.

DEFINITION OF TNM

The definitions of the T categories correspond to the several stages accepted by The Federation Internationale de Gynecologie et d'Obstetrique (FIGO). Both systems are included for comparison.

Primary Tumor (T)

TNM categories	FIGO stages	
TX		Primary tumor cannot be assessed
T0		No evidence of primary tumor
T1	I	Tumor limited to ovaries (one or both)
T1a	IA	Tumor limited to one ovary; capsule intact, no tumor on ovarian surface. No malignant cells in ascites or peritoneal washings*
T1b	IB	Tumor limited to both ovaries; capsules intact, no tumor on ovarian surface. No malignant cells in ascites or peritoneal washings*
T1c	IC	Tumor limited to one or both ovaries with any of the following: capsule ruptured, tumor on ovarian surface, malignant cells in ascites or peritoneal washings
T2	II	Tumor involves one or both ovaries with pelvic extension
T2a	IIA	Extension and/or implants on uterus and/or tube(s). No malignant cells in ascites or peritoneal washings.
T2b	IIB	Extension to other pelvic tissues. No malignant cells in ascites or peritoneal washings.
T2c	IIC	Pelvic extension (2a or 2b) with malignant cells in ascites or peritoneal washings.
T3 and/or N1	III	Tumor involves one or both ovaries with microscopically confirmed peritoneal metastasis outside the pelvis and/or regional lymph node metastasis.
T3a	IIIA	Microscopic peritoneal metastasis beyond pelvis
T3b	IIIB	Macroscopic peritoneal metastasis beyond pelvis 2 cm or less in greatest dimension
T3c and/or N1	IIIC	Peritoneal metastasis beyond pelvis more than 2 cm in greatest dimension and/or regional lymph node metastasis
M1	IV	Distant metastasis (excludes peritoneal metastasis)

**Note:* The presence of nonmalignant ascites is not classified. The presence of ascites does not affect staging unless malignant cells are present.

Note: Liver capsule metastases are T3/Stage III; liver parenchymal metastasis, M1/Stage IV. Pleural effusion must have positive cytology for M1/Stage IV.

Regional Lymph Nodes (N)

NX Regional lymph nodes cannot be assessed
N0 No regional lymph node metastasis
N1 Regional lymph node metastasis

Distant Metastasis (M)

MX Distant metastasis cannot be assessed
M0 No distant metastasis
M1 Distant metastasis (excludes peritoneal metastasis)

pTNM Pathologic Classification

The pT, pN, and pM categories correspond to the T, N, and M categories.

STAGE GROUPING

Stage IA	T1a	N0	M0
Stage IB	T1b	N0	M0
Stage IC	T1c	N0	M0
Stage IIA	T2a	N0	M0
Stage IIB	T2b	N0	M0
Stage IIC	T2c	N0	M0
Stage IIIA	T3a	N0	M0
Stage IIIB	T3b	N0	M0
Stage IIIC	T3c	N0	M0
	Any T	N1	M0
Stage IV	Any T	Any N	M1

HISTOPATHOLOGIC TYPE

The American Joint Committee on Cancer (AJCC) endorses the histologic typing of malignant ovarian tumors as presented in the World Health Organization (WHO) publication no. 9, 1973, and recommends that all ovarian epithelial tumors be subdivided according to a simplified version of this classification. The types recommended are as follows: serous tumors, mucinous tumors, endometrioid tumors, clear cell (mesonephroid) tumors, Brenner, undifferentiated tumors, and unclassified tumors.

A. Serous tumors
   1. Benign serous cystadenomas
   2. Of borderline malignancy: Serous cystadenomas with proliferating activity of the epithelial cells and nuclear abnormalities, but with no infiltrative destructive growth (carcinomas of low potential malignancy)
   3. Serous cystadenocarcinomas
B. Mucinous tumors
   1. Benign mucinous cystadenomas
   2. Of borderline malignancy: Mucinous cystadenomas with proliferating activity of the epithelial cells and nuclear abnormalities, but with no infiltrative destructive growth (carcinomas of low potential malignancy)
   3. Mucinous cystadenocarcinomas
C. Endometrioid tumors
   1. Benign endometrioid cystadenomas
   2. Endometrioid tumors with proliferating activity of the epithelial cells and nuclear abnormalities, but with no infiltrative destructive growth (carcinomas of low potential malignancy)
   3. Endometrioid adenocarcinomas
D. Clear cell tumors
   1. Benign clear cell tumors
   2. Clear cell tumors with proliferating activity of the epithelial cells and nuclear abnormalities, but with no infiltrative destructive growth (low potential malignancy)
   3. Clear cell cystadenocarcinomas
E. Brenner
   1. Benign Brenner
   2. Borderline malignancy
   3. Malignant
   4. Transitional cell
F. Undifferentiated carcinomas
   A malignant tumor of epithelial structure that is too poorly differentiated to get placed in any other group.
G. Mixed epithelial tumors
   These tumors are composed of two or more of the five major cell types of common epithelial tumors (types should be specified).
H. Cases with intraperitoneal carcinoma in which the ovaries appear to be incidentally involved and not the primary origin should be labeled as extraovarian peritoneal carcinoma.

HISTOPATHOLOGIC GRADE (G)

GX	Grade cannot be assessed
GB	Borderline malignancy
G1	Well differentiated
G2	Moderately differentiated
G3-4	Poorly differentiated or undifferentiated

PROGNOSTIC FACTORS

Histologic evaluation is an important prognostic factor. Borderline tumors (low malignant potential) stage for stage carry a considerably better prognosis than those patients with invasive cancer. Even with the invasive lesion, this tendency continues as those patients with a well-differentiated lesion do much better than those would are poorly differentiated stage for stage. Histologic type appears to be less important in regards to prognosis, although some studies have suggested endometrioid types do carry a better prognosis. Ploidy DNA index, although in some studies appear to be important, have not been found to be so uniformly.

Particularly in advanced disease, other than the stage of the disease process, the most important prognostic factor is the residual disease after the initial surgical management. Even with advanced stage, patients with no gross residual after the surgical debulking have a considerably better prognosis than those with minimal or extensive residual. Not only is the size of the residual important but the number of sites of residual tumor appears important (tumor volume).

Other factors such as age, growth factors, and oncogene amplification at this point in time do not appear to be important prognostically.

Data Form for Cancer Staging

Patient identification
Name ____________________
Address ____________________
Hospital or clinic number ____________________
Age ____ Sex ____ Race ____________________

Institution identification
Hospital or clinic ____________________
Address ____________________

Oncology Record

Anatomic site of cancer ____________________
Histologic type ____________________
Grade (G) ____________________
Date of classification ____________________

Clin	Path	TNM categories	FIGO stage	DEFINITIONS
				Primary Tumor (T)
[ ]	[ ]	TX		Primary tumor cannot be assessed
[ ]	[ ]	T0		No evidence of primary tumor
[ ]	[ ]	T1	I	Tumor limited to ovaries (one or both)
[ ]	[ ]	T1a	IA	Tumor limited to one ovary; capsule intact, no tumor on ovarian surface. No malignant cells in ascites or peritoneal washings.*
[ ]	[ ]	T1b	IB	Tumor limited to both ovaries; capsules intact, no tumor on ovarian surface. No malignant cells in ascites or peritoneal washings.*
[ ]	[ ]	T1c	IC	Tumor limited to one or both ovaries with any of the following: capsule ruptured, tumor on ovarian surface, malignant cells in ascites, or peritoneal washings.
[ ]	[ ]	T2	II	Tumor involves one or both ovaries with pelvic extension
[ ]	[ ]	T2a	IIA	Extension and/or implants on uterus and/or tube(s). No malignant cells in ascites or peritoneal washings.
[ ]	[ ]	T2b	IIB	Extension to other pelvic tissues. No malignant cells in ascites or peritoneal washings.
[ ]	[ ]	T2c	IIC	Pelvic extension (2a or 2b) with malignant cells in ascites or peritoneal washings.
[ ]	[ ]	T3 &/or N1	III	Tumor involves one or both ovaries with microscopically confirmed peritoneal metastasis outside the pelvis and/or regional lymph node metastasis
[ ]	[ ]	T3a	IIIA	Microscopic peritoneal metastasis beyond pelvis
[ ]	[ ]	T3b	IIIB	Macroscopic peritoneal metastasis beyond pelvis 2 cm or less in greatest dimension
[ ]	[ ]	T3c &/or N1	IIIC	Peritoneal metastasis beyond pelvis more than 2 cm in greatest dimension and/or regional lymph node metastasis
[ ]	[ ]	M1	IV	Distant metastasis (excludes peritoneal metastasis)

**The presence of nonmalignant ascites is not classified. The presence of ascites does not affect staging unless malignant cells are present. Liver capsule metastasis is T3/Stage III, liver parenchymal metastasis M1/Stage IV. Pleural effusion must have positive cytology for M1/Stage IV.*

Regional Lymph Nodes (N)

Clin	Path		
[ ]	[ ]	NX	Regional lymph nodes cannot be assessed
[ ]	[ ]	N0	No regional lymph node metastasis
[ ]	[ ]	N1	Regional lymph node metastasis

Distant Metastasis (M)

Clin	Path		
[ ]	[ ]	MX	Presence of distant metastasis cannot be assessed
[ ]	[ ]	M0	No distant metastasis
[ ]	[ ]	M1	Distant metastasis (Excludes peritoneal metastasis)

Stage Grouping

AJCC/UICC/FIGO

Clin	Path	Stage	T	N	M
[ ]	[ ]	IA	T1a	N0	M0
[ ]	[ ]	IB	T1b	N0	M0
[ ]	[ ]	IC	T1c	N0	M0
[ ]	[ ]	IIA	T2a	N0	M0
[ ]	[ ]	IIB	T2b	N0	M0
[ ]	[ ]	IIC	T2c	N0	M0
[ ]	[ ]	IIIA	T3a	N0	M0
[ ]	[ ]	IIIB	T3b	N0	M0
[ ]	[ ]	IIIC	T3c	N0	M0
			Any T	N1	M0
[ ]	[ ]	IV	Any T	Any N	M1

Staged by ____________________ M.D.
____________________ Registrar
Date ____________________

(continued on next page)

Histopathologic Grade (G)

[ ] GX Grade cannot be assessed
[ ] GB Borderline malignancy
[ ] G1 Well differentiated
[ ] G2 Moderately differentiated
[ ] G3-G4 Poorly differentiated or undifferentiated

Histopathologic Type

The task force of the AJCC endorses the histologic typing of malignant ovarian tumors as presented in the WHO publication no. 9, 1973, and recommends that all ovarian epithelial tumors be subdivided according to a simplified version of this classification. The types recommended are as follows: serous tumors, mucinous tumors, endometrioid tumors, clear cell (mesonephroid) tumors, Brenner, undifferentiated tumors, and unclassified tumors.

A. Serous tumors
   1. Benign serous cystadenomas
   2. Of borderline malignancy: serous cystadenomas with proliferating activity of the epithelial cells and nuclear abnormalities, but with no infiltrative destructive growth (carcinomas of low potential malignancy)
   3. Serous cystadenocarcinomas

B. Mucinous tumors
   1. Benign mucinous cystadenomas
   2. Of borderline malignancy: mucinous cystadenomas with proliferating activity of the epithelial cells and nuclear abnormalities, but with no infiltrative destructive growth (carcinomas of low potential malignancy)
   3. Mucinous cystadenocarcinomas

C. Endometrioid tumors
   1. Benign endometrioid cystadenomas
   2. Endometrioid tumors with proliferating activity of the epithelial cells and nuclear abnormalities, but with no infiltrative destructive growth (carcinomas of low potential malignancy)
   3. Endometrioid adenocarcinomas

D. Clear cell tumors
   1. Benign clear cell tumors
   2. Clear cell tumors with proliferating activity of the epithelial cells and nuclear abnormalities, but with no infiltrative destructive growth (low potential malignancy)
   3. Clear cell cystadenocarcinomas

E. Brenner
   1. Benign Brenner
   2. Borderline malignancy
   3. Malignant
   4. Transitional cell

F. Undifferentiated carcinomas
   A malignant tumor of epithelial structure that is too poorly differentiated to get placed in any other group.

G. Mixed epithelial tumors
   These tumors are composed of two or more of the five major cell types of common epithelial tumors (types should be specified).

H. Cases with intraperitoneal carcinoma in which the ovaries appear to be incidentally involved and not the primary origin should be labeled as extraovarian peritoneal carcinoma.

Illustrations

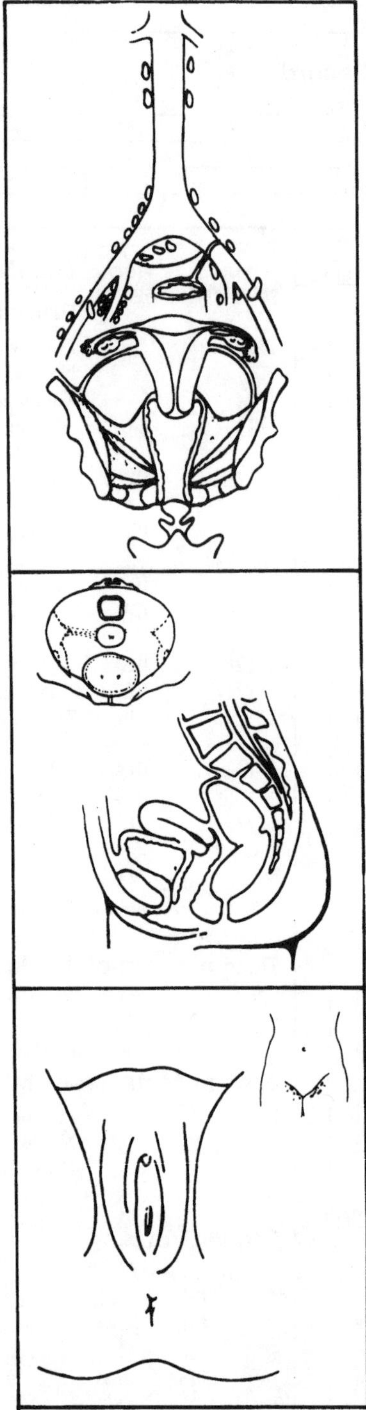

Indicate on diagrams primary tumor and regional nodes involved.

31

Fallopian Tube

C57.0 Fallopian tube

The fallopian tube extends from the posterior superior aspect of the uterine fundus laterally and anteriorly to the ovary. Its length is approximately 10 cm. The lateral end opens to the peritoneal cavity. Carcinoma of the oviduct can metastasize to the regional lymph nodes including the para-aortic nodes. The regional lymph nodes are the hypogastric (obturator), common iliac, external iliac, internal iliac, lateral sacral, para-aortic, and inguinal lymph nodes. Direct extension to surrounding organs, as well as intraperitoneal seeding, occurs frequently. Peritoneal implants may occur with an intact tube.

1. Carcinoma *in situ* of the fallopian tube is a defined entity; therefore, it is included in the staging under stage 0.
2. Since the fallopian tube is a hollow viscus and extension into the submucosa or muscularis and to and beyond the serosa can be defined (a concept similar to that of Dukes' classification for colon cancer), these are taken into consideration in stage Ia, Ib, and Ic in addition to laterality, as well as the presence or absence of ascites. As in ovarian carcinoma, peritoneal washings positive for malignant cells or malignant ascites are placed into stage IC.
3. It should be noted that in stage III the classification of the tumor is based on the findings at the time of entry into the abdominal cavity, *not* on the residual at the end of the debulking. In addition, surface involvement of the liver is in stage III, as is inguinal node metastasis. Like ovarian cancer, pleural effusion must have malignant cells to be called stage IV.

Laparotomy and resection of tubal masses, as well as hysterectomy, form the basis for staging. Biopsies of all suspicious sites, such as the omentum, mesentery, liver, diaphragm, and pelvic and para-aortic nodes, are required.

The final histologic findings after surgery (and cytologic ones when available) are to be considered in the staging.

Clinical studies, if carcinoma of the tube is diagnosed, include routine radiography of chest. Computed tomography may be helpful in both initial staging and follow-up of tumors.

Staging for fallopian tube is by the surgical pathologic system. Operative findings prior to tumor debulking may be modified by histopathologic, as well as clinical or radiologic evaluation.

DEFINITION OF TNM

Primary Tumor (T)

TNM categories	FIGO stages	
TX		Primary tumor cannot be assessed
T0		No evidence of primary tumor
Tis	0	Carcinoma *in situ* (limited to tubal mucosa)
T1	I	Tumor limited to the fallopian tube(s)
T1a	IA	Tumor limited to one tube, without penetrating the serosal surface; no ascites
T1b	IB	Tumor limited to both tubes, without penetrating the serosal surface; no ascites
T1c	IC	Tumor limited to one or both tubes with extension onto or through the tubal serosa, or with malignant cells in ascites or peritoneal washings

T2	II	Tumor involves one or both fallopian tubes with pelvic extension
T2a	IIA	Extension and/or metastasis to the uterus and/or ovaries
T2b	IIB	Extension to other pelvic structures
T2c	IIC	Pelvic extension with malignant cells in ascites or peritoneal washings
T3 and/or N1	III	Tumor involves one or both fallopian tubes, with peritoneal implants outside the pelvis and/or positive regional lymph nodes
T3a	IIIA	Microscopic peritoneal metastasis outside the pelvis
T3b	IIIB	Macroscopic peritoneal metastasis outside the pelvis 2 cm or less in greatest dimension
T3c and/or N1	IIIC	Peritoneal metastasis more than 2 cm in diameter and/or positive regional lymph nodes
M1	IV	Distant metastases (excludes peritoneal metastasis)

Note: Liver capsule metastases are T3/Stage III; liver parenchymal metastasis, M1/Stage IV. Pleural effusion must have positive cytology for M1/Stage IV.

Regional Lymph Nodes (N)

NX Regional lymph nodes cannot be assessed
N0 No regional lymph node metastasis
N1 Regional lymph node metastasis

Distant Metastasis (M)

MX Distant metastasis cannot be assessed
M0 No distant metastasis
M1 Distant metastasis

STAGE GROUPING

Stage 0	Tis	N0	M0
Stage IA	T1a	N0	M0
Stage IB	T1b	N0	M0
Stage IC	T1c	N0	M0
Stage IIA	T2a	N0	M0
Stage IIB	T2b	N0	M0
Stage IIC	T2c	N0	M0
Stage IIIA	T3a	N0	M0
Stage IIIB	T3b	N0	M0
Stage IIIC	T3c	N0	M0
	Any T	N1	M0
Stage IV	Any T	Any N	M1

HISTOPATHOLOGIC TYPES

Adenocarcinoma is the most frequent histology seen.

HISTOPATHOLOGIC GRADE

GX Grade cannot be assessed
G1 Well differentiated
G2 Moderately differentiated
G3 Poorly differentiated
G4 Undifferentiated

PROGNOSTIC FACTORS

This is one of the rarest gynecological cancers and is surgically staged. Stage appears to be the most important prognostic factor, but because of the rarity of the disease, it is unclear whether other factors may be prognostically important.

Data Form for Cancer Staging

Patient identification
Name ______
Address ______
Hospital or clinic number ______
Age ____ Sex ____ Race ______

Institution identification
Hospital or clinic ______
Address ______

Oncology Record

Anatomic site of cancer ______
Histologic type ______
Grade (G) ______
Date of classification ______

DEFINITIONS

Primary Tumor (T)

Clin	Path	TNM categories	FIGO stage	
[ ]	[ ]	TX		Primary tumor cannot be assessed
[ ]	[ ]	T0		No evidence of primary tumor
[ ]	[ ]	Tis	0	Carcinoma *in situ* (limited to tubal mucosa)
[ ]	[ ]	T1	I	Tumor limited to the fallopian tube(s)
[ ]	[ ]	T1a	IA	Tumor limited to one tube, without penetrating the serosal surface; no ascites
[ ]	[ ]	T1b	IB	Tumor limited to both tubes, without penetrating the serosal surface; no ascites
[ ]	[ ]	T1c	IC	Tumor limited to one or both tubes with extension onto or through the tubal serosa, or with malignant cells in ascites or peritoneal washings
[ ]	[ ]	T2	II	Tumor involves one or both fallopian tubes with pelvic extension
[ ]	[ ]	T2a	IIA	Extension and/or metastasis to the uterus and/or ovaries
[ ]	[ ]	T2b	IIB	Extension to other pelvic structures
[ ]	[ ]	T2c	IIC	Pelvic extension with malignant cells in ascites or peritoneal washings
[ ]	[ ]	T3 &/or N1	III	Tumor involves one or both fallopian tubes, with peritoneal implants outside the pelvis and/or positive regional lymph nodes.
[ ]	[ ]	T3a	IIIA	Microscopic peritoneal metastasis outside the pelvis
[ ]	[ ]	T3b	IIIB	Macroscopic peritoneal metastasis outside the pelvis 2 cm or less in greatest dimension
[ ]	[ ]	T3c &/or N1	IIIC	Peritoneal metastasis more than 2 cm in diameter and/or positive regional lymph nodes
[ ]	[ ]	M1	IV	Distant metastases (excludes peritoneal metastasis)

Liver capsule metastases are T3/Stage III; liver parenchymal metastasis, M1/Stage IV. Pleural effusion must have positive cytology for M1/Stage IV.

Regional Lymph Nodes (N)

Clin	Path		
[ ]	[ ]	NX	Regional lymph nodes cannnot be assessed
[ ]	[ ]	N0	No regional lymph node metastasis
[ ]	[ ]	N1	Regional lymph node metastasis

Distant Metastasis (M)

Clin	Path		
[ ]	[ ]	MX	Distant metastasis cannot be assessed
[ ]	[ ]	M0	No distant metastasis
[ ]	[ ]	M1	Distant metastasis (Pelvic lymph node metastasis is M1)

Stage Grouping

AJCC/UICC/FIGO

Clin	Path	Stage	T	N	M
[ ]	[ ]	0	Tis	N0	M0
[ ]	[ ]	IA	T1a	N0	M0
[ ]	[ ]	IB	T1b	N0	M0
[ ]	[ ]	IC	T1c	N0	M0
[ ]	[ ]	IIA	T2a	N0	M0
[ ]	[ ]	IIB	T2b	N0	M0
[ ]	[ ]	IIC	T2c	N0	M0
[ ]	[ ]	IIIA	T3a	N0	M0
[ ]	[ ]	IIIB	T3b	N0	M0
[ ]	[ ]	IIIC	T3c	N0	M0
			Any T	N1	M0
[ ]	[ ]	IV	Any T	Any N	M1

Histopathologic Grade (G)

[ ] GX Grade cannot be assessed
[ ] G1 Well differentiated
[ ] G2 Moderately differentiated
[ ] G3 Poorly differentiated
[ ] G4 Undifferentiated

Histopathologic Type

Adenocarcinoma is the most frequently seen histology.

Staged by ______ M.D.
______ Registrar
Date ______

32

Gestational Trophoblastic Tumors

C54.0 Isthmus uteri
C54.1 Endometrium
C54.2 Myometrium
C54.3 Fundus uteri
C54.8 Overlapping lesion
C54.9 Corpus uteri
C55.9 Uterus, NOSG

In 1991, Federation Internationale de Gynecologie et d'Obstetrique (FIGO) added nonsurgical-pathologic prognostic risk factors to the classic anatomic staging system. These include β-hCG levels of greater than 10^5 and the duration of disease more than 6 months from termination of the antecedent pregnancy.

Since gestational trophoblastic tumors have a very high cure rate in virtually all patients, the ultimate goal of staging is to identify patients who are likely to respond to less intensive chemotherapeutic protocols from those who will require more intensive chemotherapy in order to achieve remission.

Nodal involvement is rare in gestational trophoblastic tumors but has a very poor prognosis when evident. The outcome of patients with nodal disease is the same as those with M1 disease. Regional lymph node (N) classification does not apply to these tumors.

Staging should be based on history, clinical examination, and appropriate laboratory and radiologic studies. Since β-hCG titers accurately reflect clinical disease, histologic verification is not required for diagnosis although it may aid in therapy.

DEFINITION OF TNM

Primary Tumor (T)

TX Primary tumor cannot be assessed
T0 No evidence of primary tumor
T1 Disease limited to uterus
T2 Disease outside of uterus but is limited to genital structures (ovary, tube, vagina, broad ligaments)

Distant Metastasis (M)

M0 No clinical metastasis
M1a Lung metastasis
M1b All other distant metastasis

FIGO STAGE

Stage I	Disease confined to the uterus
Stage IA	Disease confined to the uterus with no risk factors
Stage IB	Disease confined to the uterus with one risk factor
Stage IC	Disease confined to the uterus with two risk factors
Stage II	GTT extends outside of the uterus but is limited to the genital structures (ovary, tube, vagina, broad ligament)
Stage IIA	GTT involving genital structures without risk factors
Stage IIB	GTT extends outside of the uterus but limited to genital structures with one risk factor
Stage IIC	GGT extends outside of the uterus but limited to the genital structures with two risk factors

Stage III	GTT extends to the lungs, with or without known genital tract involvement
Stage IIIA	GTT extends to the lungs, with or without genital tract involvement and with no risk factors
Stage IIIB	GTT extends to the lungs, with or without genital tract involvement and with one risk factor
Stage IIIC	GTT extends to the lungs, with or without genital tract involvement and with two risk factors
Stage IV	All other metastatic sites
Stage IVA	All other metastatic sites, without risk factors
Stage IVB	All other metastatic sites, with one risk factor
Stage IVC	All other metastatic sites, with two risk factors

Risk factors affecting staging include the following:

1. hCG > 100,000 IU/24-hour urine
2. The detection of disease more than 6 months from termination of the antecedent pregnancy

The following factors should be considered and noted in reporting:

1. Prior chemotherapy for known GTT
2. Placental site tumors should be reported separately
3. Histologic verification of disease is not required

STAGE GROUPING

Stage	T	M	Risk Factors
Stage IA	T1	M0	without
Stage IB	T1	M0	one
Stage IC	T1	M0	two
Stage IIA	T2	M0	without
Stage IIB	T2	M0	one
Stage IIC	T2	M0	two
Stage IIIA	Any T	M1a	without
Stage IIIB	Any T	M1a	one
Stage IIIC	Any T	M1a	two
Stage IVA	Any T	M1b	without
Stage IVB	Any T	M1b	one
Stage IVC	Any T	M1b	two

PROGNOSTIC FACTORS

Historically, gestational trophoblastic disease has been anatomically staged. Because of the recognition of several important prognostic factors, there have been several proposed staging classifications taking into consideration prognostic factors. One classification suggested that gestational trophoblastic disease should be categorized into three categories: nonmetastatic gestational trophoblastic disease, metastatic low-risk, and metastatic high risk. This takes into consideration anatomical as well as prognostic factors. The difference between metastatic low risk and high risk is that the latter group required a certain level of hCG, brain, or liver metastasis, and prolonged period of time since last preceding pregnancy. Some have suggested full-term pregnancy puts the patient into this category. Nonmetastatic and low-risk metastatic disease essentially have 100% survival and the high-risk metastatic disease has a varied prognosis overall approaching 80%. This did, however, vary depending upon the risk factors. For instance, liver metastases have less than 50% long-term survival whereas a patient who has only a very high hCG has almost 100% survival. Other classifications have become extremely sophisticated almost to the point that clinical application is unpractical.

In 1991, FIGO developed a staging in which the classic anatomic plus prognostic factors were included. The prognostic factors were hCG of 100,000 mIU and a period of greater than six months since the precedent pregnancy to diagnosis. Because hCG is such a sensitive marker for this disease entity and response and cure rate is determined by the hCG titer alone, histologic confirmation for this disease is not required. Because this is still a relatively rare tumor, particularly in the westernized world, other prognostic factors continue to be evaluated. With the current data, none appears to be prognostically important at this time.

GESTATIONAL TROPHOBLASTIC TUMORS

Data Form for Cancer Staging

Patient identification
Name ____________________
Address ____________________
Hospital or clinic number ____________________
Age ____ Sex ____ Race ____________________

Institution identification
Hospital or clinic ____________________
Address ____________________

Oncology Record

Anatomic site of cancer ____________________
Histologic type ____________________
Grade (G) ____________________
Date of classification ____________________

Clin	Path	DEFINITIONS	
		Primary Tumor (T)	
[ ]	[ ]	TX	Primary tumor cannot be assessed
[ ]	[ ]	T0	No evidence of primary tumor
[ ]	[ ]	T1	Disease limited to uterus
[ ]	[ ]	T2	Disease outside of uterus but is limited to genital structures (ovary, tube, vagina, broad ligaments)
		Distant Metastasis (M)	
[ ]	[ ]	M0	No clinical metastasis
[ ]	[ ]	M1a	Lung metastasis
[ ]	[ ]	M1b	All other distant metastasis
		FIGO STAGE	
[ ]	[ ]	Stage I	Disease confined to the uterus
		Stage IA	Disease confined to the uterus with no risk factors
		Stage IB	Disease confined to the uterus with one risk factor
		Stage IC	Disease confined to the uterus with two risk factors
[ ]	[ ]	Stage II	GTT extends outside of the uterus but is limited to the genital structures (ovary, tube, vagina, broad ligament)
		Stage IIA	GTT involving genital structures without risk factors
		Stage IIB	GTT extends outside of the uterus but limited to genital structures with one risk factor
		Stage IIC	GGT extends outside of the uterus but limited to the genital structures with two risk factors
[ ]	[ ]	Stage III	GTT extends to the lungs, with or without known genital tract involvement
		Stage IIIA	GTT extends to the lungs, with or without genital tract involvement and with no risk factors
		Stage IIIB	GTT extends to the lungs, with or without genital tract involvement and with one risk factor
		Stage IIIC	GTT extends to the lungs, with or without genital tract involvement and with two risk factors
[ ]	[ ]	Stage IV	All other metastatic sites
		Stage IVA	All other metastatic sites, without risk factors
		Stage IVB	All other metastatic sites, with one risk factor
		Stage IVC	All other metastatic sites, with no risk factors

Risk factors affecting staging include the following:

1. hCG > 100,000 IU/24-hour urine
2. The detection of disease more than 6 months from termination of the antecedent pregnancy

The following factors should be considered and noted in reporting:

1. Prior chemotherapy for known GTT
2. Placental site tumors should be reported separately
3. Histologic verification of disease is not required

(continued on next page)

GESTATIONAL TROPHOBLASTIC TUMORS *(continued)*

Stage Grouping

Clin	Path	Stage	T	M	Risk Factors
[ ]	[ ]	Stage IA	T1	M0	without
[ ]	[ ]	Stage IB	T1	M0	one
[ ]	[ ]	State IC	T1	M0	two
[ ]	[ ]	Stage IIA	T2	M0	without
[ ]	[ ]	Stage IIB	T2	M0	one
[ ]	[ ]	Stage IIC	T2	M0	two
[ ]	[ ]	Stage IIIA	Any T	M1a	without
[ ]	[ ]	Stage IIIB	Any T	M1a	one
[ ]	[ ]	Stage IIIC	Any T	M1a	two
[ ]	[ ]	Stage IVA	Any T	M1b	without
[ ]	[ ]	Stage IVB	Any T	M1b	one
[ ]	[ ]	Stage IVC	Any T	M1b	two

Staged by ____________________ M.D.

____________________ Registrar

Date ____________________

GENITOURINARY SITES

33

Penis

(Melanomas are not included.)

C60.0 Prepuce
C60.1 Glans penis
C60.2 Body of penis
C60.8 Overlapping lesion
C60.9 Penis, NOS

Cancers of the penis are rare in the United States, although the incidence varies in different countries of the world. Most are squamous cell carcinomas that arise in the skin or on the glans penis. Prognosis is favorable provided the lymph nodes are not involved. Melanomas can also occur. The staging classification, however, applies to carcinomas. Melanomas are staged in Chapter 24. Some cancers of the penis may be described as verrucous. These are included under this classification. An *in situ* lesion is also included and by definition should be coded as an *in situ* carcinoma of the penis.

ANATOMY

Primary Site. The penis is composed of three cylindrical masses of cavernous tissue bound together by fibrous tissue. Two masses are lateral and are known as the corpora cavernosa penis. The corpus spongiosum penis is a median mass and contains the greater part of the urethra. The penis is attached to the front and the sides of the pubic arch. The skin covering the penis is thin and loosely connected with the deeper parts of the organ. This skin at the root of the penis is continuous with that over the scrotum and perineum. Distally, the skin becomes folded upon itself to form the prepuce or foreskin. Circumcision has been associated with a decreased incidence of cancer of the penis.

Regional Lymph Nodes. The regional lymph nodes are:

Single superficial inguinal (femoral)
Multiple or bilateral superficial inguinal (femoral)
Deep inguinal: Rosenmuller's or Cloquet's node
External iliac
Internal iliac (hypogastric)
Pelvic nodes, NOS

Metastatic Sites. Lung, liver, or bone are most often involved.

RULES FOR CLASSIFICATION

Clinical Staging. Clinical examination, endoscopy where possible, and histologic confirmation are required. Imaging techniques are indicated for metastatic disease detection.

Pathologic Staging. Complete resection of the primary site with appropriate margins is required. Where regional lymph node involvement is suspected these should be included.

DEFINITION OF TNM

Primary Tumor (T)

TX Primary tumor cannot be assessed
T0 No evidence of primary tumor
Tis Carcinoma *in situ*
Ta Noninvasive verrucous carcinoma
T1 Tumor invades subepithelial connective tissue
T2 Tumor invades corpus spongiosum or cavernosum

T3 Tumor invades urethra or prostate
T4 Tumor invades other adjacent structures

Regional Lymph Nodes (N)

NX Regional lymph nodes cannot be assessed
N0 No regional lymph node metastasis
N1 Metastasis in a single superficial, inguinal lymph node
N2 Metastasis in multiple or bilateral superficial inguinal lymph nodes
N3 Metastasis in deep inguinal or pelvic lymph node(s) unilateral or bilateral

Distant Metastasis (M)

MX Distant metastasis cannot be assessed
M0 No distant metastasis
M1 Distant metastasis

STAGE GROUPING

Stage 0	Tis	N0	M0
	Ta	N0	M0
Stage I	T1	N0	M0
Stage II	T1	N1	M0
	T2	N0	M0
	T2	N1	M0
Stage III	T1	N2	M0
	T2	N2	M0
	T3	N0	M0
	T3	N1	M0
	T3	N2	M0
Stage IV	T4	Any N	M0
	Any T	N3	M0
	Any T	Any N	M1

HISTOPATHOLOGIC TYPE

Cell types are limited to carcinomas.

HISTOPATHOLOGIC GRADE (G)

GX Grade cannot be assessed
G1 Well differentiated
G2 Moderately differentiated
G3-4 Poorly differentiated or undifferentiated

BIBLIOGRAPHY

Assimos DG, Jarrow JP: Role of laparoscopic pelvic lymph node dissection in the management of patients with penile cancer and inguinal adenopathy. J Endocrol 8:365–369, 1994

Aynaud O, Ionesco M, Barrasso R: Penile intraepithelial neoplasia: specific clinical features correlate with histologic and virologic findings. Cancer 74:1762–1767, 1994

Lubke WL, Thompson IM: The case for inguinal lymph node dissection in the treatment of T2 -T4 N0 penile cancer. Semin Urol 11:80–84, 1993

Parra RO: Accurate staging of carcinoma of the penis in men with nonpalpable inguinal lymph nodes by modified inguinal lymphadenectomy. J Urol 155:560–563, 1996

Scappini P, Piscioloi F, Pusiol T, et al: Penile cancer: aspiration biopsy cytology for staging. Cancer 58:1526–1533, 1986

Wajsman Z, Gamarra M, Park JJ, et al: Transabdominal fine needle aspiration of retroperitoneal lymph nodes in staging of genitourinary tract cancer (correlation with node dissection findings). J Urol 128:1238–1240, 1982

Wajsman Z, et al: Fine needle aspiration of metastatic lesions and regional lymph nodes in genitourinary cancer. Urology 19:356, 1982

Data Form for Cancer Staging

Patient identification
Name ____________________
Address ____________________
Hospital or clinic number ____________________
Age ____ Sex ____ Race ____________________

Institution identification
Hospital or clinic ____________________
Address ____________________

Oncology Record

Anatomic site of cancer ____________________
Histologic type ____________________
Grade (G) ____________________
Date of classification ____________________

Clin	Path	DEFINITIONS	
		Primary Tumor (T)	
[ ]	[ ]	TX	Primary tumor cannot be assessed
[ ]	[ ]	T0	No evidence of primary tumor
[ ]	[ ]	Tis	Carcinoma *in situ*
[ ]	[ ]	Ta	Noninvasive verrucous carcinoma
[ ]	[ ]	T1	Tumor invades subepithelial connective tissue
[ ]	[ ]	T2	Tumor invades corpus spongiosum or cavernosum
[ ]	[ ]	T3	Tumor invades urethra or prostate
[ ]	[ ]	T4	Tumor invades other adjacent structures
		Regional Lymph Nodes (N)	
[ ]	[ ]	NX	Regional lymph nodes cannot be assessed
[ ]	[ ]	N0	No regional lymph node metastasis
[ ]	[ ]	N1	Metastasis in a single, superficial inguinal lymph node
[ ]	[ ]	N2	Metastasis in multiple or bilateral superficial inguinal lymph nodes
[ ]	[ ]	N3	Metastasis in deep inguinal or pelvic lymph node(s), unilateral or bilateral
		Distant Metastasis	
[ ]	[ ]	MX	Distant metastasis cannot be assessed
[ ]	[ ]	M0	No distant metastasis
[ ]	[ ]	M1	Distant metastasis

Stage Grouping

Clin	Path	Stage	T	N	M
[ ]	[ ]	0	Tis	N0	M0
			Ta	N0	M0
[ ]	[ ]	I	T1	N0	M0
[ ]	[ ]	II	T1	N1	M0
			T2	N0	M0
			T2	N1	M0
[ ]	[ ]	III	T1	N2	M0
			T2	N2	M0
			T3	N0	M0
			T3	N1	M0
			T3	N2	M0
[ ]	[ ]	IV	T4	Any N	M0
			Any T	N3	M0
			Any T	Any N	M1

Histopathologic Grade (G)

[ ] GX Grade cannot be assessed
[ ] G1 Well differentiated
[ ] G2 Moderately differentiated
[ ] G3–4 Poorly differentiated or undifferentiated

Histopathologic Type

Cell types are limited to carcinomas.

Staged by ____________________ M.D.
____________________ Registrar
Date ____________________

34

Prostate

(Sarcomas and transitional cell carcinomas are not included.)

C61.9 Prostate gland

Prostate cancer is the most common cancer in men, with increasing incidence in older age groups. Prostate cancer has a tendency to metastasize to bone. Earlier detection may now be possible with a blood test, prostate-specific antigen (PSA), and simplified biopsy using transrectal ultrasound (TRUS) guides. This TNM classification for carcinoma of the prostate was first proposed in 1992.

ANATOMY

Primary Site. Adenocarcinoma of the prostate usually arises within the peripheral zone and most often posteriorly in that zone, where it is usually amenable to detection by digital rectal examination (DRE) or by TRUS. A less common site of origin is the anteromedial prostate, the transition zone, which is remote from the rectal surface and is the site of origin of benign nodular hyperplasia. The central zone, which comprises most of the base of the prostate, seldom gives rise to cancer but is often invaded by the spread of large cancers. Pathologically, cancers of the prostate are often multifocal in origin.

There is agreement that the incidence of both clinical and latent carcinoma increases with age. However, this cancer is rarely diagnosed in men under 40 years of age. There are substantial limitations in the ability of both DRE and TRUS to define precisely the size or local extent of disease; DRE is currently the most common modality used to define the local stage. Heterogeneity within the T1c category resulting from inherent limitations of either DRE or imaging to quantify the cancer may be balanced by the inclusion of other prognostic factors such as histologic grade, PSA level, and possibly extent of cancer on needle biopsy that contain cancer. Diagnosis of clinically suspicious areas of the prostate can be confirmed histologically by needle biopsy.

The histologic grade of the prostate cancer is important for prognosis. The histopathologic grading of these tumors can be complex because of the morphologic heterogeneity so often encountered in surgical specimens. Either a histologic or a pattern type of grading method can be used. The Gleason score for assessing the histologic pattern of prostate cancer is widely used.

Regional Lymph Nodes. The regional lymph nodes are the nodes of the true pelvis, which essentially are the pelvic nodes below the bifurcation of the common iliac arteries. They include the following groups:

Pelvic, NOS
Hypogastric
Obturator
Iliac (internal, external, NOS)
Sacral (lateral, presacral, promontory [Gerota's], or NOS)

Laterality does not affect the "N" classification.

Distant Lymph Nodes. Distant lymph nodes lie outside the confines of the true pelvis. They can be imaged using ultrasound, computed tomography, magnetic resonance imaging, or lymphangiography. Involvement of distant lymph nodes is classified as M.

Aortic (para-aortic lumbar)
Common iliac
Inguinal, deep
Superficial inguinal (femoral)
Supraclavicular
Cervical
Scalene
Retroperitoneal, NOS

The significance of regional lymph node metastasis, pN, in staging prostate cancer lies in the presence of metastatic foci present within the lymph nodes.

Metastatic Sites. Metastasis to bone from carcinoma of the prostate is common. In addition, this tumor frequently spreads to distant lymph nodes. Lung metastases are uncommon and may be lymphangitic in pattern of spread. Liver metastases are usually identified late in the course of the disease.

RULES FOR CLASSIFICATION

Clinical Staging. Primary tumor assessment includes digital rectal examination of the prostate and histologic or cytologic confirmation of prostate carcinoma. All information available prior to first definitive treatment may be used for clinical staging. Imaging techniques may be valuable in some cases; TRUS is the most commonly used imaging tool. Tumor found in one or both lobes by needle biopsy, but not palpable or visible by imaging is classified as T1c. Considerable uncertainty exists about the ability of imaging to define the extent of a nonpalpable lesion (see definition of T1c below). For research purposes, investigators should specify if clinical staging into the T1c category is based on DRE only or DRE plus TRUS.

Pathologic Staging. Total prostatoseminal-vesiculectomy, including regional node specimen, and histologic confirmation are required for pathologic T classification. A positive biopsy of the rectum permits a pT4 classification without prostatoseminal-vesiculectomy. However, there is no pT1 category because there is insufficient tissue to assess the highest pT category. Margin positivity, potentially a consequence of surgical technique rather than anatomic extent of disease, should be specified along with pathologic stage.

Independent prognostic factors for survival in addition to pathologic stage have been identified for prostate cancer. These include age of patient, co-morbid diseases, histologic grade, Gleason score, PSA level, surgical margin status, and ploidy.

DEFINITION OF TNM

Primary Tumor, Clinical (T)

TX Primary tumor cannot be assessed
T0 No evidence of primary tumor
T1 Clinically inapparent tumor not palpable nor visible by imaging
  T1a Tumor incidental histologic finding in 5% or less of tissue resected
  T1b Tumor incidental histologic finding in more than 5% of tissue resected
  T1c Tumor identified by needle biopsy (e.g., because of elevated PSA)
T2 Tumor confined within prostate*
  T2a Tumor involves one lobe
  T2b Tumor involves both lobes
T3 Tumor extends through the prostate capsule**
  T3a Extracapsular extension (unilateral or bilateral)
  T3b Tumor invades seminal vesicle(s)
T4 Tumor is fixed or invades adjacent structures other than seminal vesicles: bladder neck, external sphincter, rectum, levator muscles, and/or pelvic wall

**Note:* Tumor found in one or both lobes by needle biopsy, but not palpable or reliably visible by imaging, is classified as T1c.

***Note:* Invasion into the prostatic apex or into (but not beyond) the prostatic capsule is not classified as T3, but as T2.

Primary Tumor, Pathologic (pT)

pT2*** Organ confined
  pT2a Unilateral
  pT2b Bilateral
pT3 Extraprostatic extension
  pT3a Extraprostatic extension
  pT3b Seminal vesicle invasion
pT4 Invasion of bladder, rectum

****Note:* There is no pathologic T1 classification.

Regional Lymph Nodes (N)

NX Regional lymph nodes cannot be assessed
N0 No regional lymph node metastasis
N1 Metastasis in regional lymph node or nodes

Distant Metastasis**** (M)

MX Distant metastasis cannot be assessed
M0 No distant metastasis
M1 Distant metastasis
- M1a Nonregional lymph node(s)
- M1b Bone(s)
- M1c Other site(s)

*****Note:* When more than one site of metastasis is present, the most advanced category is used. pM1c is most advanced.

STAGE GROUPING

Stage I	T1a	N0	M0	G1
Stage II	T1a	N0	M0	G2, 3-4
	T1b	N0	M0	Any G
	T1c	N0	M0	Any G
	T1	N0	M0	Any G
	T2	N0	M0	Any G
Stage III	T3	N0	M0	Any G
Stage IV	T4	N0	M0	Any G
	Any T	N1	M0	Any G
	Any T	Any N	M1	Any G

HISTOPATHOLOGIC TYPE

This classification applies to adenocarcinoma, but not to sarcoma or transitional cell carcinoma of the prostate. Transitional cell carcinoma of the prostate is classified as a urethral tumor. (see Chapter 39) There should be histological confirmation of the disease.

HISTOPATHOLOGIC GRADE (G)

GX Grade cannot be assessed
G1 Well differentiated (slight anaplasia)
G2 Moderately differentiated (moderate anaplasia)
G3-4 Poorly differentiated or undifferentiated (marked anaplasia)

If grouping of Gleason scores is necessary for research purposes, the following grouping is suggested:

Gleason score
2–4 well differentiated
5–6 moderately differentiated
7 moderately poorly differentiated
8–10 poorly differentiated

BIBLIOGRAPHY

Aihara M, Wheeler TM, Ohori M, et al: Heterogeneity of prostate cancer in radical prostatectomy specimens. Urology 43:60–67, 1994

Albertsen PC, Fryback DG, Storer BE, et al: Long-term survival among men with conservatively treated localized prostate cancer. JAMA 274:626–631, 1995

Bazinet M, Meshref AW, Trudel C, Aronson S, et al: Prospective evaluation of prostate-specific antigen density and systematic biopsies for early detection of prostatic carcinoma. Urology 43:44–52, 1994

Catalona WJ, Hudson MA, Scardino PT, et al: Selection of optimal prostate specific antigen cutoffs for early detection of prostate cancer: receiver operating characteristic curves. J Urol 152:2037–2042, 1994

Chodak GW, Thisted RA, Gerber GS, et al: Results of conservative management of clinically localized prostate cancer. N Engl J Med 330:242–248, 1994

Epstein JI, Pizov G, Walsh PC: Correlation of pathologic findings with progression after radical retropubic prostatectomy. Cancer 71:3582–3593, 1993

Ferguson JK, Bostwick DG, Suman V, et al: Prostate-specific antigen detected prostate cancer: pathological characteristics of ultrasound visible versus ultrasound invisible tumors. Eur Urol 27:8–12, 1995

Grignon DJ, Hammond EH: College of American Pathologists Conference XXVI on clinical relevance of prognostic markers in solid tumors. Arch Pathol Lab Med 119:December, 1995

Henson DE, Hutter RV, Farrow G: Practice protocol for the examination of specimens removed from patients with carcinoma of the prostate gland. Arch Pathol Lab Med 118:779–783, 1994

Humphrey PA, Frazier HA, Vollmer RT, et al: Stratification of pathologic features in radical prostatectomy specimens that are predictive of elevated initial postoperative serum prostate-specific antigen levels. Cancer 71:1822–1827, 1992

McNeal JE, Villers AA, Redwine EA, et al: Histologic differentiation, cancer volume, and pelvic lymph node metastasis in adenocarcinoma of the prostate. Cancer 66:1225–1233, 1990

Miller GJ: New developments in grading prostate cancer. Semin Urol 8:9–18, 1990

Montie JE: Staging of prostate cancer: current TNM classifications and future prospects for prognostic factors. Cancer Supplement 75:1814–1818, 1995

Partin AW, Oesterling JE: The clinical usefulness of prostate specific antigen: update 1994. J Urol 152:1358–1368, 1994

Pinover WH, Hanlon A, Lee WR, et al: Prostate carcinoma patients upstaged by imaging and treated with irradiation—an outcome-based analysis. Cancer 77(7):1334–1341, 1996

Rifkin MD, Zerhouni EA, Gatsonis CA, Quint LE, et al: Comparison of magnetic resonance imaging and ultrasonography in staging early prostate cancer: results of a multi-institutional cooperative trial. N Engl J Med 323:621–625, 1990

Simon R, Altman DG: Statistical aspects of prognostic factor studies in oncology. Br J Cancer 69:979–985, 1994

Smith DS, Catalona WJ: Interexaminer variability of digital rectal examination in detecting prostate cancer. Urology 45:70–74, 1995

Terris MK, McNeal JE, Freiha FS, et al: Efficacy of transrectal ultrasound-guided seminal vesicle biopsies in the detection of seminal vesicle invasion by prostate cancer. J Urol 149:1035–1039, 1993

Zagars GK, von Eschenbach AC: Prostate-specific antigen—an important marker for prostate cancer treated by external beam radiation therapy. Cancer 72:538–548, 1993

Zincke H, Bergstrahl EJ, Blute ML, et al: Radical prostatectomy for clinically localized prostate cancer: long-term results of 1,143 patients from a single institution. J Clin Oncol 12:2254–2263, 1994

Data Form for Cancer Staging

Patient identification
Name ______
Address ______
Hospital or clinic number ______
Age ____ Sex ____ Race ______

Institution identification
Hospital or clinic ______
Address ______

Oncology Record

Anatomic site of cancer ______
Histologic type ______
Grade (G) ______
Date of classification ______

Clin	Path	DEFINITIONS	
		Primary Tumor (T)	
[ ]	[ ]	TX	Primary tumor cannot be assessed
[ ]	[ ]	T0	No evidence of primary tumor
[ ]	[ ]	T1	Clinically inapparent tumor not palpable or visible by imaging
[ ]	[ ]	T1a	Tumor incidental histologic finding in 5% or less of tissue resected
[ ]	[ ]	T1b	Tumor incidental histologic finding in more than 5% of tissue resected
[ ]	[ ]	T1c	Tumor identified by needle biopsy (e.g., because of elevated PSA)
[ ]	[ ]	T2	Palpable tumor confined within prostate*
[ ]	[ ]	T2a	Tumor involves one lobe
[ ]	[ ]	T2b	Tumor involves both lobes
[ ]	[ ]	T3	Tumor extends through the prostatic capsule**
[ ]	[ ]	T3a	Extracapsular extension (unilateral or bilateral)
[ ]	[ ]	T3b	Tumor invades seminal vesicle(s)
[ ]	[ ]	T4	Tumor is fixed or invades adjacent structures other than seminal vesicles: bladder neck, external sphincter, rectum, levator muscles, and/or pelvic wall
		**Tumor found in one or both lobes by needle biopsy, but not palpable or reliably visible by imaging, is classified as T1c.*	
		***Invasion into the prostatic apex or into (but not beyond) the prostatic capsule is not classified as T3, but as T2.*	
		Primary Tumor, Pathologic (pT)	
[ ]	[ ]	pT2***	Organ confined
[ ]	[ ]	pT2a	Unilateral
[ ]	[ ]	pT2b	Bilateral
[ ]	[ ]	pT3	Extraprostatic extension
[ ]	[ ]	pT3a	Extraprostatic extension
[ ]	[ ]	pT3b	Seminal vesicle invasion
[ ]	[ ]	pT4	Invasion of bladder, rectum
		****There is no pathologic T1 classification.*	
		Regional Lymph Nodes (N)	
[ ]	[ ]	NX	Regional lymph nodes cannot be assessed
[ ]	[ ]	N0	No regional lymph node metastasis
[ ]	[ ]	N1	Metastasis in regional lymph node or nodes
		Distant Metastasis (M)****	
[ ]	[ ]	MX	Distant metastasis cannot be assessed
[ ]	[ ]	M0	No distant metastasis
[ ]	[ ]	M1	Distant metastasis
[ ]	[ ]	M1a	Nonregional lymph nodes
[ ]	[ ]	M1b	Bone(s)
[ ]	[ ]	M1c	Other site(s)
		*****When more than one site of metastasis is present, the most advanced category is used. pM1c is most advanced.*	

(continued on next page)

Stage Grouping

Clin	Path	Stage	T	N	M	G
[ ]	[ ]	I	T1a	N0	M0	G1
[ ]	[ ]	II	T1a	N0	M0	G2, 3-4
			T1b	N0	M0	Any G
			T1c	N0	M0	Any G
			T1	N0	M0	Any G
			T2	N0	M0	Any G
[ ]	[ ]	III	T3	N0	M0	Any G
[ ]	[ ]	IV	T4	N0	M0	Any G
			Any T	N1	M0	Any G
			Any T	Any N	M1	Any G

Staged by ______________________________ M.D.

______________________________ Registrar

Date ______________________________

Histopathologic Grade (G)

[ ] GX Grade cannot be assessed
[ ] G1 Well differentiated (slight anaplasia)
[ ] G2 Moderately differentiated (moderate anaplasia)
[ ] G3-4 Poorly differentiated or undifferentiated (marked anaplasia)

If grouping of Gleason scores is necessary for research purposes, the following grouping is suggested:

Gleason score		
	2–4	well differentiated
	5–6	moderately differentiated
	7	moderately poorly differentiated
	8–10	poorly differentiated

Histopathologic Type

This classification applies to adenocarcinoma, but not to sarcoma or transitional cell carcinoma of the prostate. Transitional cell carcinoma of the prostate is classified as a urethral tumor. There should be histologic confirmation of the disease.

Illustrations

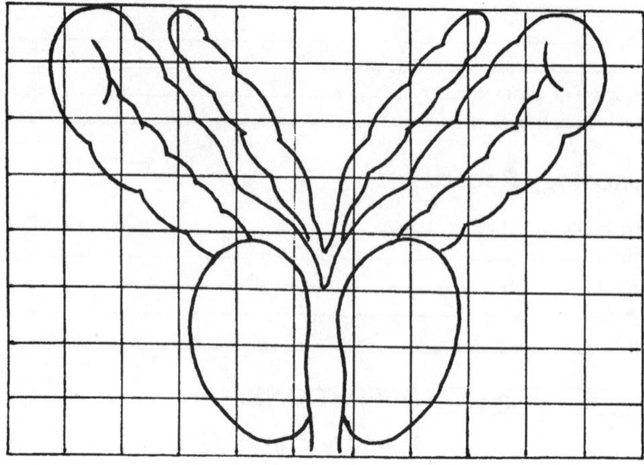

This diagram is for use with the prostate diagram. Sketch in extent of tumor.

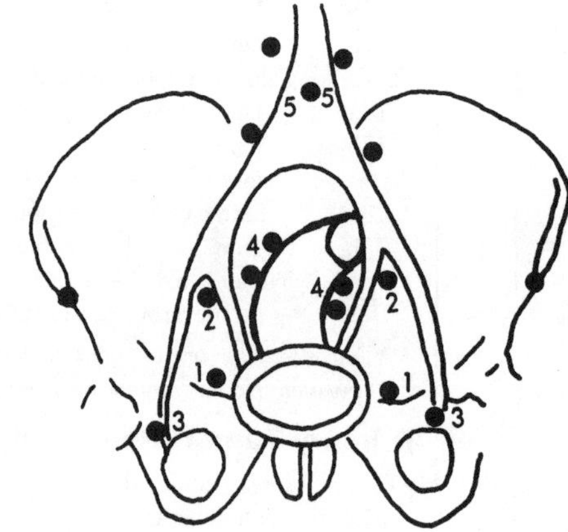

Indicate on diagram primary tumor and regional nodes involved.

35

Testis

C62.0 Undescended testis
C62.1 Descended testis
C62.9 Testis, NOS

Cancers of the testis are usually found in young adults and account for less than 1% of all malignancies in males. Cryptorchidism is a predisposing condition. Germ cell tumors of the testis are categorized into two main histologic types: seminomas and nonseminomas. The latter group is composed of either individual or combinations of histologic subtypes including embryonal carcinoma, teratoma, choriocarcinoma, and yolk sac tumor. The presence of serum markers, including alpha-fetoprotein (AFP), human chorionic gonadotropin (hCG), and lactate dehydrogenase (LDH), is frequent in this disease. Staging is based on the determination of the extent of disease and assessment of serum tumor markers. Cancer of the testis is highly curable, even in cases with advanced disease.

ANATOMY

Primary Site. The testes are composed of convoluted seminiferous tubules with a stroma containing functional endocrine interstitial cells. Both are encased in a dense capsule, the tunica albuginea, with fibrous septa extending into and separating the testes into lobules. The tubules converge and exit at the mediastinum of the testis into the rete testis and efferent ducts, which join a single duct. This duct—the epididymis—coils outside the upper and lower pole of the testicle, then joins the vas deferens, a muscular conduit that accompanies the vessels and lymphatic channels of the spermatic cord. The major route for local extension of cancer is through the lymphatic channels. The tumor emerges from the mediastinum of the testis and courses through the spermatic cord. Occasionally, the epididymis is invaded early, and then the external iliac nodes may become involved. If there has been previous scrotal or inguinal surgery or invasion of the scrotal wall is found (though this is rare), then the lymphatic spread may be to inguinal nodes.

Regional Lymph Nodes. The following nodes are considered regional:

Interaortocaval
Para-aortic (Peri-aortic)
Paracaval
Preaortic
Precaval
Retroaortic
Retrocaval

The intrapelvic, external iliac, and inguinal nodes are considered regional only after scrotal or inguinal surgery prior to the presentation of the testis tumor. All nodes outside the regional nodes are distant. Nodes along the spermatic vein are considered regional.

Metastatic Sites. Distant spread of testicular tumors occurs most commonly to the lymph nodes, followed by metastases to the lung, liver, bone, and other visceral sites. Stage is dependent on the extent of disease and the determination of serum tumor markers. Extent of disease includes assessment for involvement and size of regional lymph nodes, evidence of disease in nonregional lymph nodes and metastases to pulmonary and nonpulmonary visceral sites. The stage is subdivided based on the presence and the degree of elevation of serum tumor markers. Serum tumor markers are obtained immediately after orchiectomy and, if elevated, should be performed serially after orchiectomy according to the normal decay for the AFP (half-life < 7 days) and the hCG (half-life < 3 days) to assess for persistent serum tumor marker elevation. The serum level of lactate dehydrogenase (LDH) has prognostic value in patients with metastatic disease and is included for staging.

RULES FOR CLASSIFICATION

Clinical Staging. Staging of testis tumors includes determination of the T, N, M, and S categories. Clinical examination and radical orchiectomy are required for clinical staging. Radiographic assessment of the chest, abdomen, and pelvis are required to determine the N and M status of disease. Serum tumor markers including AFP, hCG, and LDH should be obtained to complete the status of the serum tumor markers (S).

Pathologic Staging. Histologic evaluation of the radical orchiectomy specimen must be used for the pT classification. The gross size of the tumor should be recorded. Careful gross examination should determine if the tumor is intra- or extratesticular. If intratesticular, it should be determined whether the tumor extends through the tunica albuginea, or invades the epididymis and/or spermatic cord. Tissue sections should document these findings. The tumor should be sampled extensively, including all grossly diverse areas (hemorrhagic, mucoid, solid, cystic, etc.). The junction of tumor and nonneoplastic testis and at least one section remote from the tumor should be obtained to determine if intratubular germ cell neoplasia (carcinoma *in situ*) is present. These sections will allow assessment of either the presence or absence of vascular invasion. If possible, most tissue sections should include overlying tunica albuginea. Small tumors (2 cm or less) may be submitted *in toto*. In larger tumors, a sufficient amount of tissue should be sampled, perhaps one section for each 1 or 2 cm of maximum tumor diameter.

The specimens from a defined node-bearing area (e.g., retroperitoneal lymph node dissection) must be used for the pN classification. Retroperitoneal lymph node dissection should be oriented by the surgeon. All lymph nodes should be dissected and the diameters of the largest nodes, as well as the number of lymph nodes involved by tumor should be recorded. Extranodal soft tissue extension of disease should be noted, if present. It is important to carefully examine and liberally sample the specimen, including cystic, fibrotic, hemorrhagic, necrotic, and solid areas. Laterality does not affect the N classification. In post-treatment specimens, it may be difficult to distinguish individual lymph nodes.

DEFINITION OF TNM

Primary Tumor (pT)

The extent of primary tumor is classified after radical orchiectomy.

pTX Primary tumor cannot be assessed (if no radical orchiectomy has been performed, TX is used.)
pT0 No evidence of primary tumor (e.g., histologic scar in testis)
pTis Intratubular germ cell neoplasia (carcinoma *in situ)*
pT1 Tumor limited to the testis and epididymis without vascular/lymphatic invasion; tumor may invade into the tunica albuginea but not the tunica vaginalis
pT2 Tumor limited to the testis and epididymis with vascular/lymphatic invasion, or tumor extending through the tunica albuginea with involvement of the tunica vaginalis
pT3 Tumor invades the spermatic cord with or without vascular/lymphatic invasion
pT4 Tumor invades the scrotum with or without vascular/lymphatic invasion

Regional Lymph Nodes (N)

Clinical

NX Regional lymph nodes cannot be assessed
N0 No regional lymph node metastasis
N1 Metastasis with a lymph node mass 2 cm or less in greatest dimension; or multiple lymph nodes, none more than 2 cm in greatest dimension
N2 Metastasis with a lymph node mass, more than 2 cm but not more than 5 cm in greatest dimension; or multiple lymph nodes, any one mass greater than 2 cm but not more than 5 cm in greatest dimension
N3 Metastasis with a lymph node mass more than 5 cm in greatest dimension

Pathologic (pN)

pNX Regional lymph nodes cannot be assessed
pN0 No regional lymph node metastasis

pN1 Metastasis with a lymph node mass, 2 cm or less in greatest dimension and less than or equal to 5 nodes positive, none more than 2 cm in greatest dimension

pN2 Metastasis with a lymph node mass, more than 2 cm but not more than 5 cm in greatest dimension; or more than 5 nodes positive, none more than 5 cm; or evidence of extranodal extension of tumor

pN3 Metastasis with a lymph node mass more than 5 cm in greatest dimension

Distant Metastasis (M)

MX Distant metastasis cannot be assessed
M0 No distant metastasis
M1 Distant metastasis
- M1a Nonregional nodal or pulmonary metastasis
- M1b Distant metastasis other than to nonregional lymph nodes and lungs.

Serum Tumor Markers (S)

SX Marker studies not available or not performed
S0 Marker study levels within normal limits
S1 LDH < 1.5 × N **AND**
hCG (mIu/ml) < 5000 **AND**
AFP (ng/ml) < 1000
S2 LDH 1.5–10 × N **OR**
hCG (mIu/ml) 5000–50,000 **OR**
AFP (ng/ml) 1000–10,000
S3 LDH > 10 × N **OR**
hCG (mIu/ml) > 50,000 **OR**
AFP (ng/ml) > 10,000
N indicates the upper limit of normal for the LDH assay.

STAGE GROUPING

Stage 0	pTis	N0	M0	S0
Stage I	pT1–4	N0	M0	SX
Stage IA	pT1	N0	M0	S0
Stage IB	pT2	N0	M0	S0
	pT3	N0	M0	S0
	pT4	N0	M0	S0
Stage IS	Any pT/Tx	N0	M0	S1–3
Stage II	Any pT/Tx	N1–3	M0	SX
Stage IIA	Any pT/Tx	N1	M0	S0
	Any pT/Tx	N1	M0	S1
Stage IIB	Any pT/Tx	N2	M0	S0
	Any pT/Tx	N2	M0	S1
Stage IIC	Any pT/Tx	N3	M0	S0
	Any pT/Tx	N3	M0	S1
Stage III	Any pT/Tx	Any N	M1	SX
Stage IIIA	Any pT/Tx	Any N	M1a	S0
	Any pT/Tx	Any N	M1a	S1
Stage IIIB	Any pT/Tx	N1–3	M0	S2
	Any pT/Tx	Any N	M1a	S2
Stage IIIC	Any pT/Tx	N1–3	M0	S3
	Any pT/Tx	Any N	M1a	S3
	Any pT/Tx	Any N	M1b	Any S

HISTOPATHOLOGIC TYPE

Following the guidelines of the *World Health Organization Histological Classification of Tumors,* germ cell tumors may be either seminomatous or nonseminomatous. Seminomas may be classic type or with syncytiotrophoblasts. Nonseminomatous germ cell tumors may be pure (embryonal carcinoma, yolk sac tumor, teratoma, choriocarcinoma) or mixed. Mixtures of these types (including seminoma) should be noted, starting with the most prevalent component and ending with the least represented. Similarly, gonadal stromal tumors should be classified according to the *World Health Organization Histological Classification of Tumors.*

BIBLIOGRAPHY

Bajorin DF, Mazumdar M, Vlamis V, et al: Factors predictive of response to platin-based chemotherapy in germ cell tumors (GCT): a multivariate analysis in 773 patients. Proc Am Soc Clin Oncol 12:234(Abstr), 1993

Hoskin P, Dilly S, Easton D, et al: Prognostic factors in stage I nonseminomatous germ-cell testicular tumors managed by orchiectomy and surveillance: Implications for adjuvant chemotherapy. J Clin Oncol 4:1031–1036, 1986

Klepp O, Olsson AM, Henrikson H, et al: Prognostic factors in clinical stage I nonseminomatous germ cell tumors of the testis: multivariate analysis of a prospective multicenter study. Swedish-Norwegian Testicular Cancer Group. J Clin Oncol 8:509–518, 1990

Mead GM: International Consensus prognostic classification for metastatic germ cell tumors treated with platinum-based chemotherapy: final report of the international germ cell cancer collaborative group (IGCCCG). Proc Am Soc Clin Oncol 14: 235(Abstr 615), 1995

Mostofi FK, Sesterhenn IA: Revised international classification of testicular tumors. In Jones WG, Harnden P, Appleyard I (Eds.), Germ cell tumors III. Oxford: Pergamon; 153–158, 1994

Richie JP, Kantoff PW: Is adjuvant chemotherapy necessary for patients with stage B1 testicular cancer? J Clin Oncol 9:1393–1396, 1991

Williams SD, Stablein DM, Einhorn LH, et al: Immediate adjuvant chemotherapy versus observation with treatment at relapse in pathologic stage II testicular cancer. N Engl J Med 317:1433–1438, 1987

Data Form for Cancer Staging

Patient identification
Name ______
Address ______
Hospital or clinic number ______
Age ______ Sex ______ Race ______

Institution identification
Hospital or clinic ______
Address ______

Oncology Record

Anatomic site of cancer ______
Histologic type ______
Grade (G) ______
Date of classification ______

Clin	Path	DEFINITIONS
		Primary Tumor (pT)
[ ]	[ ]	The extent of primary tumor is classified after radical orchiectomy.
[ ]	[ ]	pTX Primary tumor cannot be assessed. (If no radical orchiectomy has been performed, TX is used)
[ ]	[ ]	pT0 No evidence of primary tumor (e.g., histologic scar in testis)
[ ]	[ ]	pTis Intratubular germ cell neoplasia (carcinoma *in situ*)
[ ]	[ ]	pT1 Tumor limited to the testis and epididymis without vascular/lymphatic invasion. Tumor may invade into the tunica albuginea but not the tunica vaginalis
[ ]	[ ]	pT2 Tumor limited to the testis and epididymis with vascular/lymphatic invasion, or tumor extending through the tunica albuginea with involvement of the tunica vaginalis
[ ]	[ ]	pT3 Tumor invades the spermatic cord with or without vascular/lymphatic invasion
[ ]	[ ]	pT4 Tumor invades the scrotum with or without vascular/lymphatic invasion
		Regional Lymph Nodes (N)
		Clinical
[ ]	[ ]	NX Regional lymph nodes cannot be assessed
[ ]	[ ]	N0 No regional lymph node metastasis
[ ]	[ ]	N1 Metastasis with a lymph node mass 2 cm or less in greatest dimension; or multiple lymph nodes, none more than 2 cm in greatest dimension
[ ]	[ ]	N2 Metastasis with a lymph node mass, more than 2 cm but not more than 5 cm in greatest dimension; or multiple lymph nodes, any one mass greater than 2 cm but not more than 5 cm in greatest dimension
[ ]	[ ]	N3 Metastasis with a lymph node mass more than 5 cm in greatest dimension
		Pathologic (pN)
[ ]	[ ]	pNX Regional lymph nodes cannot be assessed
[ ]	[ ]	pN0 No regional lymph node metastasis
[ ]	[ ]	pN1 Metastasis with a lymph node mass, 2 cm or less in greatest dimension and less than or equal to 5 nodes positive, none more than 2 cm in greatest dimension
[ ]	[ ]	pN2 Metastasis with a lymph node mass, more than 2 cm but not more than 5 cm in greatest dimension; or more than 5 nodes positive; none more than 5 cm; or evidence of extranodal extension of tumor
[ ]	[ ]	pN3 Metastasis with a lymph node mass more than 5 cm in greatest dimension
		Distant Metastasis (M)
[ ]	[ ]	MX Distant metastasis cannot be assessed
[ ]	[ ]	M0 No distant metastasis
[ ]	[ ]	M1 Distant metastasis
[ ]	[ ]	M1a Nonregional nodal or pulmonary metastasis
[ ]	[ ]	M1b Distant metastasis other than to nonregional lymph nodes and lungs.

(continued on next page)

DEFINITIONS

Serum Tumor Markers (S)

Clin	Path			
[ ]	[ ]	SX	Marker studies not available or not performed	
[ ]	[ ]	S0	Marker study levels within normal limits	
[ ]	[ ]	S1	LDH	< 1.5 × N AND
[ ]	[ ]		hCG (mIu/ml)	< 5000 AND
[ ]	[ ]		AFP (ng/ml)	< 1000
[ ]	[ ]	S2	LDH	1.5–10 × N OR
[ ]	[ ]		hCG (mIu/ml)	5000–50,000 OR
[ ]	[ ]		AFP (ng/ml)	1000–10,000
[ ]	[ ]	S3	LDH	> 10 × N OR
[ ]	[ ]		hCG (mIu/ml)	> 50,000 OR
[ ]	[ ]		AFP (ng/ml)	> 10,000

N indicates the upper limit of normal for the LDH assay.

Stage Grouping

Clin	Path					
[ ]	[ ]	0	pTis	N0	M0	S0
[ ]	[ ]	I	pT1–4	N0	M0	SX
[ ]	[ ]	IA	pT1	N0	M0	S0
[ ]	[ ]	IB	pT2	N0	M0	S0
			pT3	N0	M0	S0
			pT4	N0	M0	S0
[ ]	[ ]	IS	Any pT/Tx	N0	M0	S1–3
[ ]	[ ]	II	Any pT/Tx	N1–3	M0	SX
[ ]	[ ]	IIA	Any pT/Tx	N1	M0	S0
			Any pT/Tx	N1	M0	S1
[ ]	[ ]	IIB	Any pT/Tx	N2	M0	S0
			Any pT/Tx	N2	M0	S1
[ ]	[ ]	IIC	Any pT/Tx	N3	M0	S0
			Any pT/Tx	N3	M0	S1
[ ]	[ ]	III	Any pT/Tx	Any N	M1	SX
[ ]	[ ]	IIIA	Any pT/Tx	Any N	M1a	S0
			Any pT/Tx	Any N	M1a	S1
[ ]	[ ]	IIIB	Any pT/Tx	N1–3	M0	S2
			Any pT/Tx	Any N	M1a	S2
[ ]	[ ]	IIIC	Any pT/Tx	N1–3	M0	S3
			Any pT/Tx	Any N	M1a	S3
			Any pT/Tx	Any N	M1b	Any S

Staged by ______________________________ M.D.

______________________________ Registrar

Date ______________________________

Histopathologic Type

Following the guidelines of the *World Health Organization Histological Classification of Tumors* germ cell tumors may be either seminomatous or nonseminomatous. Seminomas may be classic type or with syncytiotrophoblasts. Nonseminomatous germ cell tumors may be pure (embryonal carcinoma, yolk sac tumor, teratoma, choriocarcinoma) or mixed. Mixtures of these types (including seminoma) should be noted, starting with the most prevalent component and ending with the least represented. Similarly, gonadal stromal tumors should be classified according to the *World Health Organization Histological Classification of Tumors*.

Illustration

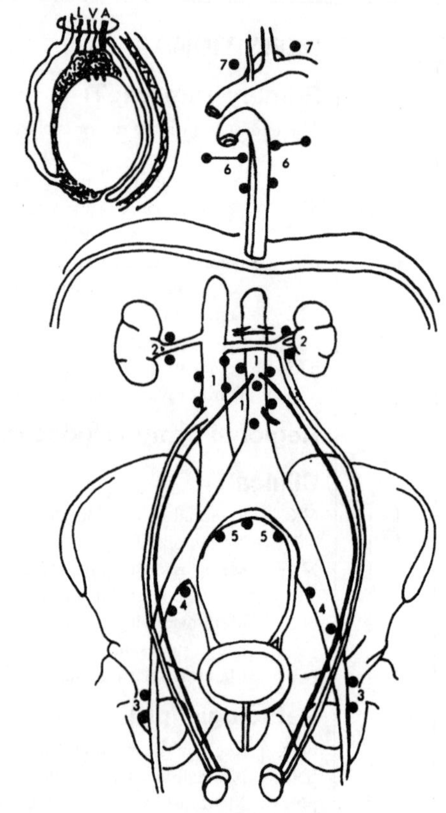

Indicate on diagram primary tumor and regional nodes involved.

36

Kidney

(Sarcomas and adenomas are not included.)

C64.9 Kidney, NOS

Cancers of the kidney are relatively rare, accounting for less than 3% of all malignancies. Nearly all malignant tumors are carcinomas arising from the renal tubular epithelium or, less frequently, from the renal pelvis (see Chapter 37). These tumors are more common in males. Pain and hematuria are usually the presenting features, but a majority of kidney tumors are now being detected incidentally in asymptomatic individuals. These carcinomas have a tendency to extend along the renal vein and even into the vena cava. Staging depends upon the size of the primary tumor, invasion of the adjacent structures, and vascular extension.

ANATOMY

Primary Site. Encased by a fibrous capsule and surrounded by perirenal fat, the kidney consists of the cortex (glomeruli, convoluted tubules) and the medulla (Henle's loops, pyramids of converging tubules). Each papilla opens into the minor calices; these in turn unite in the major calices and drain into the renal pelvis. At the hilus are the pelvis, ureter, and renal artery and vein. Gerota's fascia overlies the psoas and quadrants lumborum.

Regional Lymph Nodes. The regional lymph nodes are:

Renal hilar
Paracaval
Aortic (para-aortic, periaortic, lateral aortic)
Retroperitoneal, NOS

Metastatic Sites. Common metastatic sites include bone, liver, lung, brain, and distant lymph nodes.

RULES FOR CLASSIFICATION

The classification applies only to the renal-cell carcinomas. Adenoma is excluded. There should be histologic confirmation of the disease. Refer to Histopathologic Type.

Clinical Staging. Clinical examination, abdominal computed tomography scanning, and appropriate imaging techniques are required for assessment of the primary tumor and its extensions, both local and distant. Evaluation for distant metastases should be done by laboratory biochemical studies, chest x-rays, and, if clinically indicated, isotopic studies. Clinical staging may also include laparotomy and biopsy of distant sites.

Pathologic Staging. Histologic examination and confirmation of extent is recommended. Resection of the primary tumor, kidney, Gerota's fascia, perinephric fat, renal vein, and appropriate lymph nodes is recommended. Laterality does not affect the N classification.

DEFINITION OF TNM

Primary Tumor (T)

TX Primary tumor cannot be assessed
T0 No evidence of primary tumor
T1 Tumor 7 cm or less in greatest dimension limited to the kidney
T2 Tumor more than 7 cm in greatest dimension limited to the kidney
T3 Tumor extends into major veins or invades the adrenal gland or perinephric tissues, but not beyond Gerota's fascia

T3a Tumor invades the adrenal gland or perinephric tissues but not beyond Gerota's fascia
T3b Tumor grossly extends into the renal vein(s) or vena cava below the diaphragm
T3c Tumor grossly extends into the renal vein(s) or vena cava above the diaphragm
T4 Tumor invades beyond Gerota's fascia

Regional Lymph Nodes (N)*

NX Regional lymph nodes cannot be assessed
N0 No regional lymph node metastases
N1 Metastases in a single regional lymph node
N2 Metastasis in more than one regional lymph node

**Note:* Laterality does not affect the N classification.

Distant Metastasis (M)

MX Distant metastasis cannot be assessed
M0 No distant metastasis
M1 Distant metastasis

STAGE GROUPING

Stage I	T1	N0	M0
Stage II	T2	N0	M0
Stage III	T1	N1	M0
	T2	N1	M0
	T3a	N0	M0
	T3a	N1	M0
	T3b	N0	M0
	T3b	N1	M0
	T3c	N0	M0
	T3c	N1	M0
Stage IV	T4	N0	M0
	T4	N1	M0
	Any T	N2	M0
	Any T	Any N	M1

HISTOPATHOLOGIC TYPE

The predominant cancer is adenocarcinoma; subtypes are clear-cell and granular-cell carcinoma. A grading system as below is recommended when feasible. Sarcomas and adenomas are not included. The histopathologic types are:

Renal cell carcinoma
Adenocarcinoma
Renal papillary adenocarcinoma
Tubular carcinoma
Granular cell carcinoma
Clear cell carcinoma (hypernephroma)

HISTOPATHOLOGIC GRADE (G)

GX Grade cannot be assessed
G1 Well differentiated
G2 Moderately differentiated
G3-4 Poorly differentiated or undifferentiated

BIBLIOGRAPHY

Glazer AA, Novick AC: Long-term follow-up after surgical treatment for renal cell carcinoma extending into the right atrium. J Urol 155:448–450, 1996

Guinan PD, Vogelzang NJ, Freingen AM, et al: Renal cell carcinoma: tumor size, stage, and survival. J Urol 153:901–903, 1995

Hermanek P and Schrott KM: Evaluation of the new tumor, nodes, and metastases classification of renal cell carcinoma. J Urol 144:238–242, 1990

McDonald JR, Priestley JT: Malignant tumors of the kidney: surgical and prognostic significance of tumor thrombosis of the renal vein. Surg Gynecol Obstet 77:295, 1983

Mostafi FK, et al: Histological typing of kidney tumors. WHO international histological classification of tumours. World Health Organization: Geneva, 1981

Targonski PV, Frank W, Stuhldreher D, et al: Value of tumor size in predicting survival from renal cell carcinoma among tumors, nodes, and metastases stage I and stage II patients. J Urol 152:1389–1392, 1994

Data Form for Cancer Staging

Patient identification
Name ______
Address ______
Hospital or clinic number ______
Age ____ Sex ____ Race ______

Institution identification
Hospital or clinic ______
Address ______

Oncology Record

Anatomic site of cancer ______
Histologic type ______
Grade (G) ______
Date of classification ______

Clin	Path	DEFINITIONS	
		Primary Tumor (T)	
[ ]	[ ]	TX	Primary tumor cannot be assessed
[ ]	[ ]	T0	No evidence of primary tumor
[ ]	[ ]	T1	Tumor 7 cm or less in greatest dimension limited to the kidney
[ ]	[ ]	T2	Tumor more than 7 cm in greatest dimension limited to the kidney
[ ]	[ ]	T3	Tumor extends into major veins or invades adrenal gland or perinephric tissues but not beyond Gerota's fascia
[ ]	[ ]	T3a	Tumor invades adrenal gland or perinephric tissues but not beyond Gerota's fascia
[ ]	[ ]	T3b	Tumor grossly extends into renal vein(s) or vena cava below diaphragm
[ ]	[ ]	T3c	Tumor grossly extends into vena cava above diaphragm
[ ]	[ ]	T4	Tumor invades beyond Gerota's fascia
		Regional Lymph Nodes (N)*	
[ ]	[ ]	NX	Regional lymph nodes cannot be assessed
[ ]	[ ]	N0	No regional lymph node metastasis
[ ]	[ ]	N1	Metastasis in a single regional lymph node
[ ]	[ ]	N2	Metastasis in more than one regional lymph node
		**Laterality does not affect the N classification.*	
		Distant Metastasis (M)	
[ ]	[ ]	MX	Distant metastasis cannot be assessed
[ ]	[ ]	M0	No distant metastasis
[ ]	[ ]	M1	Distant metastasis

Clin	Path	Stage Grouping			
[ ]	[ ]	I	T1	N0	M0
[ ]	[ ]	II	T2	N0	M0
[ ]	[ ]	III	T1	N1	M0
			T2	N1	M0
			T3a	N0	M0
			T3a	N1	M0
			T3b	N0	M0
			T3b	N1	M0
			T3c	N0	M0
			T3c	N1	M0
[ ]	[ ]	IV	T4	Any N	M0
			Any T	N2	M0
			Any T	Any N	M1

Staged by ______ **M.D.**
______ **Registrar**
Date ______

(continued on next page)

Histopathologic Grade (G)

[ ] GX Grade cannot be assessed
[ ] G1 Well differentiated
[ ] G2 Moderately differentiated
[ ] G3-4 Poorly differentiated or undifferentiated

Histopathologic Type

The histopathologic types are:

Renal cell carcinoma
Adenocarcinoma
Renal papillary adenocarcinoma
Tubular carcinoma
Granular cell carcinoma
Clear cell carcinoma—Hypernephroma

The predominant cancer is adenocarcinoma; subtypes are clear-cell and granular-cell carcinoma. A grading system is recommended when feasible. The staging system does not apply to sarcomas of the kidney. A separate classification is published for nephroblastomas.

Illustrations

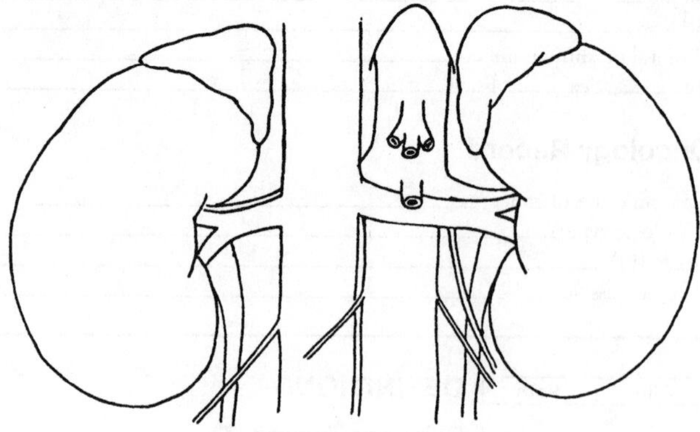

This drawing is to be used with the checklist. Sketch in the urographic, angiographic, ultrasound, or CT extent of the tumor.

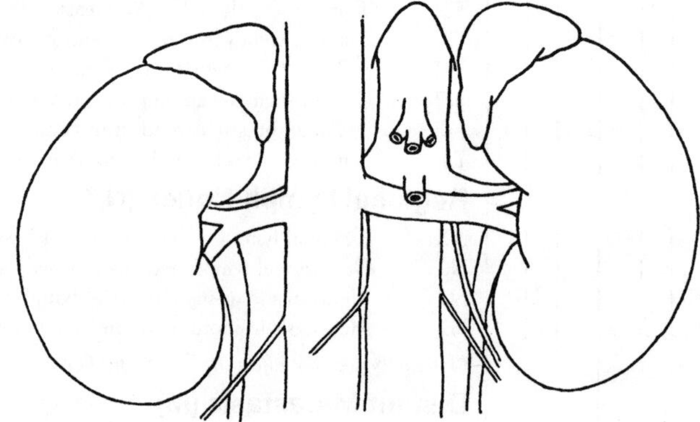

This drawing is to be used with the checklist and the upper drawing. Sketch in the pathologic extent of tumor.

37

Renal Pelvis and Ureter

C65.9 Renal pelvis
C66.9 Ureter

Transitional cell carcinoma may occur at any site within the upper urinary collecting system from the renal calyx to the ureterovesical junction. The tumors occur most commonly in adults and are rare before 40 years of age. There is a two- to three-fold increase in incidence in men compared with women. The lesions are often multiple and are more common in patients with a history of transitional cell carcinoma of the bladder. Local staging depends upon the depth of invasion. A common staging system is used regardless of tumor location within the upper urinary collecting system except for category T3, which differs between the pelvis or calyceal system and the ureter.

ANATOMY

Primary Site. The renal pelvis and ureter form a single unit that cephalad is continuous with the collecting ducts of the renal pyramides and comprises the minor and major calyces, which are continuous with the renal pelvis. The ureteropelvic junction is variable in position and location, but serves as a "landmark" that separates the renal pelvis and the ureter, which continues caudad and traverses the wall of the urinary bladder as the intramural ureter opening in the trigone of the bladder at the ureteral orifice. The renal pelvis and ureter are composed of the following layers: epithelium, subepithelial connective tissue, and muscularis, which is continuous with a connective tissue adventitial layer. It is in this outer layer that the major blood supply and lymphatics are found.

The intrarenal portion of the renal pelvis is surrounded by renal parenchyma; the extrarenal pelvis, by perihilar fat. The ureter courses through the retroperitoneum adjacent to the parietal peritoneum and rests on the retroperitoneal musculature above the pelvic vessels. As it crosses the vessels and enters the deep pelvis, the ureter is surrounded by pelvic fat until it traverses the bladder wall.

Regional Lymph Nodes. The regional lymph nodes are:

For Renal Pelvis:
- Renal hilar
- Paracaval
- Aortic
- Retroperitoneal, NOS

For Ureter:
- Renal hilar
- Iliac (common, internal [hypogastric], external)
- Paracaval
- Peri-ureteral
- Pelvic, NOS

Any amount of regional lymph node metastasis is a poor prognostic finding and outcome is minimally influenced by the number, size, or location of the regional nodes which are involved.

Metastatic Sites. Distant spread to lung, bone, or liver is most common.

RULES FOR CLASSIFICATION

Clinical Staging. Primary tumor assessment includes radiographic imaging, usually by intravenous and/or retrograde pyelography. Computerized tomography scanning can be used to assess regional nodes. Ureteroscopic visualization of the tumor is desirable and tissue biopsy through the ureteroscope may be performed if feasible. Urine cytology may help determine tumor grade if tissue is not available. Staging of tumors of the renal pelvis and ureter is not influenced by the presence of any concomitant bladder tumors which may be identified.

Pathologic Staging. Pathologic staging depends upon histologic determination of the extent of invasion by the primary tumor. Treatment frequently requires resection of the entire kidney, ureter, and a cuff of bladder surrounding the ureteral orifice. Appropriate regional nodes may be sampled. A more conservative surgical resection may be performed, especially with distal ureteral tumors or in the presence of compromised renal function.

Endoscopic resection through a ureteroscope or a percutaneous approach may be used in some circumstances. Submitted tissue may be insufficient for accurate histologic examination and pathologic staging. Laser or electrocautery coagulation or vaporization of the tumor may be performed, especially if the visible appearance is consistent with a low grade and low stage tumor. Under these circumstances, there may be no material available for histologic review.

DEFINITION OF TNM

Primary Tumor (T)

TX Primary tumor cannot be assessed
T0 No evidence of primary tumor
Ta Papillary noninvasive carcinoma
Tis Carcinoma *in situ*
T1 Tumor invades subepithelial connective tissue
T2 Tumor invades the muscularis
T3 (For renal pelvis only) Tumor invades beyond muscularis into peripelvic fat or the renal parenchyma
T3 (For ureter only) Tumor invades beyond muscularis into periureteric fat
T4 Tumor invades adjacent organs, or through the kidney into the perinephric fat.

Regional Lymph Nodes (N)*

NX Regional lymph nodes cannot be assessed
N0 No regional lymph node metastasis
N1 Metastasis in a single lymph node, 2 cm or less in greatest dimension
N2 Metastasis in a single lymph node, more than 2 cm but not more than 5 cm in greatest dimension; or multiple lymph nodes, none more than 5 cm in greatest dimension
N3 Metastasis in a lymph node more than 5 cm in greatest dimension

**Note:* Laterality does not affect the N classification.

Distant Metastasis (M)

MX Distant metastasis cannot be assessed
M0 No distant metastasis
M1 Distant metastasis

STAGE GROUPING

Stage 0a	Ta	N0	M0
Stage 0is	Tis	N0	M0
Stage I	T1	N0	M0
Stage II	T2	N0	M0
Stage III	T3	N0	M0
Stage IV	T4	N0	M0
	Any T	N1	M0
	Any T	N2	M0
	Any T	N3	M0
	Any T	Any N	M1

HISTOPATHOLOGIC TYPE

The histologic types are:

Transitional cell carcinoma
Squamous cell carcinoma
Epidermoid carcinoma
Adenocarcinoma
Urothelial carcinoma

HISTOPATHOLOGIC GRADE

GX Grade cannot be assessed
G1 Well differentiated
G2 Moderately differentiated
G3-4 Poorly differentiated or undifferentiated

BIBLIOGRAPHY

al-Abadi H, Nagel R: Transitional cell carcinoma of the renal pelvis and ureter: prognostic relevance of nuclear deoxyribonucleic acid ploidy studied by slide cytometry: an 8-year survival time study. J Urol 148(1):31–37, 1992

Anderstrom C, Johansson SL, Pettersson S, et al: Carcinoma of the ureter: a clinicopathologic study of 49 cases. J Urol 142(2 Pt 1):280–283, 1989

Borgmann V, al-Abadi H, Nagel R: Prognostic relevance of DNA ploidy and proliferative activity in urothelial carcinoma of the renal pelvis and ureter. A study on a follow-up period of 6 years. Urol Int 47(1):7–11, 1991

Corrado F, Ferri C, Mannini D, et al: Transitional cell carcinoma of the upper urinary tract: evaluation of prognostic factors by histopathology and flow cytometric analysis. J Urol 145(6):1159–1163, 1991

Huben RP, Mounzer AM, Murphy GP: Tumor grade and stage as prognostic variables in upper urothelial tumors. Cancer 62(9):2016–2020, 1988

Jinza S, Iki M, Noguchi S, et al: Nucleolar organizer regions: a new prognostic factor for upper tract urothelial cancer. J Urol 154(5):1688–1692, 1995

Williams RD: Tumors of the kidney, ureter, and bladder. West J Med 156(5):523–534, 1992

Data Form for Cancer Staging

Patient identification
Name ______
Address ______
Hospital or clinic number ______
Age ______ Sex ______ Race ______

Institution identification
Hospital or clinic ______
Address ______

Oncology Record

Anatomic site of cancer ______
Histologic type ______
Grade (G) ______
Date of classification ______

DEFINITIONS

Primary Tumor (T)

Clin	Path		
[ ]	[ ]	TX	Primary tumor cannot be assessed
[ ]	[ ]	T0	No evidence of primary tumor
[ ]	[ ]	Ta	Papillary noninvasive carcinoma
[ ]	[ ]	Tis	Carcinoma *in situ*
[ ]	[ ]	T1	Tumor invades subepithelial connective tissue
[ ]	[ ]	T2	Tumor invades muscularis
[ ]	[ ]	T3	(For renal pelvis only) Tumor invades beyond muscularis into peripelvic fat or renal parenchyma
[ ]	[ ]	T3	(For ureter only) Tumor invades beyond muscularis into periureteric fat
[ ]	[ ]	T4	Tumor invades adjacent organs or through the kidney into perinephric fat

Regional Lymph Nodes (N)*

Clin	Path		
[ ]	[ ]	NX	Regional lymph nodes cannot be assessed
[ ]	[ ]	N0	No regional lymph node metastasis
[ ]	[ ]	N1	Metastasis in a single lymph node, 2 cm or less in greatest dimension
[ ]	[ ]	N2	Metastasis in a single lymph node, more than 2 cm but not more than 5 cm in greatest dimension; or multiple lymph nodes, none more than 5 cm in greatest dimension
[ ]	[ ]	N3	Metastasis in a lymph node more than 5 cm in greatest dimension

*Laterality does not affect the N classification.

Distant Metastasis (M)

Clin	Path		
[ ]	[ ]	MX	Distant metastasis cannot be assessed
[ ]	[ ]	M0	No distant metastasis
[ ]	[ ]	M1	Distant metastasis

Stage Grouping

Clin	Path	Stage	T	N	M
[ ]	[ ]	0a	Ta	N0	M0
[ ]	[ ]	0is	Tis	N0	M0
[ ]	[ ]	I	T1	N0	M0
[ ]	[ ]	II	T2	N0	M0
[ ]	[ ]	III	T3	N0	M0
[ ]	[ ]	IV	T4	N0	M0
			Any T	N1	M0
			Any T	N2	M0
			Any T	N3	M0
			Any T	Any N	M1

Histopathologic Grade (G)

[ ] GX Grade cannot be assessed
[ ] G1 Well differentiated
[ ] G2 Moderately differentiated
[ ] G3-4 Poorly differentiated or undifferentiated

Histopathologic Type

The histopathologic types are:

Transitional cell carcinoma
Squamous cell carcinoma
Epidermoid carcinoma
Adenocarcinoma
Urothelial carcinoma

Staged by ______ M.D.
______ Registrar
Date ______

38

Urinary Bladder

C67.0 Trigone
C67.1 Dome
C67.2 Lateral wall
C67.3 Anterior wall
C67.4 Posterior wall
C67.5 Bladder neck
C67.6 Ureteric orifice
C67.7 Urachus
C67.8 Overlapping lesion
C67.9 Bladder, NOS

Bladder cancer can present as a low grade papillary lesion, as an *in situ* lesion which can occupy large areas of the mucosal surface, or as an infiltrative cancer that rapidly extends through the bladder wall. The papillary and *in situ* lesions may be associated with a malignant course, with sudden invasion of the bladder wall. Predisposing factors include the exposure to certain chemicals and smoking. Bladder cancer is more common in men. Hematuria is the most common presenting sign.

ANATOMY

Primary Site. The urinary bladder consists of three layers: the epithelium and the subepithelial connective tissue, the muscularis, and the perivesical fat (peritoneum covering the superior surface and upper part). In the male, the bladder adjoins the rectum and seminal vesicle posteriorly, the prostate inferiorly, and the pubis and peritoneum anteriorly. In the female, the vagina is located posteriorly and the uterus superiorly. The bladder is located extraperitoneally.

Regional Lymph Nodes. The regional lymph nodes are the nodes of the true pelvis, which essentially are the pelvic nodes below the bifurcation of the common iliac arteries.

The significance of regional lymph node metastasis in staging bladder cancer lies in the number and size and not in whether metastasis is unilateral or contralateral.

Regional nodes include:

Hypogastric
Obturator
Iliac (internal, external, NOS)
Perivesical
Pelvic, NOS
Sacral (lateral, sacral promontory [Gerota's])
Presacral

The common iliac nodes are considered sites of distant metastasis and should be coded as M1.

Metastatic Sites. Distant spread to lymph nodes, lung, bone, and liver is most common.

RULES FOR CLASSIFICATION

Clinical Staging. Primary tumor assessment includes bimanual examination under anesthesia before and after endoscopic surgery (biopsy or transurethral resection) and histologic verification of the presence or absence of tumor when indicated. Bimanual examination following endoscopic surgery is an indicator of clinical stage. The finding of bladder wall thickening, a mobile mass, or a fixed mass suggests the presence of T3a, T3b, and T4b disease, respectively. Add "m" for multiple tumors. Add "is" to any T to indicate associated carcinoma *in situ*.

Appropriate imaging techniques for lymph node evaluation should be used. When indicated, evaluation for distant metastases includes imaging of the chest, biochemical studies, and isotopic studies to detect common metastatic sites. Computed tomography or other modalities may subsequently be used to supply information concerning minimal requirements for staging. The primary tumor may be superficial or invasive and can be partially or totally resected with sufficient tissue from the tumor base for evaluation of full depth of tumor invasion. Visually adjacent cystoscopically normal mucosa should be considered for biopsy; urinary cytology and pyelography are important.

Pathologic Staging. Microscopic examination and confirmation of extent is required. Total cystectomy and lymph node dissection generally are required for this staging. Laterality does not affect the N classification.

DEFINITION OF TNM

Primary Tumor (T)

- TX Primary tumor cannot be assessed
- T0 No evidence of primary tumor
- Ta Noninvasive papillary carcinoma
- Tis Carcinoma *in situ:* "flat tumor"
- T1 Tumor invades subepithelial connective tissue
- T2 Tumor invades muscle
  - T2a Tumor invades superficial muscle (inner half)
  - T2b Tumor invades deep muscle (outer half)
- T3 Tumor invades perivesical tissue
  - T3a microscopically
  - T3b macroscopically (extravesical mass)
- T4 Tumor invades any of the following: prostate, uterus, vagina, pelvic wall, abdominal wall
  - T4a Tumor invades prostate, uterus, vagina
  - T4b Tumor invades pelvic wall, abdominal wall

Regional Lymph Nodes (N)

Regional lymph nodes are those within the true pelvis; all others are distant lymph nodes.

- NX Regional lymph nodes cannot be assessed
- N0 No regional lymph node metastasis
- N1 Metastasis in a single lymph node, 2 cm or less in greatest dimension
- N2 Metastasis in a single lymph node, more than 2 cm but not more than 5 cm in greatest dimension; or multiple lymph nodes, none more than 5 cm in greatest dimension
- N3 Metastasis in a lymph node more than 5 cm in greatest dimension

Distant Metastasis (M)

- MX Distant metastasis cannot be assessed
- M0 No distant metastasis
- M1 Distant metastasis

STAGE GROUPING

Stage 0a	Ta	N0	M0
Stage 0is	Tis	N0	M0
Stage I	T1	N0	M0
Stage II	T2a	N0	M0
	T2b	N0	M0
Stage III	T3a	N0	M0
	T3b	N0	M0
	T4a	N0	M0
Stage IV	T4b	N0	M0
	Any T	N1	M0
	Any T	N2	M0
	Any T	N3	M0
	Any T	Any N	M1

HISTOPATHOLOGIC TYPE

The histologic types are:

Transitional cell carcinoma (urothelial)
- *In situ*
  - Papillary
  - Flat
- With squamous metaplasia
- With glandular metaplasia
- With squamous and glandular metaplasia

Squamous cell carcinoma
Adenocarcinoma
Undifferentiated carcinoma

The predominant cancer is transitional cell carcinoma.

HISTOPATHOLOGIC GRADE (G)

- GX Grade cannot be assessed
- G1 Well differentiated

G2 Moderately differentiated
G3-4 Poorly differentiated or undifferentiated

BIBLIOGRAPHY

deVere White RW, Olsson CA, Deitch AD: Flow cytometry: role in monitoring transitional cell carcinoma of bladder. Urology 28:15–20, 1986

Herr HW: Staging invasive bladder tumors. J Surg Oncol 51:217–220, 1992

Jewett HJ, Strong GH: Infiltrating carcinoma of the bladder: Relation of depth of penetration of the bladder wall to incidence of local extension and metastasis. J Urol 55:366–372, 1946

Pagano F, Bassi P, Ferrante GL, et al: Is stage pT4 (D1) reliable in assessing transitional cell carcinoma involvement of the prostate in patients with a concurrent bladder cancer? A necessary distinction for contiguous or noncontiguous involvement. J Urology 155:244–247, 1996

Pagano F, Guazzieri S, Artibani W, et al: Prognosis of bladder cancer. III. The value of radical cystectomy in the management of invasive bladder cancer. European Urology 15:166–170, 1988

Sarkis AS, Dalbagni G, Cordon-Cardo C, et al: Association of p53 nuclear overexpression and tumor progression in carcinoma in situ of the bladder. J Urol 152:388–392, 1994

Siemiatycki J, Dewar R, Nadon L, et al: Occupational risk factors for bladder cancer: results from a case-control study in Montreal, Quebec, Canada. Am J Epidemiol 140:1061–1080, 1994

Wishnow KI, Levinson AK, Johnson DE: Stage B (P2/3aN0) transitional cell carcinoma of the bladder highly curable by radical cystectomy. Urology 39:12–16, 1992

Data Form for Cancer Staging

Patient identification
Name ____
Address ____
Hospital or clinic number ____
Age ____ Sex ____ Race ____

Institution identification
Hospital or clinic ____
Address ____

Oncology Record

Anatomic site of cancer ____
Histologic type ____
Grade (G) ____
Date of classification ____

Clin	Path	DEFINITIONS	
		Primary Tumor (T)	
[ ]	[ ]	TX	Primary tumor cannot be assessed
[ ]	[ ]	T0	No evidence of primary tumor
[ ]	[ ]	Ta	Noninvasive papillary carcinoma
[ ]	[ ]	Tis	Carcinoma *in situ:* "flat tumor"
[ ]	[ ]	T1	Tumor invades subepithelial connective tissue
[ ]	[ ]	T2	Tumor invades muscle
[ ]	[ ]	T2a	Tumor invades superficial muscle (inner half)
[ ]	[ ]	T2b	Tumor invades deep muscle (outer half)
[ ]	[ ]	T3	Tumor invades perivesical tissue
[ ]	[ ]	T3a	microscopically
[ ]	[ ]	T3b	macroscopically (extravesical mass)
[ ]	[ ]	T4	Tumor invades any of the following: prostate, uterus, vagina, pelvic wall, abdominal wall
[ ]	[ ]	T4a	Tumor invades prostate, uterus, vagina
[ ]	[ ]	T4b	Tumor invades pelvic wall, abdominal wall
		Regional Lymph Nodes (N)	
		Regional lymph nodes are those within the true pelvis; all others are distant lymph nodes.	
[ ]	[ ]	NX	Regional lymph nodes cannot be assessed
[ ]	[ ]	N0	No regional lymph node metastasis
[ ]	[ ]	N1	Metastasis in a single lymph node, 2 cm or less in greatest dimension
[ ]	[ ]	N2	Metastasis in a single lymph node, more than 2 cm but not more than 5 cm in greatest dimension, or multiple lymph nodes, none more than 5 cm in greatest dimension
[ ]	[ ]	N3	Metastasis in a lymph node more than 5 cm in greatest dimension
		Distant Metastasis (M)	
[ ]	[ ]	MX	Distant metastasis cannot be assessed
[ ]	[ ]	M0	No distant metastasis
[ ]	[ ]	M1	Distant metastasis

Clin	Path	Stage Grouping			
[ ]	[ ]	0a	Ta	N0	M0
[ ]	[ ]	0is	Tis	N0	M0
[ ]	[ ]	I	T1	N0	M0
[ ]	[ ]	II	T2a	N0	M0
			T2b	N0	M0
[ ]	[ ]	III	T3a	N0	M0
			T3b	N0	M0
			T4a	N0	M0
[ ]	[ ]	IV	T4b	N0	M0
			Any T	N1	M0
			Any T	N2	M0
			Any T	N3	M0
			Any T	Any N	M1

Staged by ____ **M.D.**
____ **Registrar**
Date ____

(continued on next page)

Histopathologic Grade (G)

[ ] GX Grade cannot be assessed
[ ] G1 Well differentiated
[ ] G2 Moderately differentiated
[ ] G3-4 Poorly differentiated or undifferentiated

Histopathologic Type

The histologic types are:

Transitional cell carcinoma (urothelial)
- *In situ*
  - Papillary
  - Flat
- With squamous metaplasia
- With glandular metaplasia
- With squamous and glandular metaplasia

Squamous cell carcinoma
Adenocarcinoma
Undifferentiated carcinoma

The predominant cancer is a transitional cell cancer.

Illustrations

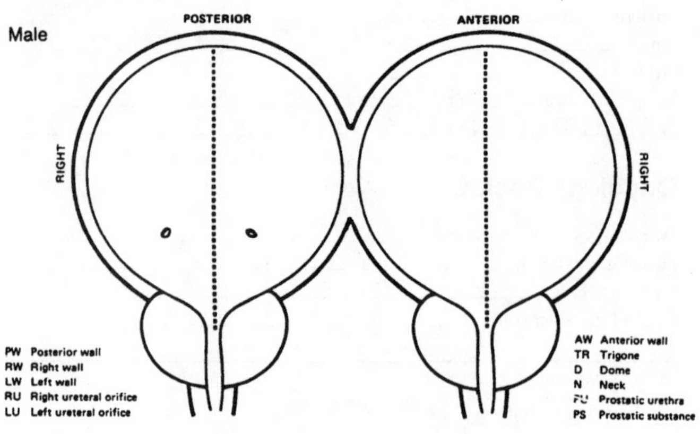

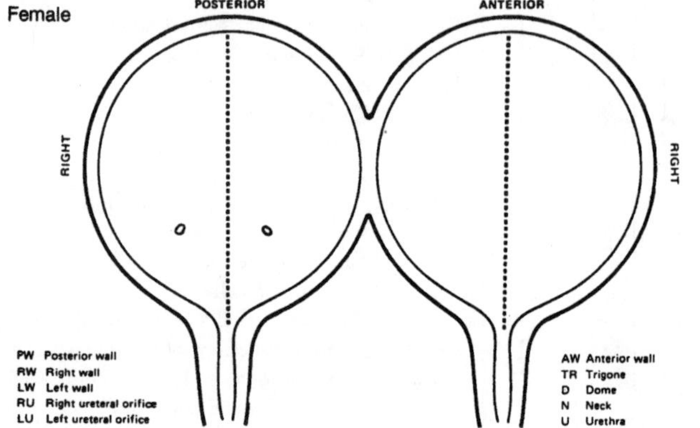

Indicate on diagrams primary tumor and regional nodes involved.

39

Urethra

C68.0 Urethra
C68.1 Paraurethral gland
C68.8 Overlapping lesion of urinary organs
C68.9 Urinary system, NOS

Cancer of the urethra is a rare neoplasia, found in both sexes, but more common in females. In males, the cancer may be associated with chronic stricture disease and in females with urethral diverticula. Tumors of the urethra may be of primary origin from the urethral epithelium or ducts, or may be associated with multifocal urothelial neoplasia. Histologically, these tumors may represent the spectrum of epithelium neoplasms including squamous, adeno- or transitional carcinoma. Prostatic urethral neoplasms arising from the prostatic urethral epithelium or from the periurethral portion of the prostatic ducts are considered urethral neoplasms as distinct from those arising elsewhere in the prostate (see Chapter 34).

ANATOMY

Primary Site. The male urethra consists of mucosa, submucosal stroma, and the surrounding corpus spongiosum. Histologically, the meatal and parameatal urethra are lined with squamous epithelium; the penile and bulbomembranous urethra, with pseudostratified or stratified columnar epithelium, and the prostatic urethra is lined by transitional epithelium. There are scattered islands of stratified squamous epithelium and glands of Littre' liberally situated throughout the entire urethra distal to the prostate portion.

The epithelium of the female urethra is supported on subepithelial connective tissue. The periurethral glands of Skene are concentrated near the meatus but extend along the entire urethra. The urethra is surrounded by a longitudinal layer of smooth muscle continuous with the bladder. The urethra is contiguous to the vaginal wall. The distal two-thirds of the urethra is lined with squamous epithelium; the proximal one-third, with transitional epithelium. The periurethral glands are lined with pseudostratified and stratified columnar epithelium.

Regional Lymph Nodes. The regional lymph nodes are:

Inguinal (superficial or deep)
Iliac (common, internal [hypogastric], obturator, external)
Presacral
Sacral, NOS
Pelvic, NOS

The significance of regional lymph node metastasis in staging urethral cancer lies in the number and size and not in whether unilateral or bilateral.

Metastatic Sites. Distant spread to lung, liver, or bone is most common.

RULES FOR CLASSIFICATION

Clinical Staging. Radiographic imaging, cystourethroscopy, palpation, and biopsy or cytology of the tumor prior to definitive treatment are desirable. The site of origin should be confirmed to exclude metastatic disease.

Pathologic Staging. The assignment of stage for nonprostatic urethral tumors is based on depth of invasion. Prostatic urethral tumors may arise from the prostatic epithelium or from the distal portions of the prostatic ducts and will be classified as prostatic urethral neoplasms. Other prostatic malignancies will be classified under prostate.

DEFINITION OF TNM

Primary Tumor (T) (male and female)

TX Primary tumor cannot be assessed
T0 No evidence of primary tumor
Ta Noninvasive papillary, polypoid, or verrucous carcinoma
Tis Carcinoma *in situ*
T1 Tumor invades subepithelial connective tissue
T2 Tumor invades any of the following: corpus spongiosum, prostate, periurethral muscle
T3 Tumor invades any of the following: corpus cavernosum, beyond prostatic capsule, anterior vagina, bladder neck
T4 Tumor invades other adjacent organs

Transitional Cell Carcinoma of the Prostate

Tis pu Carcinoma *in situ,* involvement of the prostatic urethra
Tis pd Carcinoma *in situ,* involvement of the prostatic ducts
T1 Tumor invades subepithelial connective tissue
T2 Tumor invades any of the following: prostatic stroma, corpus spongiosum, periurethral muscle
T3 Tumor invades any of the following: corpus cavernosum, beyond prostatic capsule, bladder neck (extraprostatic extension)
T4 Tumor invades other adjacent organs (invasion of the bladder)

Regional Lymph Nodes (N)

NX Regional lymph nodes cannot be assessed
N0 No regional lymph node metastasis
N1 Metastasis in a single lymph node, 2 cm or less in greatest dimension
N2 Metastasis in a single node more than 2 cm in greatest dimension, or in multiple nodes

Distant Metastasis (M)

MX Distant metastasis cannot be assessed
M0 No distant metastasis
M1 Distant metastasis

STAGE GROUPING

Stage 0a	Ta	N0	M0
Stage 0is	Tis	N0	M0
	Tis pu	N0	M0
	Tis pd	N0	M0
Stage I	T1	N0	M0
Stage II	T2	N0	M0
Stage III	T1	N1	M0
	T2	N1	M0
	T3	N0	M0
	T3	N1	M0
Stage IV	T4	N0	M0
	T4	N1	M0
	Any T	N2	M0
	Any T	Any N	M1

HISTOPATHOLOGIC TYPE

The classification applies to transitional, squamous, and glandular carcinomas of the urethra, and transitional cell carcinomas of the prostate and prostatic urethra. There should be histologic or cytologic confirmation of the disease.

HISTOPATHOLOGIC GRADE (G)

GX Grade cannot be assessed
G1 Well differentiated
G2 Moderately differentiated
G3-4 Poorly differentiated or undifferentiated

BIBLIOGRAPHY

Levine RL: Urethral cancer. Cancer 45:1965–1972, 1980
Matzkin H, Soloway MS, Hardeman S: Transitional cell carcinoma of the prostate. J Urol 146:1207–1212, 1991
Rogers RE, Burns B: Carcinoma of the female urethra. Obstet Gynecol 33:54–57, 1969
Vernon HK, Wilkins RD: Primary carcinoma of the male urethra. Br J Urol 21:232–235, 1950
Wishnow KI and Ro JY: Importance of early treatment of transitional cell carcinoma of the bladder. J Urol 140:289, 1988

Data Form for Cancer Staging

Patient identification
Name ______
Address ______
Hospital or clinic number ______
Age ____ Sex ____ Race ______

Institution identification
Hospital or clinic ______
Address ______

Oncology Record

Anatomic site of cancer ______
Histologic type ______
Grade (G) ______
Date of classification ______

DEFINITIONS

Primary Tumor (T) (male and female)

Clin	Path		
[ ]	[ ]	TX	Primary tumor cannot be assessed
[ ]	[ ]	T0	No evidence of primary tumor
[ ]	[ ]	Ta	Noninvasive papillary, polypoid, or verrucous carcinoma
[ ]	[ ]	Tis	Carcinoma *in situ*
[ ]	[ ]	T1	Tumor invades subepithelial connective tissue
[ ]	[ ]	T2	Tumor invades any of the following: corpus spongiosum, prostate, periurethral muscle
[ ]	[ ]	T3	Tumor invades any of the following: corpus cavernosum, beyond prostate capsule, anterior vagina, bladder neck
[ ]	[ ]	T4	Tumor invades other adjacent organs
		Transitional cell carcinoma of the prostate:	
[ ]	[ ]	Tis pu	Carcinoma *in situ*, involvement of the prostatic urethra
[ ]	[ ]	Tis pd	Carcinoma *in situ*, involvement of the prostatic ducts
[ ]	[ ]	T1	Tumor invades subepithelial connective tissue
[ ]	[ ]	T2	Tumor invades any of the following: prostatic stroma, corpus spongiosum, periurethral muscle
[ ]	[ ]	T3	Tumor invades any of the following: corpus cavernosum, beyond prostatic capsule, bladder neck (extraprostatic extension)
[ ]	[ ]	T4	Tumor invades other adjacent organs (invasion of the bladder)

Regional Lymph Nodes (N)

Clin	Path		
[ ]	[ ]	NX	Regional lymph nodes cannot be assessed
[ ]	[ ]	N0	No regional lymph node metastasis
[ ]	[ ]	N1	Metastasis in a single lymph node, 2 cm or less in greatest dimension
[ ]	[ ]	N2	Metastasis in a single lymph node, more than 2 cm in greatest dimension, or in multiple lymph nodes

Distant Metastasis (M)

Clin	Path		
[ ]	[ ]	MX	Distant metastasis cannot be assessed
[ ]	[ ]	M0	No distant metastasis
[ ]	[ ]	M1	Distant metastasis

Stage Grouping

Clin	Path	Stage	T	N	M
[ ]	[ ]	0a	Ta	N0	M0
[ ]	[ ]	0is	Tis	N0	M0
			Tis pu	N0	M0
			Tis pd	N0	M0
[ ]	[ ]	I	T1	N0	M0
[ ]	[ ]	II	T2	N0	M0
[ ]	[ ]	III	T1	N1	M0
			T2	N1	M0
			T3	N0	M0
			T3	N1	M0
[ ]	[ ]	IV	T4	N0	M0
			T4	N1	M0
			Any T	N2	M0
			Any T	Any N	M1

Staged by ______ M.D.
______ Registrar
Date ______

Histopathologic Type

The classification applies to transitional, squamous, and glandular carcinomas of the urethra, and transitional cell carcinomas of the prostate and prostatic urethra. There should be histologic or cytologic confirmation of the disease.

Histopathologic Grade (G)

[ ]	GX	Grade cannot be assessed
[ ]	G1	Well differentiated
[ ]	G2	Moderately differentiated
[ ]	G3-4	Poorly differentiated or undifferentiated

OPHTHALMIC SITES

The orbit and its contents—primarily the eye—contain many types of tissues. Consequently, a wide variety of malignant tumors occur in this anatomic area. Included in this section are recommendations for staging these cancers based on data available in the literature and knowledge of the experts serving on the Task Force for Staging of Cancer of the Eye of the American Joint Committee on Cancer.

The following sites are included:

Carcinoma of the Eyelid
Conjunctiva
Uvea
Retina
Orbit
Lacrimal gland

Staging of malignant melanoma of the eyelid is included under melanoma of the skin (see Chapter 24).

40

Carcinoma of the Eyelid

C44.1 Eyelid

ANATOMY

Primary Site. The eyelid is covered externally by epidermis and internally by conjunctiva, which becomes continuous with the conjunctiva that covers the eyeball. Basal cell carcinoma and squamous cell carcinoma arise from the epidermal surface. Sebaceous cell carcinoma arises from the meibomian glands in the tarsus, the glands of Zeis at the lid margin, and the sebaceous glands of the caruncle. Other adnexal carcinomas arise from the sweat glands of Moll and the hair follicles.

Regional Lymph Nodes. The eyelids are supplied with lymphatics that drain into the pre- and infra-auricular, facial, submandibular, and cervical lymph nodes. For pN, histologic examination of a regional lymphadenectomy specimen will ordinarily include 6 or more regional lymph nodes.

Metastatic Sites. Tumors of the eyelids not only metastasize to distant sites by way of the regional lymphatics and bloodstream but also spread directly into the orbit, including the lacrimal gland, and into the eyeball.

RULES FOR CLASSIFICATION

The classification applies only to carcinoma. There should be histologic verification of the cancer. This verification permits a division of cases by histologic type (i.e., basal cell, squamous cell, and sebaceous carcinoma). Any unconfirmed case must be reported separately.

Clinical Staging. The assessment of the cancer is based on inspection, slit-lamp examination, palpation of the regional lymph nodes, and, when indicated, radiologic (including computed tomography and magnetic resonance imaging) and ultrasonographic examination of the orbit, paranasal sinuses, brain, and chest.

Pathologic Staging. Complete resection of the primary site is indicated. Histologic study of the margins and the deep aspect of resected tissues is necessary. Resection or needle biopsy of enlarged regional lymph nodes or orbital masses is desirable. Extensive orbital involvement may require exenteration.

DEFINITION OF TNM

The following definitions apply to both clinical and pathologic staging.

Primary Tumor (T)

TX Primary tumor cannot be assessed
T0 No evidence of primary tumor
Tis Carcinoma *in situ*
T1 Tumor of any size, not invading the tarsal plate or, at the eyelid margin, 5 mm or less in greatest dimension
T2 Tumor invades tarsal plate or, at the eyelid margin, more than 5 mm but not more than 10 mm in greatest dimension
T3 Tumor involves full eyelid thickness or, at the eyelid margin, more than 10 mm in greatest dimension
T4 Tumor invades adjacent structures

Regional Lymph Nodes (N)

NX Regional lymph nodes cannot be assessed
N0 No regional lymph node metastasis
N1 Regional lymph node metastasis

Distant Metastasis (M)

MX Distant metastasis cannot be assessed
M0 No distant metastasis
M1 Distant metastasis

STAGE GROUPING

No stage grouping is presently recommended.

HISTOPATHOLOGIC TYPE

Basal cell carcinoma
Squamous cell carcinoma
Sebaceous cell carcinoma
Eccrine gland carcinoma

HISTOPATHOLOGIC GRADE (G)

GX Grade cannot be assessed
G1 Well differentiated
G2 Moderately differentiated
G3 Poorly differentiated
G4 Undifferentiated

BIBLIOGRAPHY

Doxanas MT, Green WR, Iliff CE: Factors in the successful surgical management of basal cell carcinoma of the eyelid. Am J Ophthalmol 91:726–736, 1981

Font RL: Eyelids and lacrimal drainage system tumors. In Spencer WH (Ed.), Ophthalmic pathology. An atlas and textbook, 4th ed, Volume 4. Philadelphia: WB Saunders; 2226–2333, 1996

Grizzard WS, Torcynski ET, Edwards WC: Adenocarcinoma of eccrine sweat glands. Arch Ophthalmol 94:2119–2123, 1976

Kwitko ML, Boniuk M, Zimmerman LE: Eyelid tumors with reference to lesions confused with squamous cell carcinoma. 1. Incidence and errors in diagnosis. Arch Ophthalmol 69:693–697, 1963

Ni C, Searl SS, Kuo P: Sebaceous gland carcinoma of the ocular adnexa. Int Ophthalmol Clin 22:23–61, 1982

Wolfe JTI, Campbell RJ, Yeatts RP, et al: Sebaceous carcinoma of the eyelid: errors in clinical and pathologic diagnosis. Am J Surg Pathol 8:597–606, 1984

CARCINOMA OF THE EYELID

Data Form for Cancer Staging

Patient identification
Name ______
Address ______
Hospital or clinic number ______
Age ____ Sex ____ Race ______

Institution identification
Hospital or clinic ______
Address ______

Oncology Record

Anatomic site of cancer ______
Histologic type ______
Grade (G) ______
Date of classification ______

Clin	Path	DEFINITIONS	
		Primary Tumor (T)	
[ ]	[ ]	TX	Primary tumor cannot be assessed
[ ]	[ ]	T0	No evidence of primary tumor
[ ]	[ ]	Tis	Carcinoma *in situ*
[ ]	[ ]	T1	Tumor of any size, not invading the tarsal plate or, at the eyelid margin, 5 mm or less in greatest dimension
[ ]	[ ]	T2	Tumor invades tarsal plate or, at the eyelid margin, more than 5 mm but not more than 10 mm in greatest dimension
[ ]	[ ]	T3	Tumor involves full eyelid thickness or, at the eyelid margin, more than 10 mm in greatest dimension
[ ]	[ ]	T4	Tumor invades adjacent structures
		Regional Lymph Nodes (N)	
[ ]	[ ]	NX	Regional lymph nodes cannot be assessed
[ ]	[ ]	N0	No regional lymph node metastasis
[ ]	[ ]	N1	Regional lymph node metastasis
		Distant Metastasis (M)	
[ ]	[ ]	MX	Distant metastasis cannot be assessed
[ ]	[ ]	M0	No distant metastasis
[ ]	[ ]	M1	Distant metastasis

Stage Grouping

No stage grouping is presently recommended.

Staged by ______ M.D.
______ Registrar
Date ______

Histopathologic Type

Basal cell carcinoma
Squamous cell carcinoma
Sebaceous carcinoma
Eccrine gland carcinoma

Histopathologic Grade (G)

[ ] GX Grade cannot be assessed
[ ] G1 Well differentiated
[ ] G2 Moderately differentiated
[ ] G3 Poorly differentiated
[ ] G4 Undifferentiated

Illustration

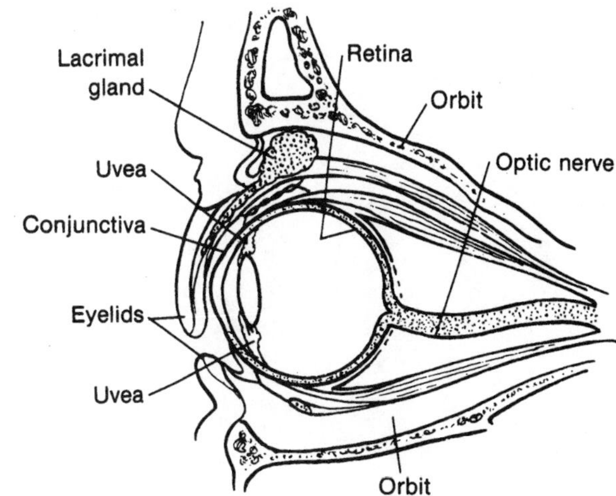

Indicate on diagram and describe exact location and characteristics of tumor.

41

Carcinoma of the Conjunctiva

C69.0 Conjunctiva

ANATOMY

Primary Site. The conjunctiva consists of stratified epithelium that contains mucus-secreting goblet cells; these cells are most numerous in the fornices. Palpebral conjunctiva lines the eyelid; bulbar conjunctiva covers the eyeball. Conjunctival epithelium merges with that of the cornea at the limbus. It is at this site, particularly at the temporal limbus, that carcinoma is most likely to arise. Conjunctival intraepithelial neoplasia (C.I.N.) embraces all forms of intraepithelial dysplasia, including *in situ* carcinoma. Mucinous adenocarcinoma is a rare form of adenocarcinoma of the conjunctival goblet cells.

Regional Lymph Nodes. The regional lymph nodes are:

Pre-auricular (parotid)
Submandibular
Cervical

For pN, histologic examination of a regional lymphadenectomy specimen will ordinarily include 6 or more regional lymph nodes.

Metastatic Sites. Tumors of the conjunctiva, in addition to spread by way of regional lymphatics, may also involve the eyelid proper, the orbit, lacrimal gland, and brain.

RULES FOR CLASSIFICATION

Clinical Staging. The assessment of the cancer is based on inspection, slit-lamp examination, palpation of the regional lymph nodes, and, when indicated, radiologic examination (including computed tomography and magnetic resonance imaging) and ultrasonographic examination of the orbit, paranasal sinuses, brain, and chest.

Pathologic Staging. Complete resection of the primary site is indicated. Cryotherapy and/or topical chemotherapy may be considered as adjunctive therapies. Extensive local involvement of orbital spread requires exenteration. Histologic study of the margins of the deep aspect of resected tissues is necessary.

DEFINITION OF TNM

These definitions apply to both clinical and pathologic staging.

Primary Tumor (T)

TX Primary tumor cannot be assessed
T0 No evidence of primary tumor
Tis Carcinoma *in situ*
T1 Tumor 5 mm or less in greatest dimension
T2 Tumor more than 5 mm in greatest dimension, without invasion of adjacent structures
T3 Tumor invades adjacent structures, excluding the orbit
T4 Tumor invades the orbit

Regional Lymph Nodes (N)

NX Regional lymph nodes cannot be assessed
N0 No regional lymph node metastasis
N1 Regional lymph node metastasis

Distant Metastasis (M)

MX Distant metastasis cannot be assessed
M0 No distant metastasis
M1 Distant metastasis

STAGE GROUPING

No stage grouping is presently recommended.

HISTOPATHOLOGIC TYPE

This classification applies only to carcinoma of the conjunctiva.

HISTOPATHOLOGIC GRADE (G)

GX Grade cannot be assessed
G1 Well differentiated
G2 Moderately differentiated
G3 Poorly differentiated
G4 Undifferentiated

BIBLIOGRAPHY

Buuns DR, Folberg R: Microscopically controlled excision of conjunctival squamous cell carcinoma. Am J Ophthalmol 117:97–109, 1994

Campbell RJ: Tumors of eyelid, conjunctiva and cornea. In Klintworth (Ed.). Pathobiology of ocular disease garner, 2nd ed. New York: Marcel Dekker; 1367–1403, 1994

Cohen BH, Green W, Iliff NT, et al: Spindle cell carcinoma of the conjunctiva. Arch J Ophthalmol 98:1809–1813, 1980

Husain SE, Patrinely JR, Zimmerman LE, et al: Primary basal cell carcinoma of the limbal conjunctiva. Ophthalmology 100:1720–1722, 1993

Jakobiec FA, Folberg R, Iwamoto T: Clinicopathologic characteristics of premalignant and malignant lesions of the conjunctiva. Ophthalmology 96:147–166, 1989

Data Form for Cancer Staging

Patient identification
Name ______________________
Address ______________________
Hospital or clinic number ______________________
Age ____ Sex ____ Race ______________________

Institution identification
Hospital or clinic ______________________
Address ______________________

Oncology Record

Anatomic site of cancer ______________________
Histologic type ______________________
Grade (G) ______________________
Date of classification ______________________

Clin	Path	DEFINITIONS	
		Primary Tumor (T)	
[ ]	[ ]	TX	Primary tumor cannot be assessed
[ ]	[ ]	T0	No evidence of primary tumor
[ ]	[ ]	Tis	Carcinoma *in situ*
[ ]	[ ]	T1	Tumor 5 mm or less in greatest dimension
[ ]	[ ]	T2	Tumor more than 5 mm in greatest dimension, without invasion of adjacent structures
[ ]	[ ]	T3	Tumor invades adjacent structures, excluding the orbit
[ ]	[ ]	T4	Tumor invades the orbit
		Regional Lymph Nodes (N)	
[ ]	[ ]	NX	Regional lymph nodes cannot be assessed
[ ]	[ ]	N0	No regional lymph node metastasis
[ ]	[ ]	N1	Regional lymph node metastasis
		Distant Metastasis (M)	
[ ]	[ ]	MX	Distant metastasis cannot be assessed
[ ]	[ ]	M0	No distant metastasis
[ ]	[ ]	M1	Distant metastasis

Stage Grouping

No stage grouping is presently recommended.

Staged by ______________________ M.D.
______________________ Registrar
Date ______________________

Histopathologic Type

This classification applies only to carcinoma of the conjunctiva.

Histopathologic Grade (G)

[ ] GX Grade cannot be assessed
[ ] G1 Well differentiated
[ ] G2 Moderately differentiated
[ ] G3 Poorly differentiated
[ ] G4 Undifferentiated

Illustration

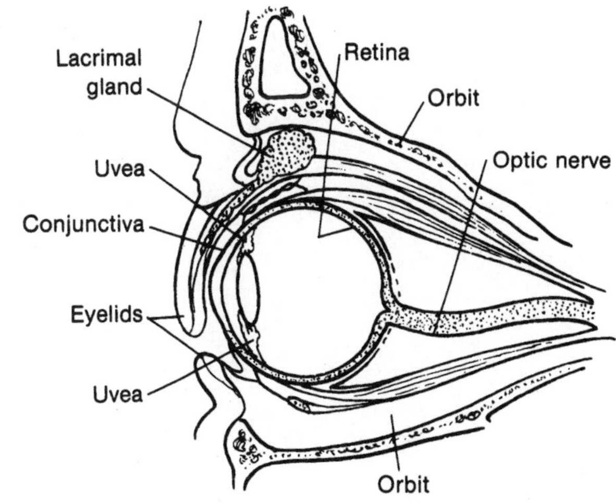

Indicate on diagram and describe exact location and characteristics of tumor.

42

Malignant Melanoma of the Conjunctiva

C69.0 Conjunctiva

ANATOMY

Primary Site. In addition to mucus-secreting goblet cells within the stratified epithelium, melanocytic cells exist in the basal layer. These are of neuroectodermal origin, and melanocytic tumors may arise from these cells. Melanomas may arise from junctional and compound nevi, from primary acquired melanosis, or *de novo*. Tumors must be distinguished from nontumorous pigmentation.

Regional Lymph Nodes. The regional lymph nodes are:

Parotid
Pre-auricular
Submandibular
Cervical

For pN, histologic examination of a regional lymphadenectomy specimen will ordinarily include 6 or more regional lymph nodes.

Metastatic Sites. In addition to spread by lymphatics and the bloodstream, direct extension to the eyeball and orbit occur.

RULES FOR CLASSIFICATION

The classification applies only to melanoma. There should be histologic verification of the melanocytic lesion.

Clinical Staging. The assessment of the cancer is based on inspection, slit-lamp examination, palpation of the regional lymph nodes, and, when indicated, radiologic (including computed tomography) and ultrasonographic examination of the orbit, paranasal sinuses, and chest.

Pathologic Staging. Complete resection of the primary site is indicated. Histologic study of the margins and the deep aspect of resected tissues is necessary. Resection or needle biopsy of enlarged regional lymph nodes or orbital masses is desirable.

DEFINITION OF TNM

Clinical Classification (cTNM)

Primary Tumor (T)

TX Primary tumor cannot be assessed
T0 No evidence of primary tumor
T1 Tumor(s) of bulbar conjunctiva occupying one quadrant or less
T2 Tumor(s) of bulbar conjunctiva occupying more than one quadrant
T3 Tumor(s) of conjunctival fornix and/or palpebral conjunctiva and/or caruncle
T4 Tumor invades eyelid, cornea, and/or orbit

Regional Lymph Nodes (N)

NX Regional lymph nodes cannot be assessed
N0 No regional lymph node metastasis
N1 Regional lymph node metastasis

Distant Metastasis (M)

MX Distant metastasis cannot be assessed
M0 No distant metastasis
M1 Distant metastasis

Pathologic Classification (pTNM)

Primary Tumor (pT)

pTX Primary tumor cannot be assessed
pT0 No evidence of primary tumor
pT1 Tumor(s) of bulbar conjunctiva occupying one quadrant or less and 2 mm or less in thickness
pT2 Tumor(s) of bulbar conjunctiva occupying more than one quadrant and 2 mm or less in thickness
pT3 Tumor(s) of the conjunctival fornix and/or palpebral conjunctiva and/or caruncle or tumor(s) of the bulbar conjunctiva, more than 2 mm in thickness
pT4 Tumor invades eyelid, cornea, and/or orbit

Regional Lymph Nodes (pN)

pNX Regional lymph nodes cannot be assessed
pN0 No regional lymph node metastasis
pN1 Regional lymph node metastasis

Distant Metastasis (pM)

pMX Distant metastasis cannot be assessed
pM0 No distant metastasis
pM1 Distant metastasis

STAGE GROUPING

No stage grouping is presently recommended.

HISTOPATHOLOGIC TYPE

This categorization applies only to melanoma of the conjunctiva.

HISTOPATHOLOGIC GRADE (G)

Histopathologic grade represents the origin of the primary tumor.

GX Origin cannot be assessed
G0 Primary acquired melanosis
G1 Malignant melanoma arises from a nevus
G2 Malignant melanoma arises from primary acquired melanosis
G3 Malignant melanoma arises *de novo*

BIBLIOGRAPHY

DePotter P, Shields CL, Shields JA, et al: Clinical predictive factors for development of recurrence and metastasis in conjunctival melanoma: a review of 68 cases. Br J Ophthalmol 77:624–630, 1993

Folberg R, McLean IW: Primary acquired melanosis and melanoma of the conjunctiva: terminlogy, classification, and biologic behaviour. Hum Path 17:652–655, 1986

Paridaens ADA, McCartney ACE, Hungerford H: Multifocal amelanotic conjunctival melanosis sine pigmento. Br J Ophthalmol 76:163–165, 1992

Silvers D, Jakobiec FA, Freeman T, et al: Melanoma of the conjunctiva: a clinicopathologic study. In Jakobiec FA (Ed.), Ocular and adnexal tumors. Birmingham: Aesculapius; 583–599, 1978

Data Form for Cancer Staging

Patient identification
Name ____________________
Address ____________________
Hospital or clinic number ____________________
Age ______ Sex ______ Race ____________________

Institution identification
Hospital or clinic ____________________
Address ____________________

Oncology Record

Anatomic site of cancer ____________________
Histologic type ____________________
Grade (G) ____________________
Date of classification ____________________

DEFINITIONS

Clinical Classification (cTNM)

Primary Tumor (T)

Clin	Path		
[ ]	[ ]	TX	Primary tumor cannot be assessed
[ ]	[ ]	T0	No evidence of primary tumor
[ ]	[ ]	T1	Tumor(s) of bulbar conjunctiva occupying one quadrant or less
[ ]	[ ]	T2	Tumor(s) of bulbar conjunctiva occupying more than one quadrant
[ ]	[ ]	T3	Tumor(s) of conjunctival fornix and/or palpebral conjunctiva and/or caruncle
[ ]	[ ]	T4	Tumor invades eyelid, cornea, and/or orbit

Regional Lymph Nodes (N)

Clin	Path		
[ ]	[ ]	NX	Regional lymph nodes cannot be assessed
[ ]	[ ]	N0	No regional lymph node metastasis
[ ]	[ ]	N1	Regional lymph node metastasis

Distant Metastasis (M)

Clin	Path		
[ ]	[ ]	MX	Distant metastasis cannot be assessed
[ ]	[ ]	M0	No distant metastasis
[ ]	[ ]	M1	Distant metastasis

Pathologic Classification (pTNM)

Primary Tumor (pT)

Clin	Path		
[ ]	[ ]	pTX	Primary tumor cannot be assessed
[ ]	[ ]	pT0	No evidence of primary tumor
[ ]	[ ]	pT1	Tumor(s) of bulbar conjunctiva occupying one quadrant or less and 2 mm or less in thickness
[ ]	[ ]	pT2	Tumor(s) of bulbar conjunctiva occupying more than one quadrant and 2 mm or less in thickness
[ ]	[ ]	pT3	Tumor(s) of conjunctival fornix and/or palpebral conjunctiva and/or caruncle and/or tumor(s) of the bulbar conjunctiva, more than 2 mm in thickness
[ ]	[ ]	pT4	Tumor invades eyelid, cornea, and/or orbit

Regional Lymph Nodes (N)

Clin	Path		
[ ]	[ ]	pNX	Regional lymph nodes cannot be assessed
[ ]	[ ]	pNO	No regional lymph node metastasis
[ ]	[ ]	pN1	Regional lymph node metastasis

Distant Metastasis (pM)

Clin	Path		
[ ]	[ ]	pMX	Distant metastasis cannot be assessed
[ ]	[ ]	pM0	No distant metastasis
[ ]	[ ]	pM1	Distant metastasis

Stage Grouping

No stage grouping is presently recommended.

Staged by ____________________ M.D.
____________________ Registrar

Date ____________________

(continued on next page)

Histopathologic Type

This categorization applies only to melanoma of the conjunctiva.

Histopathologic Grade (G)

Histopathologic grade represents the origin of the primary tumor.

[ ] GX Origin cannot be assessed
[ ] G0 Primary acquired melanosis
[ ] G1 Malignant melanoma arising from a nevus
[ ] G2 Malignant melanoma arising from primary acquired melanosis
[ ] G3 Malignant melanoma arising *de novo*

Illustration

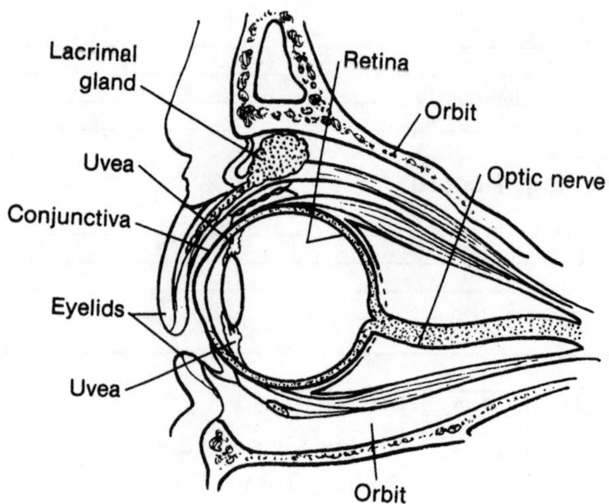

Indicate on diagram and describe exact location and characteristics of tumor.

43

Malignant Melanoma of the Uvea

C69.3 Choroid
C69.4 Ciliary body and iris

The classification applies only to melanoma.

ANATOMY

Primary Site. The uvea (uveal tract) is the middle layer of the eyeball, situated between the cornea and sclera externally and the retina and its analogues internally. The uveal tract is divided into three regions: iris, ciliary body, and choroid. It is a highly vascular structure, with the choroid in particular being composed of large blood vessels with little intervening connective tissue. There are no lymphatic channels in the uvea. Systemic metastasis from uveal melanomas occurs by hematogenous routes. Uveal melanomas are believed to arise from uveal melanocytes and are, therefore, of neural crest origin. Melanomas may spread by local extension through Bruch's membrane to involve the retina and vitreous, or by extension through the sclera or optic nerve into the orbit.

Most uveal melanomas occur in the choroid. The ciliary body is less commonly the site of origin, and the iris is least commonly involved. Iris melanomas are relatively benign and slow growing, and they rarely metastasize. Melanomas of the ciliary body and choroid are cytologically more malignant and metastasize more frequently, most commonly to the liver.

It may be clinically impossible to distinguish a large nevus from a small melanoma.

Regional Lymph Nodes. Since there are no intra-ocular lymphatics, this category applies only to extrascleral extension anteriorly. The regional lymph nodes are:

Parotid
Pre-auricular
Submandibular
Cervical

Involvement implies subconjunctival extension of the primary tumor. For pN, histologic examination of a regional lymphadenectomy specimen will ordinarily include 6 or more regional lymph nodes.

Metastatic Sites. Uveal melanomas can metastasize through hematogenous routes to various organs. The liver is most commonly involved and is usually the first site of clinically detectable metastasis. Less commonly, the lung, pleura, subcutaneous tissues, bone, and other sites may be involved.

RULES FOR CLASSIFICATION

There should be histologic verification of the disease. Any unconfirmed case must be reported separately.

Clinical Staging. The assessment of the tumor is based on clinical examination including slit-lamp examination and direct and indirect ophthalmoscopy. Additional methods such as ultrasonography, computerized stereometry, fluorescein angiography, and isotope examination may enhance the accuracy of appraisal.

Pathologic Staging. Complete resection of the primary site is indicated, either by eye wall reflection or enucleation. Histologic study of the margins and the deep aspect of resected tissues is necessary. Resection or needle biopsy of enlarged regional lymph nodes or orbital masses is desirable.

DEFINITION OF TNM

These definitions apply to both clinical and pathologic staging.

ANATOMIC SITES

Iris
Ciliary body
Choroid

Iris

Primary Tumor (T)

TX Primary tumor cannot be assessed
T0 No evidence of primary tumor
T1 Tumor limited to the iris
T2 Tumor involves one quadrant or less, with invasion into the anterior chamber angle
T3 Tumor involves more than one quadrant, with invasion into the anterior chamber angle, ciliary body, and/or choroid
T4 Tumor with extraocular extension

Regional Lymph Nodes (N)

NX Regional lymph nodes cannot be assessed
N0 No regional lymph node metastasis
N1 Regional lymph node metastasis

Distant Metastasis (M)

MX Distant metastasis cannot be assessed
M0 No distant metastasis
M1 Distant metastasis

Ciliary Body

Primary Tumor (T)

TX Primary tumor cannot be assessed
T0 No evidence of primary tumor
T1 Tumor limited to the ciliary body
T2 Tumor invades into anterior chamber and/or iris
T3 Tumor invades choroid
T4 Tumor with extraocular extension

Regional Lymph Nodes (N)

NX Regional lymph nodes cannot be assessed
N0 No regional lymph node metastasis
N1 Regional lymph node metastasis

Distant Metastasis (M)

MX Distant metastasis cannot be assessed
M0 No distant metastasis
M1 Distant metastasis

Choroid

Primary Tumor (T)

TX Primary tumor cannot be assessed
T0 No evidence of primary tumor
T1* Tumor 10 mm or less in greatest dimension with an elevation 3 mm or less
T1a Tumor 7 mm or less in greatest dimension with an elevation 2 mm or less
T1b Tumor more than 7 mm but not more than 10 mm in greatest dimension with an elevation more than 2 mm but not more than 3 mm
T2* Tumor more than 10 mm but not more than 15 mm in greatest dimension with an elevation of more than 3 mm but not more than 5 mm
T3* Tumor more than 15 mm in greatest dimension or with an elevation more than 5 mm
T4 Tumor with extraocular extension

Note: When dimension and elevation show a difference in classification, the highest category should be used for classification.

**Note:* In clinical practice the tumor base may be estimated in optic disc diameters (dd) (average: 1 dd = 1.5 mm). The elevation may be estimated in diopters (average: 3 diopters = 1 mm). Other techniques used, such as ultrasonography and computerized stereometry, may provide a more accurate measurement.

Regional Lymph Nodes (N)

NX Regional lymph nodes cannot be assessed
N0 No regional lymph node metastasis
N1 Regional lymph node metastasis

Distant Metastasis (M)

MX Distant metastasis cannot be assessed
M0 No distant metastasis
M1 Distant metastasis

STAGE GROUPING

The classification of the structure most affected is used when more than one of the uveal structures is involved by tumor.

Iris and Ciliary Body

Stage I	T1	N0	M0
Stage II	T2	N0	M0
Stage III	T3	N0	M0
Stage IVA	T4	N0	M0
Stage IVB	Any T	N1	M0
	Any T	Any N	M1

STAGE GROUPING

Choroid

Stage IA	T1a	N0	M0
Stage IB	T1b	N0	M0
Stage II	T2	N0	M0
Stage III	T3	N0	M0
Stage IVA	T4	N0	M0
Stage IVB	Any T	N1	M0
	Any T	Any N	M1

HISTOPATHOLOGIC TYPE

The histopathologic types are:

Spindle cell melanoma
Mixed cell melanoma
Epithelioid cell melanoma

HISTOPATHOLOGIC GRADE (G)

GX Grade cannot be assessed
G1 Spindle cell melanoma
G2 Mixed cell melanoma
G3 Epithelioid cell melanoma

Venous Invasion (V)

VX Venous invasion cannot be assessed
V0 Veins do not contain tumor
V1 Veins in melanoma contain tumor
V2 Vortex veins contain tumor

Scleral Invasion (S)

SX Scleral invasion cannot be assessed
S0 Sclera does not contain tumor
S1 Intrascleral invasion of tumor*
S2 Extrascleral extension of tumor

**Note:* Includes perineural and perivascular tumor invasion of scleral canals.

BIBLIOGRAPHY

Coleman DJ, Rondeau MJ, Silverman RH, et al: Correlation of microcirculation architecture with ultrasound backscatter parameters of uveal melanoma. Eur J Ophthalmol 5(2):96–106, 1995

Folberg R: Tumor progression in ocular melanomas. J Invest Dermatol 100 (3):326S–331S, 1993

Pe'er J, Rummelt V, Mawn L, et al: Mean of the ten largest nucleoli, microcirculation architecture, and prognosis of ciliochoroidal melanomas. Ophthalmology 101(7):1227–1235, 1994

Rummelt V, Folberg R, Woolson RF, et al: Relation between the microcirculation architecture and the aggressive behavior of ciliary body melanomas. Ophthalmology 102:(5):844–851, 1995

Rummelt V, Gardner LM, Folberg R, et al: Three-dimensional relationships between tumor cells and microcirculation with double cyanine immunolabeling, laser scanning confocal microscopy, and computer-assisted reconstruction: an alternative to cast corrosion preparations. J Histochem Cytochem 42(5):681–686, 1994

Shield JA, Shields CL: Intra-ocular tumors. A text and atlas. Philadelphia: Saunders, 1992

Data Form for Cancer Staging

Patient identification
Name ______
Address ______
Hospital or clinic number ______
Age ____ Sex ____ Race ______

Institution identification
Hospital or clinic ______
Address ______

Oncology Record

Anatomic site of cancer ______
Histologic type ______
Grade (G) ______
Date of classification ______

Clin	Path	DEFINITIONS	
		Primary Tumor (T)	
[ ]	[ ]	TX	Primary tumor cannot be assessed
[ ]	[ ]	T0	No evidence of primary tumor
		Iris	
[ ]	[ ]	T1	Tumor limited to the iris
[ ]	[ ]	T2	Tumor involves one quadrant or less, with invasion into the anterior chamber angle
[ ]	[ ]	T3	Tumor involves more than one quadrant, with invasion into the anterior chamber angle, ciliary body, and/or choroid
[ ]	[ ]	T4	Tumor with extraocular extension
		Ciliary Body	
[ ]	[ ]	T1	Tumor limited to ciliary body
[ ]	[ ]	T2	Tumor invades into anterior chamber and/or iris
[ ]	[ ]	T3	Tumor invades choroid
[ ]	[ ]	T4	Tumor with extraocular extension
		Choroid	
[ ]	[ ]	T1*	Tumor 10 mm or less in greatest dimension with an elevation 3 mm or less
[ ]	[ ]	T1a	Tumor 7 mm or less in greatest dimension with an elevation 2 mm or less
[ ]	[ ]	T1b	Tumor more than 7 mm but not more than 10 mm in greatest dimension with an elevation more than 2 mm but not more than 3 mm
[ ]	[ ]	T2*	Tumor more than 10 mm but not more than 15 mm in greatest dimension with an elevation of more than 3 mm but not more than 5 mm
[ ]	[ ]	T3*	Tumor more than 15 mm in greatest dimension or with an elevation more than 5 mm
[ ]	[ ]	T4	Tumor with extraocular extension

When dimension and elevation show a difference in classification, the highest category should be used for classification.

**In clinical practice the tumor base may be estimated in optic disc diameters (dd) (average: 1 dd = 1.5 mm). The elevation may be estimated in diopters (average: 3 diopters = 1 mm). Other techniques used, such as ultrasonography and computerized stereometry, may provide a more accurate measurement.*

Clin	Path		
		Regional Lymph Nodes (N)	
[ ]	[ ]	NX	Regional lymph nodes cannot be assessed
[ ]	[ ]	N0	No regional lymph node metastasis
[ ]	[ ]	N1	Regional lymph node metastasis
		Distant Metastasis (M)	
[ ]	[ ]	MX	Distant metastasis cannot be assessed
[ ]	[ ]	M0	No distant metastasis
[ ]	[ ]	M1	Distant metastasis

(continued on next page)

Stage Grouping

The classification of the structure most affected is used when more than one of the uveal structures is involved by tumor.

Iris and Ciliary Body

Clin	Path	Stage	T	N	M
[ ]	[ ]	I	T1	N0	M0
[ ]	[ ]	II	T2	N0	M0
[ ]	[ ]	III	T3	N0	M0
[ ]	[ ]	IVA	T4	N0	M0
[ ]	[ ]	IVB	Any T	N1	M0
			Any T	Any N	M1

Choroid

Clin	Path	Stage	T	N	M
[ ]	[ ]	IA	T1a	N0	M0
[ ]	[ ]	IB	T1b	N0	M0
[ ]	[ ]	II	T2	N0	M0
[ ]	[ ]	III	T3	N0	M0
[ ]	[ ]	IVA	T4	N0	M0
[ ]	[ ]	IVB	Any T	N1	M0
			Any T	Any N	M1

Staged by ______________________________ M.D.

______________________________ Registrar

Date ______________________________

Histopathologic Type

Spindle cell melanoma
Mixed cell melanoma
Epithelioid cell melanoma

Histopathologic Grade (G)

[ ] GX Grade cannot be assessed
[ ] G1 Spindle cell melanoma
[ ] G2 Mixed cell melanoma
[ ] G3 Epithelioid cell melanoma

Venous Invasion (V)

[ ] VX Venous invasion cannot be assessed
[ ] V0 Veins do not contain tumor
[ ] V1 Veins in melanoma contain tumor
[ ] V2 Vortex veins contain tumor

Scleral Invasion (S)

[ ] SX Scleral invasion cannot be assessed
[ ] S0 Sclera does not contain tumor
[ ] S1 Intrascleral invasion of tumor*
[ ] S2 Extrascleral invasion of tumor

* Includes perineural and perivascular invasion of scleral canals.

Illustrations

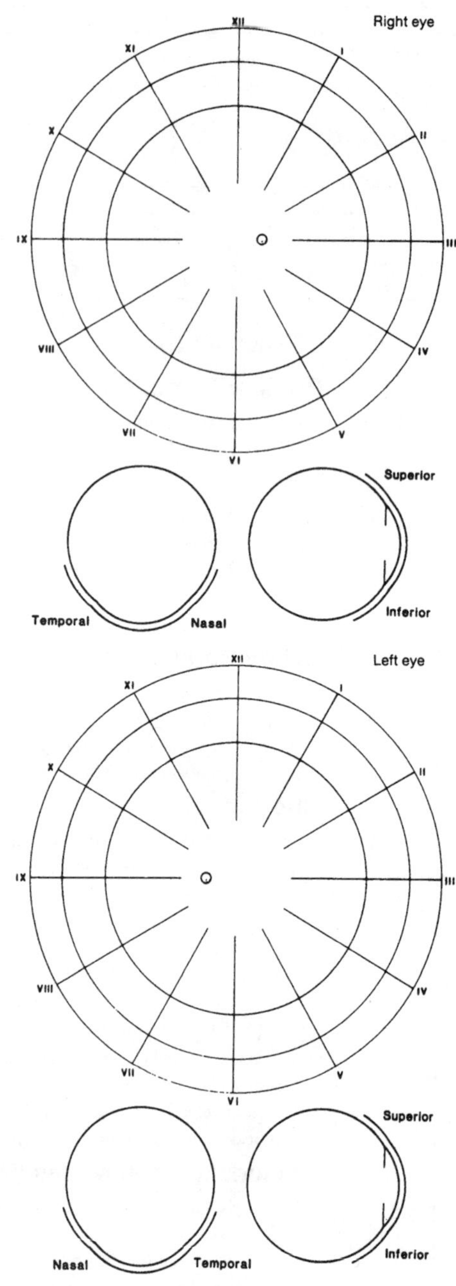

Indicate on diagrams and describe exact location and characteristics of tumor.

44

Retinoblastoma

C69.2 Retina

ANATOMY

Primary Site. The retina is composed of neurons and glial cells. The neurons give rise to retinoblastoma, whereas the glial cells give rise to astrocytomas, which in the retina are benign and extremely rare. The retina is limited internally by a membrane that separates it from the vitreous cavity. Externally, it is limited by the retinal pigment epithelium and Bruch's membrane, which separate it from the choroid and act as natural barriers to extension of retinal tumors into the choroid. The continuation of the retina with the optic nerve allows direct extension of retinoblastomas into the optic nerve and then to the subarachnoid space. Since the retina has no lymphatics, spread of retinal tumors is either by direct extension into adjacent structures or by distant metastasis through hematogenous routes.

Regional Lymph Nodes. Since there are no intra-ocular lymphatics, the category applies only to anterior extrascleral extension. The regional lymph nodes are:

Parotid
Pre-auricular
Submandibular
Cervical

Involvement implies subconjunctival extension of the tumor. For pN, histologic examination of a regional lymphadenectomy specimen will ordinarily include 6 or more regional lymph nodes.

Metastatic Sites. Retinoblastoma can metastasize through hematogenous routes to various sites, most notably the skull, long bones, brain, lymph nodes, and viscera.

RULES FOR CLASSIFICATION

Clinical Staging. In bilateral cases, each eye must be classified separately. The classification does not apply to complete spontaneous regression of the tumor. There should be histologic verification of the disease in an enucleated eye. Any unconfirmed case must be reported separately. The extent of retinal involvement is indicated as a percentage.

Pathologic Staging. All clinical and pathologic data from the resected specimen are to be used.

DEFINITION OF TNM

Clinical Classification (cTNM)

Primary Tumor (T)

TX Primary tumor cannot be assessed
T0 No evidence of primary tumor
T1 Tumor(s) limited to 25% or less of the retina
T2 Tumor(s) involve(s) more than 25% but not more than 50% of the retina
T3 Tumor(s) involve(s) more than 50% of the retina and/or invade(s) beyond the retina but remain(s) intra-ocular
  T3a Tumor(s) involve(s) more than 50% of the retina and/or tumor cells in the vitreous
  T3b Tumor(s) involve(s) optic disc
  T3c Tumor(s) involve(s) anterior chamber and/or uvea
T4 Tumor with extra-ocular invasion
  T4a Tumor invades retrobulbar optic nerve

T4b Extra-ocular extension other than invasion of optic nerve

Note: The following suffixes may be added to the appropriate T categories: "m" indicates multiple tumors (e.g., T2 [m2]); "f" indicates cases with a known family history; and "d" indicates diffuse retinal involvement without the formation of discrete masses.

Regional Lymph Nodes (N)

NX Regional lymph nodes cannot be assessed
N0 No regional lymph node metastasis
N1 Regional lymph node metastasis

Distant Metastasis (M)

MX Distant metastasis cannot be assessed
M0 No distant metastasis
M1 Distant metastasis

Pathologic Classification (pTNM)

Primary Tumor (pT)

pTX Primary tumor cannot be assessed
pT0 No evidence of primary tumor
pT1 Tumor(s) limited to 25% or less of the retina
pT2 Tumor(s) involve(s) more than 25% but not more than 50% of the retina
pT3 Tumor(s) involve(s) more than 50% of the retina and/or invade(s) beyond the retina but remain(s) intra-ocular
pT3a Tumor(s) involve(s) more than 50% of the retina and/or tumor cells in the vitreous
pT3b Tumor invades optic nerve as far as the lamina cribrosa
pT3c Tumor in anterior chamber and/or invasion with thickening of the uvea and/or intrascleral invasion
pT4 Tumor with extra-ocular invasion
pT4a Intraneural tumor beyond the lamina cribrosa but not at the line of resection
pT4b Tumor at the line of resection or other extra-ocular extension

Regional Lymph Nodes (pN)

pNX Regional lymph nodes cannot be assessed
pN0 No regional lymph node metastasis
pN1 Regional lymph node metastasis

Distant Metastasis (pM)

pMX Distant metastasis cannot be assessed
pM0 No distant metastasis
pM1 Distant metastasis

STAGE GROUPING

In cases of bilateral disease the more affected eye is used for the stage grouping.

Stage IA	T1	N0	M0
Stage IB	T2	N0	M0
Stage IIA	T3a	N0	M0
Stage IIB	T3b	N0	M0
Stage IIC	T3c	N0	M0
Stage IIIA	T4a	N0	M0
Stage IIIB	T4b	N0	M0
Stage IV	Any T	N1	M0
	Any T	Any N	M1

Note: Pathologic stage grouping corresponds to the clinical stage grouping.

HISTOPATHOLOGIC TYPE

This classification applies only to retinoblastoma.

BIBLIOGRAPHY

McLean IW: Retinoblastomas, retinocytomas and pseudoretinoblastomas. In Spencer WH (Ed.), Ophthalmic pathology. An atlas and textbook, 4th ed. Volume 2. Philadelphia: WB Saunders; 1332–1380, 1996

McLean IW, Burnier MN, Zimmerman LE, et al: Tumors of the eye and ocular adnexa. Atlas of tumor pathology, 3rd Series, Fascicle 12. Washington, D.C.: Armed Forces Institute of Pathology, 1994

RETINOBLASTOMA

Data Form for Cancer Staging

Patient identification
Name ______
Address ______
Hospital or clinic number ______
Age ____ Sex ____ Race ______

Institution identification
Hospital or clinic ______
Address ______

Oncology Record

Anatomic site of cancer ______
Histologic type ______
Grade (G) ______
Date of classification ______

Clin	Path	DEFINITIONS	
		Clinical Classification (cTNM)	
		Primary Tumor (T)	
[ ]	[ ]	TX	Primary tumor cannot be assessed
[ ]	[ ]	T0	No evidence of primary tumor
[ ]	[ ]	T1	Tumor(s) limited to 25% or less of the retina
[ ]	[ ]	T2	Tumor(s) involve(s) more than 25% but not more than 50% of the retina
[ ]	[ ]	T3	Tumor(s) involve(s) more than 50% of the retina and/or invade(s) beyond the retina but remain(s) intra-ocular
[ ]	[ ]	T3a	Tumor(s) involve(s) more than 50% of the retina and/or tumor cells in the vitreous
[ ]	[ ]	T3b	Tumor(s) involve(s) optic disc
[ ]	[ ]	T3c	Tumor(s) involve(s) anterior chamber and/or uvea
[ ]	[ ]	T4	Tumor with extra-ocular invasion
[ ]	[ ]	T4a	Tumor invades retrobulbar optic nerve
[ ]	[ ]	T4b	Extra-ocular extension other than invasion of optic nerve
		The following suffixes may be added to the appropriate T categories: "m" indicates multiple tumors (e.g., m T2 [m2]); "f" indicates cases with a known family history; and "d" indicates diffuse retinal involvement without the formation of discrete masses.	
		Regional Lymph Nodes (N)	
[ ]	[ ]	NX	Regional lymph nodes cannot be assessed
[ ]	[ ]	N0	No regional lymph node metastasis
[ ]	[ ]	N1	Regional lymph node metastasis
		Distant Metastasis (M)	
[ ]	[ ]	MX	Distant metastasis cannot be assessed
[ ]	[ ]	M0	No distant metastasis
[ ]	[ ]	M1	Distant metastasis
		Pathologic Classification (pTNM)	
		Primary Tumor (pT)	
[ ]	[ ]	pTX	Primary tumor cannot be assessed
[ ]	[ ]	pT0	No evidence of primary tumor
[ ]	[ ]	pT1	Tumor(s) limited to 25% or less of the retina
[ ]	[ ]	pT2	Tumor(s) involve(s) more than 25% but not more than 50% of the retina
[ ]	[ ]	pT3	Tumor(s) involve(s) more than 50% of the retina and/or invade(s) beyond the retina but remain(s) intra-ocular
[ ]	[ ]	pT3a	Tumor(s) involve(s) more than 50% of the retina and/or tumor cells in the vitreous
[ ]	[ ]	pT3b	Tumor invades optic nerve as far as the lamina cribrosa
[ ]	[ ]	pT3c	Tumor in anterior chamber and/or invasion with thickening of the uvea and/or intrascleral invasion
[ ]	[ ]	pT4	Tumor with extra-ocular invasion
[ ]	[ ]	pT4a	Intraneural tumor beyond the lamina cribrosa but not at the line of resection
[ ]	[ ]	pT4b	Tumor at the line of resection or other extra-ocular extension
		Regional Lymph Nodes (pN)	
[ ]	[ ]	pNX	Regional lymph nodes cannot be assessed
[ ]	[ ]	pN0	No regional lymph node metastasis
[ ]	[ ]	pN1	Regional lymph node metastasis

(continued on next page)

DEFINITIONS

Distant Metastasis (pM)

pMX Distant metastasis cannot be assessed
pM0 No distant metastasis
pM1 Distant metastasis

Stage Grouping

In cases of bilateral disease the more affected eye is used for the stage grouping.

Clin	Path	Stage	T	N	M
[ ]	[ ]	IA	T1	N0	M0
[ ]	[ ]	IB	T2	N0	M0
[ ]	[ ]	IIA	T3a	N0	M0
[ ]	[ ]	IIB	T3b	N0	M0
[ ]	[ ]	IIC	T3c	N0	M0
[ ]	[ ]	IIIA	T4a	N0	M0
[ ]	[ ]	IIIB	T4b	N0	M0
[ ]	[ ]	IV	Any T	N1	M0
			Any T	Any N	M1

Pathologic stage grouping corresponds to the clinical stage grouping.

Staged by ______________________ M.D.

______________________ Registrar

Date ______________________

Histopathologic Type

This classification applies only to retinoblastoma.

Illustrations

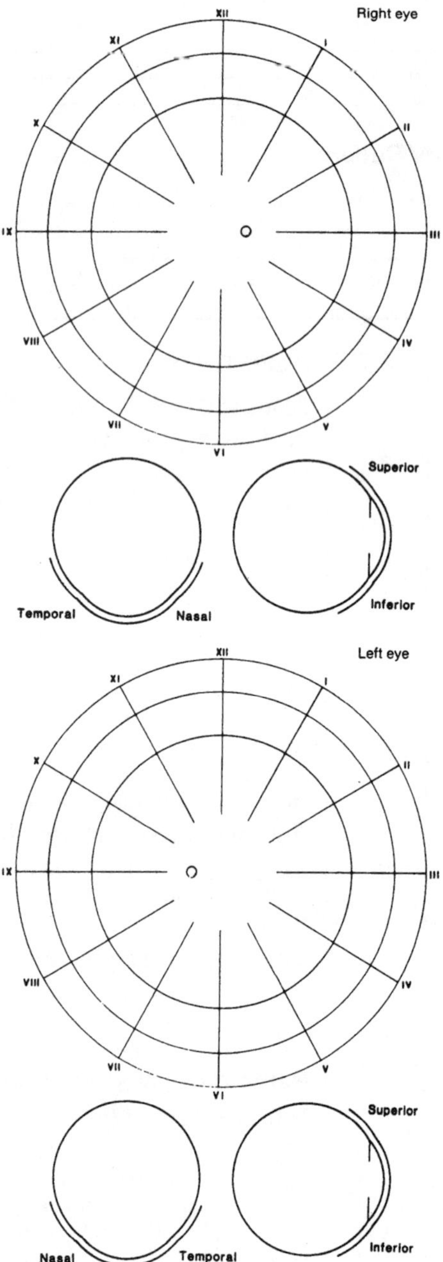

Indicate on diagrams and describe exact location and characteristics of tumor.

____

____

____

____

45

Carcinoma of the Lacrimal Gland

C69.5 Lacrimal gland

A retrospective study of 265 epithelial tumors of the lacrimal gland has been completed from material on file in the Registry of Ophthalmic Pathology at the Armed Forces Institute of Pathology. The histologic classification used is a modification of the World Health Organization (WHO) classification of salivary gland tumors. The lacrimal gland includes both lobules: the superficial (palpebral lobe) portion and the deep intra-orbital portion.

ANATOMY

Primary Site. The lacrimal gland lies in a bony excavation that is covered by periosteum. It is located in the lateral orbital wall (the fossa of the lacrimal gland). The smaller palpebral portion projects into the lateral portion of the upper lid between the palpebral fascia and the conjunctiva.

Regional Lymph Nodes. The regional lymph nodes include:

Pre-auricular
Submandibular
Cervical

For pN, histologic examination of a regional lymphadenectomy specimen will ordinarily include 6 or more regional lymph nodes.

Metastatic Sites. The lung is the most common metastatic site, followed by bone and remote viscera.

RULES FOR CLASSIFICATION

Clinical Staging. A complete physical examination, imaging of the orbit (including computed tomography [CT], magnetic resonance imaging, ultrasonography, and plane films), and CT of the adjacent paranasal sinuses should be done. Chest x-ray films, radionuclide bone scans, and blood chemistries should also be available.

Pathologic Staging. After complete resection of the mass, the entire specimen should be evaluated to determine the type of tumor and the grade of malignancy.

DEFINITION OF TNM

This classification applies to both clinical and pathologic staging of lacrimal gland carcinomas.

Primary Tumor (T)

- TX Primary tumor cannot be assessed
- T0 No evidence of primary tumor
- T1 Tumor 2.5 cm or less in greatest dimension limited to the lacrimal gland
- T2 Tumor 2.5 cm or less in greatest dimension invading the periosteum of the fossa of the lacrimal gland
- T3 Tumor more than 2.5 cm but not more than 5 cm in greatest dimension
  - T3a Tumor limited to the lacrimal gland
  - T3b Tumor invades the periosteum of the fossa of the lacrimal gland
- T4 Tumor more than 5 cm in greatest dimension
  - T4a Tumor invades the orbital soft tissues, optic nerve, or globe without bone invasion
  - T4b Tumor invades the orbital soft tissues, optic nerve, or globe with bone invasion

Regional Lymph Nodes (N)

NX Regional lymph nodes cannot be assessed
N0 No regional lymph node metastasis
N1 Regional lymph node metastasis

Distant Metastasis (M)

MX Distant metastasis cannot be assessed
M0 No distant metastasis
M1 Distant metastasis

STAGE GROUPING

No stage grouping is presently recommended.

HISTOPATHOLOGIC TYPE

The major malignant primary epithelial tumors include the following:

Carcinoma in pleomorphic adenoma (malignant mixed tumor), which includes adenocarcinoma and adenoid cystic carcinoma arising in benign mixed tumor (BMT)

Adenoid cystic carcinoma (cylindroma), arising *de novo*

Adenocarcinoma, arising *de novo*

Mucoepidermoid carcinoma

Squamous cell carcinoma

HISTOPATHOLOGIC GRADE (G)

GX Grade cannot be assessed
G1 Well differentiated
G2 Moderately differentiated: includes adenoid cystic carcinoma without baseloid (solid) pattern
G3 Poorly differentiated: includes adenoid cystic carcinoma with basaloid (solid) pattern
G4 Undifferentiated

BIBLIOGRAPHY

Henderson JW: Orbital tumors, 3rd ed. New York: Raven Press, 1993

Jakobiec FA, Bilyk JR, Font RL: Lacrimal gland tumors. In Spencer WH (Ed.), Ophthalmic pathology. An atlas and textbook, 4th ed, Volume 4. Philadelphia: WB Saunders; 2485–2524, 1996

CARCINOMA OF THE LARCRIMAL GLAND

Data Form for Cancer Staging

Patient identification
Name ______
Address ______
Hospital or clinic number ______
Age ____ Sex ____ Race ______

Institution identification
Hospital or clinic ______
Address ______

Oncology Record

Anatomic site of cancer ______
Histologic type ______
Grade (G) ______
Date of classification ______

DEFINITIONS

Primary Tumor (T)

Clin	Path		
[ ]	[ ]	TX	Primary tumor cannot be assessed
[ ]	[ ]	T0	No evidence of primary tumor
[ ]	[ ]	T1	Tumor 2.5 cm or less in greatest dimension limited to the lacrimal gland
[ ]	[ ]	T2	Tumor 2.5 cm or less in greatest dimension invading the periosteum of the fossa of the lacrimal gland
[ ]	[ ]	T3	Tumor more than 2.5 cm but not more than 5 cm in greatest dimension
[ ]	[ ]	T3a	Tumor limited to the lacrimal gland
[ ]	[ ]	T3b	Tumor invades the periosteum of the fossa of the lacrimal gland
[ ]	[ ]	T4	Tumor more than 5 cm in greatest dimension
[ ]	[ ]	T4a	With invasion of orbital soft tissues, optic nerve, or globe, *without* bone invasion
[ ]	[ ]	T4b	With invasion of orbital soft tissues, optic nerve, or globe, *with* bone invasion

Regional Lymph Nodes (N)

Clin	Path		
[ ]	[ ]	NX	Regional lymph nodes cannot be assessed
[ ]	[ ]	N0	No regional lymph node metastasis
[ ]	[ ]	N1	Regional lymph node metastasis

Distant Metastasis (M)

Clin	Path		
[ ]	[ ]	MX	Distant metastasis cannot be assessed
[ ]	[ ]	M0	No distant metastasis
[ ]	[ ]	M1	Distant metastasis

Stage Grouping

No stage grouping is presently recommended.

Staged by ______ M.D.
______ Registrar
Date ______

Histopathologic Type

The major malignant primary epithelial tumors include the following:

Carcinoma in pleomorphic adenoma (malignant mixed tumor), which includes adenocarcinoma and adenoid cystic carcinoma arising in benign mixed tumor (BMT)
Adenoid cystic carcinoma (cylindroma) arising *de novo*
Adenocarcinoma (arising *de novo*)
Mucoepidermoid carcinoma
Squamous cell carcinoma

Histopathologic Grade (G)

[ ] GX Grade cannot be assessed
[ ] G1 Well differentiated
[ ] G2 Moderately differentiated: includes adenoid cystic carcinoma without basaloid (solid) pattern
[ ] G3 Poorly differentiated: includes adenoid cystic carcinoma with basaloid (solid) pattern
[ ] G4 Undifferentiated

Illustration

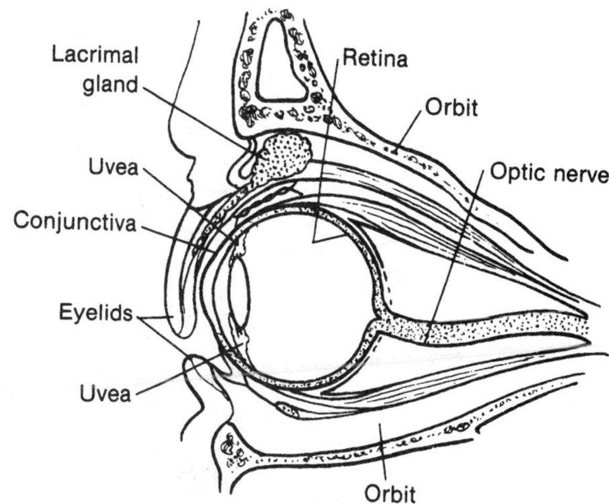

Indicate on diagrams and describe exact location and characteristics of tumor.

46

Sarcoma of the Orbit

C69.6 Orbit, NOS
C69.8 Overlapping lesion

Sarcomas of the orbit include a broad spectrum of soft-tissue tumors and sarcomas of bone.

ANATOMY

Primary Site. Sarcoma of the orbit occurs in the soft tissues and bone of the orbital fossa.

Regional Lymph Nodes. The regional lymph nodes are:

Submandibular
Parotid (pre-auricular)
Cervical

For pN, histologic examination of a regional lymphadenectomy specimen will ordinarily include 6 or more regional lymph nodes.

Metastatic Sites. Metastatic spread occurs by way of the bloodstream to distant sites.

RULES FOR CLASSIFICATION

Clinical Staging. Clinical classification is based on symptoms and signs relating to visual loss, degree of proptosis or displacement, papilledema, and optic atrophy. Diagnostic tests include radiographs of the orbit, computed tomography, and angiography.

Pathologic Staging. Pathologic classification is based on the histopathology of the tumor, its grade, and the extent of removal.

DEFINITION OF TNM

Primary Tumor (T)

TX Primary tumor cannot be assessed
T0 No evidence of primary tumor
T1 Tumor 15 mm or less in greatest dimension
T2 Tumor more than 15 mm in greatest dimension
T3 Tumor of any size with diffuse invasion of orbital tissues and/or bony walls
T4 Tumor invades beyond the orbit to adjacent sinuses and/or to cranium

Regional Lymph Nodes (N)

NX Regional lymph nodes cannot be assessed
N0 No regional lymph node metastasis
N1 Regional lymph node metastasis

Distant Metastasis (M)

MX Distant metastasis cannot be assessed
M0 No distant metastasis
M1 Distant metastasis

STAGE GROUPING

No stage grouping is presently recommended.

HISTOPATHOLOGIC TYPE

Sarcomas of the orbit include a broad spectrum of soft-tissue tumors and sarcomas of bone.

HISTOPATHOLOGIC GRADE (G)

GX Grade cannot be assessed
G1 Well differentiated
G2 Moderately differentiated
G3 Poorly differentiated
G4 Undifferentiated

BIBLIOGRAPHY

Henderson JW: Orbital tumors, 3rd ed. New York: Raven Press, 1993

Jakobiec FA, Bilyk JR, Font RL: Orbit. In Spencer WH (Ed.), Ophthalmic pathology. An atlas and textbook, 4th ed, Volume 4. Philadelphia: WB Saunders; 2569–2628, 1996

Data Form for Cancer Staging

Patient identification
Name ______________________
Address ______________________
Hospital or clinic number ______________________
Age _____ Sex _____ Race ______________________

Institution identification
Hospital or clinic ______________________
Address ______________________

Oncology Record

Anatomic site of cancer ______________________
Histologic type ______________________
Grade (G) ______________________
Date of classification ______________________

DEFINITIONS

Primary Tumor (T)

Clin	Path		
[ ]	[ ]	TX	Primary tumor cannot be assessed
[ ]	[ ]	T0	No evidence of primary tumor
[ ]	[ ]	T1	Tumor 15 mm or less in greatest dimension
[ ]	[ ]	T2	Tumor more than 15 mm in greatest dimension
[ ]	[ ]	T3	Tumor of any size with diffuse invasion of orbital tissues and/or bony walls
[ ]	[ ]	T4	Tumor invades beyond the orbit to adjacent sinuses and/or to cranium

Lymph Node (N)

Clin	Path		
[ ]	[ ]	NX	Regional lymph nodes cannot be assessed
[ ]	[ ]	N0	No regional lymph node metastasis
[ ]	[ ]	N1	Regional lymph node metastasis

Distant Metastasis (M)

Clin	Path		
[ ]	[ ]	MX	Distant metastasis cannot be assessed
[ ]	[ ]	M0	No distant metastasis
[ ]	[ ]	M1	Distant metastasis

Illustration

Indicate on diagram and describe exact location and characteristics of tumor.

Stage Grouping

No stage grouping is presently recommended.

Staged by ______________________ M.D.
______________________ Registrar
Date ______________________

Histopathologic Type

Sarcomas of the orbit include a broad spectrum of soft-tissue tumors and sarcomas of bone.

Histopathologic Grade (G)

[ ] GX Grade cannot be assessed
[ ] G1 Well differentiated
[ ] G2 Moderately differentiated
[ ] G3 Poorly differentiated
[ ] G4 Undifferentiated

CENTRAL NERVOUS SYSTEM

47

Brain and Spinal Cord

C70.0 Cerebral meninges

C71.0 Cerebrum
C71.1 Frontal lobe
C71.2 Temporal lobe
C71.3 Parietal lobe
C71.4 Occipital lobe
C71.5 Ventricle, NOS
C71.6 Cerebellum, NOS
C71.7 Brain stem
C71.8 Overlapping lesion of brain
C71.9 Brain, NOS

C72.0 Spinal cord
C72.1 Cauda equina
C72.2 Olfactory nerve
C72.3 Optic nerve
C72.4 Acoustic nerve
C72.5 Cranial nerve, NOS
C72.8 Overlapping lesion of brain and central nervous system

Attempts at developing a TNM-based classification and staging system for tumors of the central nervous system (CNS) have largely been unsuccessful. Previous editions of this manual have suggested a system that was utilized with poor compliance and proved not to be particularly useful as a predictor of outcome in clinical trials for the management of patients with primary CNS tumors. The reasons for this frustration are several, but have to do with the fact that the tumor size is much less important than tumor histology and the location of the tumor, so that the "T" classification becomes much less important than the actual biologic nature of the tumor tissue itself. Because the brain and spinal cord have no lymphatics, the "N" classification does not apply at all, as there are no lymph nodes that can be utilized in either classification or staging. An "M" classification is really not pertinent to the majority of neoplasms that affect the central nervous system, because most patients with tumors of the central nervous system do not live long enough to develop metastatic disease, except in some pediatric tumors which tend to "seed" through the spinal fluid spaces.

Many important studies have been done regarding the most common tumors affecting the brain and spinal cord, and so a variety of prognostic factors have been identified. Unfortunately, these factors do not easily fall into the usual categories that have traditionally been part of the American Joint Committee on Cancer (AJCC) TNM system.

For those reasons, it was the recommendation of the CNS Tumor Task Force that a formal classification and staging system not be attempted at this time. This chapter, however, will attempt to highlight what is known about prognostic factors in tumors of the central nervous system.

PROGNOSTIC FACTORS IN CNS TUMORS (TABLE 47-1)

Tumor Histology. The histology of tumors that affect the brain and spinal cord is by far the most important variable with regard to prognosis, and in many cases determines the treatment modalities that are employed. The latest World Health Organization (WHO) classifica-

Table 47-1. Prognostic Factors in CNS Tumors

Histology
Age of patient
Functional neurologic status (Karnofsky)
Extent of resection
Location of tumor
Metastatic spread

tion system has combined a tumor nomenclature with an implied grading system so that the actual histologic diagnosis directly correlates with the histologic grade of the tumor. Hopefully, this will clarify some of the inconsistencies that have existed in the past with regard to the utilization of a number of different grading systems, each slightly different from another. The most common histologies for brain and spinal cord tumors are given in Table 47-2, along with a general estimate of the tumor grades involved in each different diagnostic category.

Age of the Patient. Most retrospective studies of the outcome of brain tumor therapy show that the age of the patient at the time of diagnosis is one of the most powerful predictors of outcome. This fact holds true for the gliomas, which are the most common primary brain tumors, and for most other tumors that affect the adult population, including most metastatic tumors to the brain. There are, however, some childhood tumors that have a very poor prognosis and are inherently high grade, and rapidly progressive to a fatal outcome. There are some metastatic tumors, such as melanoma, that occur in younger patients that also violate this general statement with regard to the specific effect of age on prognosis.

Extent of Tumor Residual. In patients who are treated surgically for tumors of the central nervous system, the extent of resection is very frequently correlated with the outcome. This is a less powerful predictor than tumor histology or age, but most retrospective studies confirm that extent of removal is positively correlated with survival. For this reason, documentation of whether a surgical tumor removal is "gross total," "subtotal," or "biopsy only," is useful in determining the future therapy and prognosis. Any staging system to be developed for CNS tumors should take into account in a systematic fashion, extent of removal or tumor residual.

Tumor Location. Because of the differential importance of various areas of the brain, the location of a given tumor affecting the brain can have a major impact on the functional outcome, survival, and nature of therapy. The location codes available for tumors affecting the central nervous system in the ICD-9 manual are generally satisfactory, and offer the advantage of consistency to the records of patients with CNS tumors.

Functional Neurologic Status. Another important prognostic factor in most retrospective studies of CNS tumors is the functional neurologic status. This traditionally has been estimated using the Karnofsky performance scale, which is reproducible, well-known by most investigators, and in common use for stratification of patients entering clinical trials for the treatment of brain tumors. The outcome and prognosis of patients is correlated fairly well with functional neurologic status and, once again, any staging system should include a validated and reliable measure of this parameter.

Metastatic Spread. Tumors affecting the central nervous system rarely develop extraneural metastases, probably due to inherent biologic characteristics of these tumors, and also because of the fact that the brain has no lymphatic drainage system. It is true that certain tumors do spread through the cerebrospinal fluid (CSF) pathways, and such spread has a major impact on survival. Spread through the CSF pathway is a hallmark of certain childhood tumors, many of which carry a poor prognosis; however, this phenomenon is rarely seen in adult patients with the more common CNS tumors. Although of importance in certain instances, the overall importance of metastatic spread in staging is relatively minor. The "M" category however, should be

Table 47-2. Tumor Histology (WHO Classification)

MOST COMMON TUMORS	GRADE (WHO)
Pilocytic astrocytoma	1
Astrocytoma	1-2
Anaplastic (malignant) astrocytoma	3-4
Glioblastoma	4
Oligodendroglioma	1-2
Anaplastic Oligodendroglioma	3-4
Mixed Oligodendroglioma/Astrocytoma	1-4
Ependymoma	1-2
Anaplastic (malignant) ependymoma	3-4
Primitive Neuroectodermal Tumors (PNETs)	4
a) Medulloblastoma	
b) Cerebral or spinal PNET	
Schwannoma	1
Neurofibroma	1
Meningioma	1
Atypical meningioma	2-3
Anaplastic (malignant) meningioma	4
Primary malignant lymphoma	3-4
Pituitary adenoma	1

Table 47-3. Prognostic Biogenetic Markers (Under Investigation)

Proliferation index–Ki-67
DNA ploidy–flow cytometry
Loss of tumor suppressor genes–p53
Presence of oncogenes–ras, myc
Allelic loss–loss of heterozygosity (LOH)
Other chromosomal abnormalities–double minutes

part of any classification and staging system that is developed in the future for CNS tumors.

PROGNOSTIC BIOGENETIC MARKERS (UNDER INVESTIGATION)

The field of molecular neuropathology has provided us with a number of potential biogenetic markers that may be useful in the staging of CNS tumors and in making recommendations for therapy. The discovery of the pivotal role in the tumorigenesis of CNS tumors of oncogenes and the loss of tumor suppressor genes has led to a flurry of activity which may prove quite fruitful in providing valid biologic markers in these difficult tumors. Table 47-3 provides a glimpse of some of the current markers and techniques under investigation. There is room for optimism with regard to possible practical application of these methods of scientific analysis of tumor growth potential to better predict survival and, hopefully, someday response to treatments that are far more effective than those of today.

BIBLIOGRAPHY

Curran WJ, Scott CB, Horton J, et al: Recursive partitioning analysis of prognostic factors in three Radiation Therapy Oncology Group malignant glioma trials. J Natl Cancer Inst 85:704–710, 1993

Guthrie BL, Laws ER Jr: Prognostic factors in patients with brain tumors. In Morantz RA, Walsh JW (Eds.), Brain tumors. New York: Marcel Dekker; 799–808, 1994

Jelsma R, Bucy PC: Glioblastoma multiforme: its treatment and some factors affecting survival. Arch Neurol 20:161–171, 1969

Kaye AH, Laws ER Jr: Brain tumors. London: Churchill Livingstone, 1995

Kleihues P, Burger PC, Scheithauer BW: Histological typing of tumors of the central nervous system. WHO international histological classification of tumors. Berlin-Heidelberg: Springer-Verlag, 1993

Salcman M: Survival in glioblastoma: historical perspective. Neurosurgery 7:435–439, 1980

Scanlon PW, Taylor WF: Radiotherapy of intracranial astrocytomas: analysis of 417 cases treated from 1960 through 1969. Neurosurgery 5:301–308, 1979

Shaw EG, Scheithauer BW, O'Fallon JR, et al: Oligodendrogliomas: The Mayo Clinic Experience. J Neurosurg 76:428–434, 1992

VandenBerg SR: Current diagnostic concepts of astrocytic tumors. J Neuropathol Exp Neurol 51:644–657, 1992

Werner-Wasik M, Scott CB, Nelson DF, et al: Final report of a phase I/II trial of hyperfractionated and accelerated hyperfractionated radiation therapy with carmustine for adults with supratentorial malignant gliomas. Cancer 77:1535–1543, 1996

LYMPHOMAS

48 Hodgkin's Disease

A distinctive form of lymphoma, Hodgkin's disease has served as a model for treatment trials, for great strides have been made in the therapy of this disease. Staging of Hodgkin's lymphoma is not based on the local extent of disease but on its distribution and symptomatology. The classic TNM system is not useful for staging Hodgkin's disease. It is usually not possible to determine the primary tumor site. When the patient presents, the disease is often widely disseminated. Important for staging is the evaluation of many organs and groups of lymph nodes for tumor involvement. The disease is often associated with unusual immunologic abnormalities and a diversity of histologic changes. Staging is considered critical for patient management.

ANATOMY

The major lymphatic structures include groups and chains of lymph nodes, the spleen, and the thymus gland. The digestive system is also an important lymphoid organ that has collections of lymphoid tissue known as Waldeyer's ring in the oropharynx, Peyer's patches in the ileum, and lymphoid nodules in the appendix. Hodgkin's disease can involve almost any organ or tissue, especially the liver, bone marrow, and spleen, in addition to the lymph nodes.

RULES FOR CLASSIFICATION

Clinical Staging. The clinical stage is determined by obtaining an adequate initial biopsy, history, physical examination, laboratory tests, imaging studies, and gallium scanning. Such studies usually establish the diagnosis and histologic type of Hodgkin's disease. Histologic confirmation is essential. All symptoms should be recorded, especially fever and weight loss.

Pathologic Staging. Pathologic staging depends on one or more lymph node biopsies, bone marrow biopsy, and if the result will influence therapy, a laparotomy, which would include liver biopsy, splenectomy, and multiple nodal biopsies to assess distribution of the abdominal disease. Involved organs and sites should be listed.

STAGE GROUPING

Stage I	Involvement of a single lymph node region (I) or localized involvement of a single extralymphatic organ or site (I_E).
Stage II	Involvement of two or more lymph node regions on the same side of the diaphragm (II) or localized involvement of a single associated extralymphatic organ or site and its regional lymph node(s) with or without involvement of other lymph node regions on the same side of the diaphragm (II_E).

Note: The number of lymph node regions involved may be indicated by a subscript (e.g., II_3).

Stage III	Involvement of lymph node regions on both sides of the diaphragm (III), which may also be accompanied by localized involvement of an associated extralymphatic organ or site (III_E), by involvement of the spleen (III_S), or both (III_{E+S}).
Stage IV	Disseminated (multifocal) involvement of one or more extralymphatic organs, with or without associated lymph node involvement, or isolated extralymphatic organ involvement with distant (nonregional) nodal involvement.

SYSTEMIC SYMPTOMS

Each stage is subdivided into "A" and "B" categories, "B" for those with defined systemic symptoms and "A" for those without. The B designation is given to those patients with (1) unexplained loss of more than 10% of body weight in the 6 months before diagnosis; (2) unexplained fever with temperatures above 38°C; and (3) drenching night sweats. Pruritus alone does not qualify for B classification,* nor does a short febrile illness associated with an infection.

**Note:* Pruritus as a systemic symptom remains controversial. This symptom is hard to define quantitatively and uniformly, but when it is recurrent, generalized, and otherwise unexplained, and when it ebbs and flows parallel to disease activity, it may be the equivalent of a B symptom.

HISTOPATHOLOGIC TYPE

Hodgkin's disease is divided into four major histologic types and "unclassified." These types should be recorded because they have prognostic significance. They are:

Nodular sclerosis
Lymphocyte predominance
Mixed cellularity
Lymphocyte depletion
Unclassified

Histologic classification should be based on paraffin-embedded hematoxylin and eosin-stained sections.

BIBLIOGRAPHY

Aragon de la Cruz G, Cardenes H, Otero J, et al: Individual risk of abdominal disease in patients with stages I and II dupradiaphragmatic Hodgkin's disease: a rule index based on 341 laparotomized patients. Cancer 63:1799–1803, 1989

Boyd NF, Feinstein AR: Symptoms as an index of growth rates and prognosis in Hodgkin's disease. Clin Invest Med 1:25–31, 1978

Carbonne PP, Kaplan HS, Musshoff K, et al: Report of the committee on Hodgkin's disease staging classification. Cancer Res 31:1860–1861, 1971

Castellino RA, Hoppe RT, Blank N, et al: Computed tomography, lymphography, and staging laparotomy: correlations in initial staging of Hodgkin's disease. Am J Roentgenol 143:37–41, 1984

Cooper DL, Caride VJ, Zloty M, et al: Gallium scans in patients with mediastinal Hodgkin's disease treated with chemotherapy. J Clin Oncol 11:1092–1098, 1993

DeVita VT Jr., Mauch PM, Harris NL: Hodgkin's disease. In DeVita VT Jr., Hellman S, Rosenberg SA (Eds.), Cancer: principles and practice of oncology, 5th ed. Philadelphia: Lippincott–Raven Publishers; 2242–2283, 1997

Kaplan HS: Hodgkin's disease, 2nd ed. Cambridge: Harvard University Press, 1980

King SC, Reiman RJ, Prosnitrz LR: Prognostic importance of restaging gallium scans following induction chemotherapy for advanced Hodgkin's disease. J Clin Oncol 12:306–311, 1994

Leibenhaut MH, Hoppe RT, Efron B, et al: Prognostic indicators of laparotomy findings in clinical stage I-II supradiaphragmatic Hodgkin's disease. J Clin Oncol 7:81–91, 1989

Lister TA, Crowther D, Sutcliffe SB, et al: Report of a committee convened to discuss the evaluation and staging of patients with Hodgkin's disease: Cotswolds Meeting. J Clin Oncol 7:1630–1636, 1989

Mauch P, Larson D, Osteen R, et al: Prognostic factors for positive surgical staging in patients with Hodgkin's disease. J Clin Oncol 8:257–265, 1990

Regula DP Jr, Hoppe RT, Weiss LM: Nodular and diffuse types of lymphocyte predominance Hodgkin's disease. N Engl J Med 318:214–219, 1988

Smithers DW: Summary of papers delivered at the Conference on staging of Hodgkin's Disease (Ann Arbor, Michigan). Cancer Res 31:1869–1870, 1971

Taylor MA, Kaplan HS, Nelsen TS: Staging laparotomy with splenectomy for Hodgkin's disease: The Stanford Experience. World J Surg 9:449–460, 1985

Weinshel EL, Peterson BA: Hodgkin's Disease. CA Cancer J Clin 43:327–371, 1993

Data Form for Cancer Staging

Patient identification
Name ______
Address ______
Hospital or clinic number ______
Age ____ Sex ____ Race ______

Institution identification
Hospital or clinic ______
Address ______

Oncology Record

Anatomic site of cancer ______
Histologic type ______
Grade (G) ______
Date of classification ______

Clin	Path	DEFINITIONS	
		Stage Grouping	
[ ]	[ ]	Stage I	Involvement of a single lymph node region (I) or localized involvement of a single extralymphatic organ or site (I_E).
[ ]	[ ]	Stage II	Involvement of two or more lymph node regions on the same side of the diaphragm (II) or localized involvement of a single associated extralymphatic organ or site and its regional lymph node(s) with or without involvement of other lymph node regions on the same side of the diaphragm (II_E). NOTE: The number of lymph node regions involved may be indicated by a subscript (e.g., II_3).
[ ]	[ ]	Stage III	Involvement of lymph node regions on both sides of the diaphragm (III), which may also be accompanied by localized involvement of an associated extralymphatic organ or site (III_E), by involvement of the spleen (III_S), or both (III_{E+S}).
[ ]	[ ]	Stage IV	Disseminated (multifocal) involvement of one or more extralymphatic organs with or without associated lymph node involvement, or isolated extralymphatic organ involvement with distant (nonregional) nodal involvement.

Staged by ______ M.D.
______ Registrar
Date ______

Histopathologic Type

Hodgkin's disease is divided into four major histologic types and "unclassified." These types should be recorded because they have prognostic significance. They are:

Nodular sclerosis
Lymphocyte predominance
Mixed cellularity
Lymphocyte depletion
Unclassified

Histologic classification should be based on paraffin-embedded hematoxylin and eosin-stained sections.

49

Non-Hodgkin's Lymphoma

Long-term survival and even cure can be achieved in patients with non-Hodgkin's lymphomas. This requires correctly classifying the lymphoma according to the specific morphologic criteria, defining the extent of disease through staging, and selecting the appropriate therapy for the morphologic subtype and stage.

The histologic classification of the non-Hodgkin's lymphomas has been an area of considerable controversy. A number of competing classifications are in use, including those of Rappaport, Lukes and Collins, the World Health Organization (WHO), Dorfman, Kiel, and the British National Lymphoma Investigation Group. In an effort to bring some uniformity to the classification of these disorders, an international panel of expert pathologists generated a *Working Formulation,* which attempts to provide a means of interpretation of these somewhat divergent classification schemes. This formulation provides a useful format in which to discuss the staging and workup of these lymphomas.

The anatomic staging system currently employed was developed for Hodgkin's disease and has been extended to the non-Hodgkin's lymphomas, although it is more directly applicable to Hodgkin's disease. As a result, some difficulties arise in some instances when attempting to apply traditional staging systems to non-Hodgkin's lymphomas. However, in the main it has proved to be a workable system and has the advantage of being familiar and similar to that used in Hodgkin's disease.

The TNM classification, however, is not a workable system for staging the malignant lymphomas. The site of origin of these diseases is often unclear, and there is no way to differentiate T, N, and M from each other. In the non-Hodgkin's lymphomas, the pattern of node involvement (follicular versus diffuse) and the bulk of disease at individual sites is often more important than anatomic considerations.

ANATOMY

The major lymphatic structures include groups and chains (regions) of lymph nodes, the spleen, thymus, Waldeyer's ring, appendix, and Peyer's patches. Minor lymphoid collections are widely dispersed in other viscera and tissues, such as the bone marrow, liver, skin, bone, lung, pleura, and gonads. Involvement of extranodal sites is more commonly seen in the non-Hodgkin's lymphomas than in Hodgkin's disease.

RULES FOR CLASSIFICATION

The diagnosis of malignant lymphoma requires the biopsy of lymph nodes or of an extranodal lymphoid tumor in order to clarify histology based on architecture or cytologic subtype. Frozen sections are never to be used as a definitive diagnostic source, and confirmation rests on the review of the fixed specimen.

Clinical Staging. Staging generally involves the use of a combination of clinical, radiologic, and surgical procedures, progressing sequentially from less invasive to more invasive, necessary to define final stage and to provide a sound basis for planning and monitoring therapy. Clinical staging includes a carefully recorded medical history, a physical examination, urinalysis, chest roentgenograms, blood chemistry determinations, a complete blood examination, and bilateral biopsies of the bone marrow. In addition, most investigators use an abdominal computed tomography (CT) scan to fulfill the mandatory staging requirements. Other procedures often useful in full staging of patients include bone roentgenograms, technetium 99m-labeled polyphosphate bone scans, or CT scans of the thorax (if the initial chest x-ray is abnormal). Additional procedures helpful under certain circumstances include upper GI series (if Waldeyer's ring is involved or if patients have GI symptoms), lumbar puncture (if patients have diffuse histologies and bone marrow involvement), ultrasound, gallium scans, and radioisotopic scans of the spleen and liver. Surface marker studies and studies of immunoglobulin gene rearrangement are often essential for determining the correct diagnosis.

Pathologic Staging. Initial diagnosis is almost always made by surgical biopsy. In addition, biopsy of accessible extranodal primary tumors is desirable. Extranodal sites of disease at presentation are seen in about 30% of patients. About 25% of patients with non-Hodgkin's lymphomas present with evidence of abdominal disease requiring laparotomy for diagnosis. However, staging laparotomy is not routinely used in this disease and should only be used when treatment changes would result from the findings of the surgery. If liver involvement is suspected, it may be biopsied by a percutaneous needle procedure, or multiple directed biopsies of both lobes may be obtained using laparoscopy. Although a staging laparotomy is employed selectively and only after careful consideration of its impact on both staging and subsequent therapy, when employed it should include splenectomy, wedge liver biopsy, and biopsies of the perisplenic, mesenteric, portahepatic, para-aortic, and bilateral iliac nodes, unless underlying medical problems prohibit such biopsies.

Retreatment Evaluation. Suspected recurrence or relapses require biopsy confirmation, particularly if a complete remission of greater than one year has occurred. Patients may be reevaluated for extent of disease at this juncture using the procedures previously outlined for staging.

STAGE GROUPING

Stage I	Involvement of a single lymph node region (I) or localized involvement of a single extralymphatic organ or site (I_E).
Stage II	Involvement of two or more lymph node regions on the same side of the diaphragm (II), or localized involvement of a single associated extralymphatic organ or site and its regional nodes with or without other lymph node regions on the same side of the diaphragm (II_E).

Note: The number of lymph node regions involved may be indicated by a subscript (e.g., II_3).

Stage III	Involvement of lymph node regions on both sides of the diaphragm (III) that may also be accompanied by localized involvement of an extralymphatic organ or site (III_E), by involvement of the spleen (III_S), or both (III_{E+S}).
Stage IV	Disseminated (multifocal) involvement of one or more extralymphatic organs with or without associated lymph node involvement, or isolated extralymphatic organ involvement with distant (nonregional) nodal involvement.

SYSTEMIC SYMPTOMS

Systemic symptoms are not as commonly associated with the non-Hodgkin's lymphomas as with Hodgkin's disease, and patients with non-Hodgkin's lymphomas often have remarkably few symptoms, even though many node areas and/or extranodal sites are involved. However, when systemic symptoms are seen, they do have prognostic significance.

Each stage is subdivided into "A" and "B" categories: "B" for those with defined systematic symptoms and "A" for those without. The B designation is given to those patients with (1) unexplained loss of more than 10% of body weight in the 6 months before diagnosis; (2) unexplained fever with temperatures above 38°C; and (3) drenching night sweats. Pruritus alone does not qualify for B classification,* nor does a short febrileillness associated with an infection. In addition, an accurate assessment of the performance status (ECOG or Karnofsky) with allowances for unrelated diseases is most important.

**Note:* Pruritus as a systemic symptom remains controversial. This symptom is hard to define quantitatively and uniformly, but when it is recurrent, generalized, and otherwise unexplained, and when it ebbs and flows parallel to disease activity, it may be the equivalent of a B symptom.

GENERAL CONSIDERATIONS

The anatomic extent of disease in the non-Hodgkin's lymphomas is defined by the appropriate sequence of diagnostic procedures selected for a given histologic subset and a particular individual. The exact sequence of staging procedures and the magnitude of invasive staging will rest upon the patient's histology, the therapeutic approach contemplated, as well as the stage of disease. No invasive staging procedure should be employed merely to change the patient's stage, if that change of stage will not alter the therapy selected or the outcome of treatment. There is always some variation, often with good reason, in the degree of completeness and adequacy of the data used for final staging.

In general, the yield from particular staging procedures is dependent upon the histology of the patient's lymphoma. For instance, in the low grade or indolent follicular lymphomas (see Histopathologic Type) some 80% to 90% of patients will have positive lymphangiograms, 40% will have liver involvement, and more than 40% will have bone marrow involvement as well. When comprehensive staging is done on these patients, over 90% have Stage III-IV disease. This high frequency of advanced disease makes staging laparotomy rarely, if ever, required in the workup of follicular lymphoma because treatment decisions are rarely influenced by the findings in the majority of patients.

In contrast, in the intermediate or high grade lymphomas, a much lower incidence of visceral disease is generally found at initial staging. As an example, some 30% to 40% of patients have positive lymphangiograms, the frequency of positive bone marrows is about 15% to 20%, and about 15% to 20% of liver biopsies are positive. After final comprehensive staging, about 25% to 30% of patients with diffuse aggressive lymphoma appear to have localized (Stage I and II) disease. Again, the importance of the extent of staging rests upon the subsequent therapeutic approaches taken and the success of that therapy. Comprehensive staging is required if a localized form of therapy (i.e., involved field irradiation) is being considered.

CT scans are a useful addition to the staging procedures. They should be done before lymphangiography, since after lymphangiography the increase in size of nodes may lead to a false CT. Moreover, foci of lymphoreticular disease in the para-aortic region above the level of the second lumbar vertebra, in the portahepatic, splenic hilus, mesentery, gut wall, and retrocrural nodes and in other sites in the abdomen cannot be demonstrated by lymphangiography. On the other hand, CT scanning is unable to detect small defects in otherwise normal-sized nodes. Thus, a complementary role of CT scanning and lymphangiography is seen in the non-Hodgkin's lymphomas.

HISTOPATHOLOGIC TYPE

The Working Formulation is a useful classification for the majority of non-Hodgkin's lymphomas. While individual institutions and particular pathologists may use one of the many classifications of these lymphomas mentioned earlier, the corresponding Working Formulation equivalent should be identified so that inter-institutional comparisons can be made and accurate staging approaches selected. The Working Formulation is listed below. It should be noted that the term non-Hodgkin's lymphoma is not used; follicular is employed rather than nodular; and surface markers are not required.

With new diagnostic tools, new types of lymphomas (or new terminology) have become recognized. The importance of immunology, cytogenetics, and molecular genetic markers for diagnosis have resulted in identification of new subtypes of lymphoma. In an attempt to include some of these, a new classification system has been proposed, the Revised European-American Classification of Lymphoid Neoplasms (REAL).

Working Formulation

I. Low-Grade Malignant Lymphoma
- A. Small lymphocytic
- B. Follicular, predominantly small cleaved cell
- C. Follicular, mixed small cleaved and large cell

II. Intermediate-Grade Malignant Lymphoma
- D. Follicular, predominantly large cell
- E. Diffuse, small cleaved cell
- F. Diffuse, mixed, small and large cell
- G. Diffuse, large cell, cleaved or noncleaved

III. High-Grade Malignant Lymphoma
- H. Diffuse large cell immunoblastic
- I. Lymphoblastic (convoluted and/or nonconvoluted)
- J. Small noncleaved cell (Burkitt's or non-Burkitt's)

IV. Miscellaneous
  Composite
  Histiocytic
  Mycosis fungoides
  Other

Revised European-American Lymphoma Classification

B-Cell Neoplasms

I. Precursor B-cell neoplasm: Precursor B-lymphoblastic leukemia/lymphoma
II. Peripheral B-cell neoplasms
  1. B-cell chronic lymphocytic leukemia/prolymphocytic lekemia/small lymphocytic lymphoma
  2. Lymphoplasmacytoid lymphoma/immunocytoma
  3. Mantle cell lymphoma
  4. Follicle center lymphoma, follicular
     Provisional cytologic grades: I (small cell), II (mixed and large cell), III (Large cell)
     Provisional subtype: diffuse, predominantly small cell type
  5. Marginal zone B-cell lymphoma
     Extranodal (MALT-type +/− monocytoid B cells)
     Provisional subtype: Nodal (+/− monocytoid B cells)
  6. Provisional entity: Splenic marginal zone lymphoma (+/− villous lymphocytes)
  7. Hairy cell leukemia
  8. Plasmacytoma/plasma cell myeloma
  9. Diffuse Large B-cell lymphoma
     Subtype: Primary mediastinal (thymic) B-cell lymphoma
  10. Burkitt's lymphoma
  11. Provisional entity: High-grade B-cell lymphoma, Burkitt's-like

T-Cell and Putative NK-Cell Neoplasms

I. Precursor T-cell neoplasm: Precursor T-lymphoblastic lymphoma/leukemia
II. Peripheral T-cell and NK-cell neoplasms
  1. T-cell chronic lymphocytic leukemia/prolymphocytic leukemia
  2. Large granular lymphocytic leukemia (LGL)
     T-cell type
     NK-cell type
  3. Mycosis fungoides/Sezary syndrome
  4. Peripheral T-cell lymphomas, unspecified
     Provisional cytologic categories: medium sized cell, mixed medium and large cell, large cell, lymphoepithelioid cell
     Provisional subtype: Hepatosplenic gamma-delta T-cell lymphoma
     Provisional subtype: Subcutaneous panniculitic T-cell lymphoma
  5. Angioimmunoblastic T-cell lymphoma (AILD)
  6. Angiocentric lymphoma
  7. Intestinal T-cell lymphoma (+/− enteropathy associated)
  8. Adult T-cell lymphoma/leukemia (ATL/L)
  9. Anaplastic large cell lymphoma (ALCL), CD30, T- and null-cell types
  10. Provisional entity: Anaplastic large-cell lymphoma, Hodgkin's-like

PROGNOSTIC FACTORS

Using only age, Ann Arbor stage, number of extranodal sites, performance status, and serum LDH, patients with large cell lymphoma can be grouped into four prognostic classes (International Index) with widely disparate response rates and survival.

BIBLIOGRAPHY

Harris NL, Jaffe ES, Stein H, et al: A revised European-American classification of lymphoid neoplasms: a proposal from the International Lymphoma Study Group. Blood 84:1361–1392, 1994

Hermanek P, Gospodarowicz MK, Henson DE, et al: Prognostic factors in cancer. Berlin-Heidelberg-New York: Springer-Verlag, 1995

Rosenberg SA: National Cancer Institute sponsored study of classifications of non-Hodgkin's lymphomas. Summary and description of a working formulation for clinical usage. Cancer 49:2112–2135, 1982

The International Non-Hodgkin's Lymphoma Prognostic Factors Project: a predictive model for aggressive non-Hodgkin's lymphoma. N Engl J Med 329:987–994, 1993

Data Form for Cancer Staging

Patient identification
Name ______
Address ______
Hospital or clinic number ______
Age ____ Sex ____ Race ______

Institution identification
Hospital or clinic ______
Address ______

Oncology Record

Anatomic site of cancer ______
Histologic type ______
Grade (G) ______
Date of classification ______

Clin	Path	DEFINITIONS	
		Stage Grouping	
[ ]	[ ]	Stage I	Involvement of a single lymph node region (I) or localized involvement of a single extralymphatic organ or site (I_E).
[ ]	[ ]	Stage II	Involvement of two or more lymph node regions on the same side of the diaphragm (II), or localized involvement of a single associated extralymphatic organ or site and its regional nodes with or without other lymph node regions on the same side of the diaphragm (II_E). NOTE: The number of lymph node regions involved may be indicated by a subscript (e.g., II_3).
[ ]	[ ]	Stage III	Involvement of lymph node regions on both sides of the diaphragm (III), which may also be accompanied by localized involvement of an extralymphatic organ or site (III_E), by involvement of the spleen (III_S), or both (III_{E+S}).
[ ]	[ ]	Stage IV	Disseminated (multifocal) involvement of one or more extralymphatic organs with or without associated lymph node involvement, or isolated extralymphatic organ involvement with distant (nonregional) nodal involvement.

Histopathologic Type

The Working Formulation is a useful classification for the majority of non-Hodgkin's lymphomas. While individual institutions and particular pathologists may use one of the many classifications of these lymphomas mentioned earlier (see Introduction), the corresponding Working Formulation equivalent should be identified so that interinstitutional comparisons can be made and accurate staging approaches selected. The modified Working Formulation is listed below. It should be noted that the term *non-Hodgkin's lymphoma* is not used, *follicular* is employed rather than *nodular*, and surface markers are not required.

With new diagnostic tools, new types of lymphomas (or new terminology) have become recognized. The importance of immunology, cytogenetics, and molecular genetic markers for diagnosis have resulted in identification of new subtypes of lymphoma. In an attempt to include some of these, a new classification system has been proposed, the Revised European-American Classification of Lymphoid Neoplasms (REAL).

Working Formulation

I. Low-Grade Malignant Lymphoma
  A. Small lymphocytic
  B. Follicular, predominantly small cleaved cell
  C. Follicular mixed, small and large cell
II. Intermediate-Grade Malignant Lymphoma
  D. Follicular, predominantly large cell
  E. Diffuse small cleaved cell
  F. Diffuse mixed, small and large cell
  G. Diffuse large cell, cleaved/noncleaved
III. High-Grade Malignant Lymphoma
  H. Diffuse large cell immunoblastic
  I. Lymphoblastic (convoluted/nonconvoluted)
  J. Small noncleaved cell (Burkitt's/non-Burkitt's)
IV. Miscellaneous
  Composite
  Mycosis fungoides
  Other

(continued on next page)

Revised European-American Lymphoma Classification

B-Cell Neoplasms

I. Precursor B-cell neoplasm: Precursor B-lymphoblastic leukemia/lymphoma
II. Peripheral B-cell neoplasms
  1. B-cell chronic lymphocytic leukemia/prolymphocytic leukemia/small lymphocytic lymphoma
  2. Lymphoplasmacytoid lymphoma/immunocytoma
  3. Mantle cell lymphoma
  4. Follicle center lymphoma, follicular
     Provisional cytologic grades: I (small cell), II (mixed and large cell), III (Large cell)
     Provisional subtype: diffuse, predominantly small cell type
  5. Marginal zone B-cell lymphoma
     Extranodal (MALT-type +/− monocytoid B cells)
     Provisional subtype: Nodal (+/− monocytoid B cells)
  6. Provisional entity: Splenic marginal zone lymphoma (+/− villous lymphocytes)
  7. Hairy cell leukemia
  8. Plasmacytoma/plasma cell myeloma
  9. Duffuse Large B-cell lymphoma
     Subtype: Primary mediastinal (thymic) B-cell lymphoma
  10. Burkitt's lymphoma
  11. Provisional entity: High-grade B-cell lymphoma, Burkitt's-like

T-Cell and Putative NK-Cell Neoplasms

I. Precursor T-cell neoplasm: Precursor T-lymphoblastic lymphoma/leukemia
II. Peripheral T-cell and NK-cell neoplasms
  1. T-cell chronic lymphocytic leukemia/prolymphocytic leukemia
  2. Large granular lymphocytic leukemia (LGL)
     T-cell type
     NK-cell type
  3. Mycosis fungoides/Sezary syndrome
  4. Peripheral T-cell lymphomas, unspecified
     Provisional cytologic categories: medium sized cell, mixed medium and large cell, large cell, lymphoepithelioid cell
     Provisional subtype: Hepatosplenic gamma-delta T-cell lymphoma
     Provisional subtype: Subcutaneous panniculitic T-cell lymphoma
  5. Angioimmunoblastic T-cell lymphoma (AILD)
  6. Angiocentric lymphoma
  7. Intestinal T-cell lymphoma (+/− enteropathy associated)
  8. Adult T-cell lymphoma/leukemia (ALT/L)
  9. Anaplastic large cell lymphoma (ALCL), CD30, T- and null-cell types
  10. Provisional entity: Anaplastic large-cell lymphoma, Hodgkin's-like

Staged by ______________________________ **M.D.**
______________________________ **Registrar**
Date ______________________________

PART III

Personnel and Contributors

PAST AND PRESENT PERSONNEL OF THE AMERICAN JOINT COMMITTEE ON CANCER (1959–1997)

W.A.D. Anderson, M.D.
Harvey W. Baker, M.D.
Oliver H. Beahrs, M.D. (Ex-officio)
Robert W. Beart, Jr., M.D.
Harold E. Bowman, M.D.
David G. Bragg, M.D.
Weldon K. Bullock, M.D.
*Blake Cady, M.D.
Paul R. Cannon, M.D.
Paul Carbone, M.D.
David T. Carr, M.D. (Ex-officio)
William M. Christopherson, M.D.
*Jay S. Cooper, M.D.
Murray M. Copeland, M.D.
Michael P. Corder, M.D.
*Myles P. Cunningham, M.D.
Anthony R. Curreri, M.D.
Sidney J. Cutler, Sc.D.
Herbert Derman, M.D.
Theodore P. Eberhard, M.D.
Jack Edeiken, M.D.
Harmon J. Eyre, M.D.
George M. Farrow, M.D.
*Irvin D. Fleming, M.D.
Eugene P. Frenkel, M.D.
Karen K. Fu, M.D.
Alfred Gellhorn, M.D.
Eli Glatstein, M.D.
*Frederick L. Greene, M.D.
*Donald E. Henson, M.D. (Ex-officio)
Howard B. Hunt, M.D.
*Robert V.P. Hutter, M.D. (Ex-officio)
*B.J. Kennedy, M.D.
Alfred S. Ketcham, M.D.
Howard B. Latourette, M.D.
Edward R. Laws, Jr., M.D.
Louis A. Leone, M.D.
Seymour H. Levitt, M.D.
Robert D. Lindberg, M.D.
Virgil Loeb, Jr., M.D.
*Robert J. Mayer, M.D.
*Robert J. McKenna, M.D.
William A. Meissner, M.D.
William C. Moloney, M.D.
Rodney R. Million, M.D.
William T. Moss, M.D.
Clifton F. Mountain, M.D.
*Gerald P. Murphy, M.D.
Max H. Myers, Ph.D.
*Gerald Nash, M.D.
Gregory T. O'Conor, M.D.
*David L. Page, M.D.
*Harvey I. Pass, M.D.
John W. Pickren, M.D.
H. Marvin Pollard, M.D.
William E. Powers, M.D.
Antolin Raventos, M.D.
*Mack Roach, III, M.D.
Guy F. Robbins, M.D.
William L. Ross, M.D.
Philip Rubin, M.D.
R. Wayne Rundles, M.D.
William O. Russell, M.D.
Edward F. Scanlon, M.D.
Robert L. Schmitz, M.D.
Milford D. Schultz, M.D.
*Robert J. Schweitzer, M.D.
Wendell G. Scott, M.D.
Robert E. Scully, M.D.
Paul Sherlock, M.D.
Danely Slaughter, M.D.
Charles R. Smart, M.D.
Robert R. Smith, M.D.
Edward H. Soule, M.D.
*Sudhir Srivastava, Ph.D., M.P.H.
Samuel G. Taylor III, M.D.
Willis J. Taylor, M.D.
*Joel E. Tepper, M.D.

*Current Members of the AJCC Full Committee

Louis B. Thomas, M.D.
*Edward L. Trimble, M.D.
Frank Vellios, M.D.
*Mark R. Wick, M.D.
*David P. Winchester, M.D. (Ex-officio)
Morris J. Wizenberg, M.D.
David A. Wood, M.D.
*John W. Yarbro, M.D.
John L. Young, Dr.P.H.
Robert C. Young, M.D.
John Ziegler, M.D.

CURRENT MEMBERS OF THE FULL COMMITTEE OF THE AMERICAN JOINT COMMITTEE ON CANCER (1997)

Blake Cady, M.D.
*Jay S. Cooper, M.D.
*Myles P. Cunningham, M.D.
*Irvin D. Fleming, M.D. (Chairman)
Frederick L. Greene, M.D.
Donald E. Henson, M.D. (Ex-officio)
*Robert V.P. Hutter, M.D. (Ex-officio)
*B.J. Kennedy, M.D.
Robert J. Mayer, M.D.
Robert J. McKenna, M.D.
*Gerald P. Murphy, M.D. (Ex-officio and Executive Secretary)
Gerald Nash, M.D.
*David L. Page, M.D.
Harvey I. Pass, M.D.
Mack Roach, III, M.D.
Robert J. Schweitzer, M.D.
Sudhir Srivastava, Ph.D., M.P.H.
Joel E. Tepper, M.D.
*Edward L. Trimble, M.D.
Mark R. Wick, M.D.
*David P. Winchester, M.D. (Ex-officio and Executive Director)
*John W. Yarbro, M.D. (Vice-Chairman)

*Current members of the AJCC Executive Committee

1997 LIAISON MEMBERS OF THE AMERICAN JOINT COMMITTEE ON CANCER

AMERICAN SOCIETY OF CLINICAL ONCOLOGY	Derek Raghavan, M.D. Roswell Park Cancer Institute
AMERICAN UROLOGICAL ASSOCIATION	Andrew C. von Eshenbach, M.D. M. D. Anderson Cancer Center
ASSOCIATION OF AMERICAN CANCER INSTITUTES	Stephen B. Edge, M.D. Roswell Park Cancer Institute
CENTERS FOR DISEASE CONTROL AND PREVENTION	Daniel S. Miller, M.D. Centers for Disease Control and Prevention
NATIONAL CANCER REGISTRARS ASSOCIATION	Carol S. Venuti, C.T.R. Massachusetts General Hospital
NORTH AMERICAN ASSOCIATION OF CENTRAL CANCER REGISTRIES	Sue Watkins, C.T.R. Santa Barbara, California
THE AMERICAN SOCIETY OF COLON AND RECTAL SURGEONS	Mark L. Welton, M.D. University of California at San Francisco
THE SOCIETY OF GYNECOLOGIC ONCOLOGISTS	Howard W. Jones, III, M.D. Vanderbilt University Medical Center
THE SOCIETY OF UROLOGIC ONCOLOGY	Ian M. Thompson, M.D. Brooke Army Medical Center

1992–1997 EDITORIAL BOARD, TASK FORCE CHAIRMEN AND SITE CURATORS

David G. McLeod, M.D.
Walter Reed Army Medical Center

James E. Montie, M.D.
University of Michigan Medical Center

Gerald P. Murphy, M.D.
Pacific Northwest Cancer Foundation, Northwest Hospital

Andrew C. Novick, M.D.
Cleveland Clinic

Jerome P. Richie, M.D.
Brigham and Women's Hospital

Peter T. Scardino, M.D.
Baylor College of Medicine

Donald G. Skinner, M.D.
University of Southern California Medical Center

Joseph A. Smith, Jr., M.D.
Vanderbilt University Medical Center

Ian M. Thompson, M.D.
Brooke Army Medical Center

David P. Wood, M.D.
Harper Hospital

Special Task Force on Testis Cancer

Dean F. Bajorin, M.D., Task Force Chairman
Memorial Sloan Kettering Cancer Center

Andrew C. von Eschenbach, M.D.
M. D. Anderson Cancer Center

Mary Gospodarowicz, M.D.
Princess Margaret Hospital
University of Toronto

B. J. Kennedy, M.D.
University of Minnesota Hospitals and Clinics

Paul Lange, M.D.
University of Washington Medical Center

Howard Levin, M.D.
Cleveland Clinic Foundation

James E. Montie, M.D.
The University of Michigan

Craig R. Nichols, M.D.
Indiana University Medical Center

Derek Raghavan, M.D.
Roswell Park Cancer Institute

Victor Reuter, M.D.
Memorial Sloan Kettering Cancer Center

Jerome Richie, M.D.
Brigham and Women's Hospital

Nicholas Vogelzang, M.D.
University of Chicago Cancer Research Center

Gunar Zagars, M.D.
M. D. Anderson Cancer Center

Gynecological Sites

William T. Creasman, M.D.
Medical University of South Carolina

Howard W. Jones, III, M.D.
Vanderbilt University Medical Center

Head and Neck Sites

Elliot W. Strong, M.D., Task Force Chairman
Memorial Sloan Kettering Cancer Center

John G. Batsakis, M.D.
M. D. Anderson Cancer Center

Nicholas J. Cassisi, M.D.
University of Florida College of Medicine

Jay S. Cooper, M.D.
New York University Medical Center

Irvin D. Fleming, M.D.
University of Tennessee

Helmuth Goepfert, M.D.
M. D. Anderson Cancer Center

Oscar M. Guillamondegui, M.D.
M. D. Anderson Cancer Center

H. Ric Harnsberger, M.D.
University of Utah Health Sciences Center

Jonas T. Johnson, M.D.
University of Pittsburgh Medical Center

Robert D. Lindberg, M.D.
Retired, University of Louisville Hospital

Jesus E. Medina, M.D.
University of Oklahoma Health Sciences Center

Brian O'Sullivan, M.D.
Princess Margaret Hospital, University of Toronto

Jatin P. Shah, M.D.
Memorial Sloan Kettering Cancer Center

Lung

Clifton F. Mountain, M.D.
University of California at San Diego

John W. Yarbro, M.D.
Professor Emeritus, University of Missouri

Skin

Jay S. Cooper, M.D.
New York University Medical Center

Melanoma

Mark R. Wick, M.D.
Barnes Hospital

Carcinoma of the Skin

Charles J. McDonald, M.D.
Roger Williams Medical Center

Ophthalmic Sites

R. Jean Campbell, M.D., Ch.B., Task Force Chairman
The Mayo Clinic, Rochester

Irvin D. Fleming, M.D.
University of Tennessee

R. L. Font, M.D.
Baylor College of Medicine

Lois M. McNally, M.D.
The New York Eye and Ear Infirmary

Jerry A. Shields, M.D.
Wills Eye Hospital

Lorenz E. Zimmerman
Armed Forces Institute of Pathology

Soft Tissue Sarcoma

Murray F. Brennan, M.D., Task Force Chairman
Memorial Sloan Kettering Cancer Center

Lawrence Baker, M.D.
University of Michigan Comprehensive Cancer Center

Donald E. Henson, M.D.
National Cancer Institute

Robert V. P. Hutter, M.D.
St. Barnabas Medical Center

Brian O'Sullivan, M.D.
Princess Margaret Hospital
University of Toronto

David Panicek, M.D.
Memorial Sloan Kettering Cancer Center

Derek Raghavan, M.D.
Roswell Park Cancer Institute

Robert J. Schweitzer, M.D.
University of California/Davis-East Bay

James Woodruff, M.D.
Memorial Sloan Kettering Cancer Center